THE SEED SIST@S

Fiona Heckels & Kaz Goodweather

THE SENSORY HERBAL HANDBOOK

Illustrated by
BELLE BENFIELD

Foreword by
BRUCE PARRY

CONNECT WITH THE MEDICINAL POWER OF YOUR LOCAL PLANTS

WATKINS
1893

WE WISH TO DEDICATE THIS
PUBLICATION TO OUR SUPER-STAR
MENTOR, A TRUE TIME-TRAVELLING
WIZARD: *Christopher Hedley*

THE SENSORY HERBAL HANDBOOK — Seed SistAs

First published in the UK and USA in 2019 by
Watkins, an imprint of Watkins Media Limited
Unit 11, Shepperton House, 83–93 Shepperton Road
London N1 3DF

enquiries@watkinspublishing.com

Commissioning Editor: Fiona Robertson
Editor: Sophie Elletson
Senior Designer: Francesca Corsini
Commissioned Body Artwork: Barking Dog Art
Picture Research: Jennifer Veall and Francesca Corsini
Proofreading and Index: James Hodgson
Production: Uzma Taj

A CIP record for this book is available from the British
Library

ISBN: 978-1-78678-211-3

Publisher's notes:
The information in this book is not intended as a substitute
for professional medical advice and treatment. If you are
pregnant or are suffering from any medical conditions or
health problems, it is recommended that you consult a
medical professional before following any of the advice or
practice suggested in this book. Watkins Media Limited,
or any other persons who have been involved in working
on this publication, cannot accept responsibility for any
injuries or damage incurred as a result of following the
information, exercises or therapeutic techniques contained
in this book.

The availability of some over-the-counter herbal remedies
may be affected by the 2004 EU Directive on Traditional
Herbal Medicines. Consult a pharmacist or qualified herbal
practitioner for advice on this subject.

10 9 8 7 6 5

Typeset in Times New Roman Harman
Colour reproduction by XY Digital
Printed in China

www.watkinspublishing.com

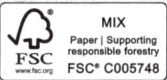

CONTENTS

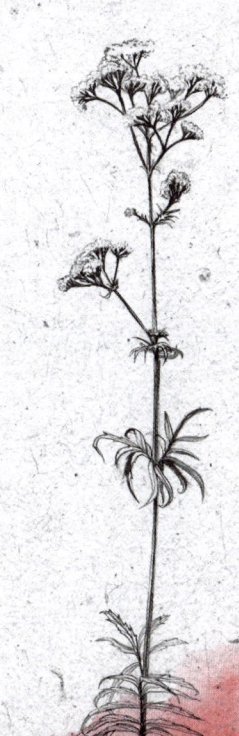

FOREWORD BY BRUCE PARRY

I first met the Seed Sistas on one of their famous witches' brew circles and was instantly struck by their unique mix of knowledge and wisdom, respect and irreverence. Over the course of a day brimming with mythology, science, anecdote and fun we were collectively enlightened and informed, reassured and transformed. Here was real magic at play. Here, indeed, I was in the company of modern-day alchemists and herbalists who could leap between worlds with confidence and dexterity.

As we stirred agaric with nightshade, mugwort with henbane, we explored the origins of lycanthropy, enchantment, flying ointments and broomsticks, and I was left in no doubt as to who I was with and the power that they held.

What I love most about these contemporary witchy herbalists is that beneath their exuberance and playfulness is a solid understanding of plants. Their pharmacological and ethnobotanical knowledge, Latin nomenclature and letters after their names offer the credibility that many of us in today's urban worlds (sadly) need in order to relax, trust and open up. But what is so special about these wonderfully wicked witchy sistas is that they have gone way beyond this structured, linear, disenchanted realm into something much more profound. In our world of categories and pigeonholes, labels and certainty we are in desperate need of those who know how to skilfully break out of the confines of our narrow way of thinking into the realms of embodied feelings and the deeper understanding that can come through intuition, myth, storytelling and the wisdom of experience.

To my mind, the best healers and shamans are fully grounded beings who live in this world but can journey into the other realms. It is the moving between the worlds and finding that balance which is the real test and testament of wisdom today. It is all too simple to abide in one space or another. Everything can be a poison, and everything can be a medicine – it is all about context and degree, relationship and dose.

Relationship is key. Plants exist within us and outside of us. Plants nourish and cure us, they propel and sustain us. An important element of the Seed Sistas' approach is the understanding that plants also have character and are imbued with an essence or spirit, just as we are. Each herb is unique while also being a part of the whole. If we can get to know the plants around us, make friends with them, honour and respect them, listen to them and see ourselves as akin to them, then the real journey of relationship can begin. With this book as a guide we can discover how we each individually relate to the world of plants and herbs.

We were all great herbalists once, and many an indigenous person still is today. I have met with people who are fully embodied in the subtle realms of communication, who can listen to and commune with the plant world. For them, the knowledge they receive in this manner is as real as any spoken or written word.

What appeals to me about the Seed Sistas' approach to herbs is that it uses the tools we all have – our own senses. Through engaging them and exploring with them, we can experience herbs and their ability to heal in new ways, and the world opens out to us, afresh, vibrant, alive. It is a deeply personal yet universally accessible pursuit. And as we learn to trust and deepen our senses, we also begin to come into contact with the hidden senses that our forest friends live by.

Intuition is not something mystical, it is within us all if we can build a relationship with our physical body, our spiritual edges and our inner realms. Meeting the plants in

this way is enriching, a tonic for our times, in which we seem so disconnected from our feelings and environment.

This book contains a wealth of wisdom and will be a great companion to us all in our tentative explorations into these otherly realms. We are all already gifted with the tools we need for this exploration – our own hearts, senses, bodies and minds – and this book will guide us on this important journey of reconnection.

I wish you well on this important venture. I am full of gratitude to the wonderful Seed Sistas for compiling this book and sharing some of what they have learned. Go well on your investigations, be safe and, above all, enjoy the trip.

Bruce Parry
Dologau, Wales

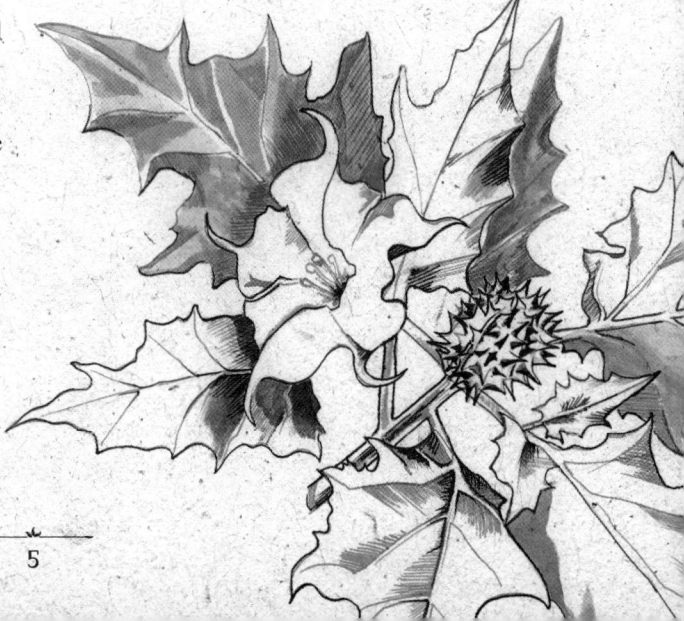

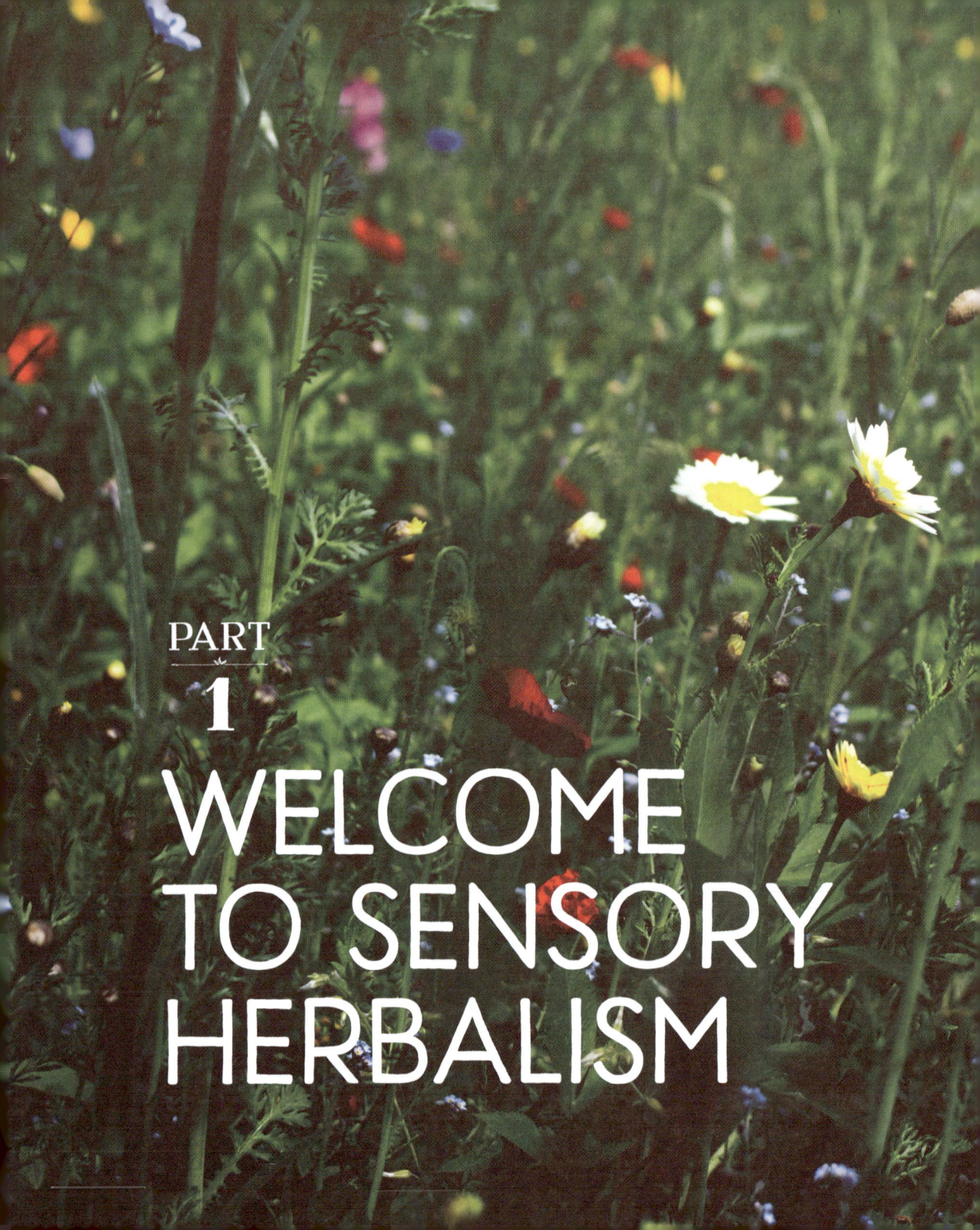

PART

1

WELCOME TO SENSORY HERBALISM

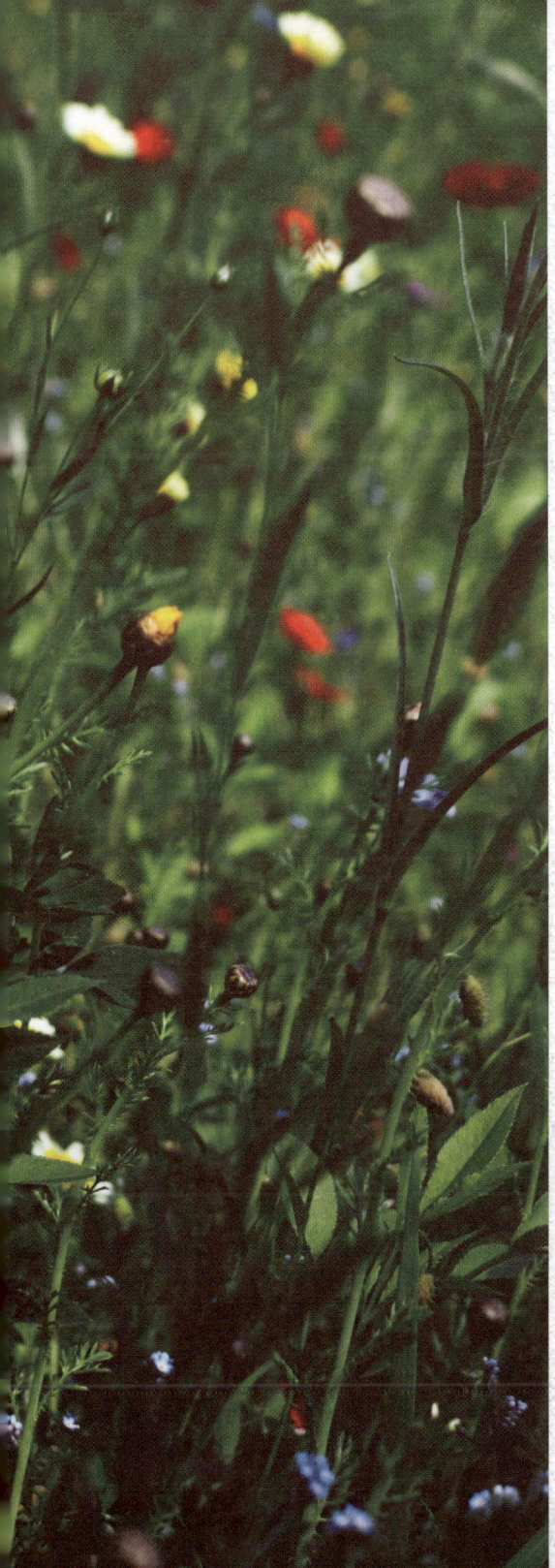

The Sensory Herbal Handbook is a guide to connecting with the plant world and the seasons, in order to create more balance, good health and wellbeing in your life. It will take you on a poetic, seasonal journey to help you form deep and lasting relationships with nature, as you rediscover the important, secret language of plants.

This book has been written for anyone who has heard the whispers of the wild and has been stirred to know more, for all people with a political conscience, and lovers of the outdoors. It is for those who want to take their health into their own hands by deepening their knowledge of the plant world.

The aim is to inspire as many people as possible to learn about their local and native herbs, and revive the history and practice of using herbs for medicine, for spiritual growth – and for fun!

WHAT IS SENSORY HERBALISM?

Sensory Herbalism is based on the Western Herbal Medicine tradition, drawing on tools and energetic language that have traditionally been used to connect with and understand plants and people. Western Herbal Medicine is a holistic system focused on returning a person's health back to a state of homeostasis or balance. It has become a practice informed by rigorous medical training but sometimes with little connection to the plants themselves. In Sensory Herbalism, the focus is on getting to know plants intimately using our senses and intuition as well as the analytical brain.

Sensory Herbalism has a strong political ethos. It is clear that plant habitats and diversity are under threat. Areas that can be harvested for wild herbs and plants have reduced in number since the introduction of modern farming practices, such as the use of pesticides. Sensory Herbalism aims to encourage the rewilding of green spaces, to protect plants and to pass on knowledge that will reignite people's interest in these most valuable, beautiful and medicinally rich beings. Working with plants is an act of political activism, a statement of self-empowerment and belief in protecting nature. The more we understand about herbs, the more we want to create the environments in which they can grow and flourish.

In Sensory Herbalism there is a focus on how we as humans can restore our own health by interacting with the plants themselves through energetic doses and through the growing and harvesting of them. Sensory Herbalism has a strong focus on creativity, placing great emphasis on connection to nature or spirit through storytelling, drawing and poetry. It asks you to draw on the power of intention as you grow, craft and take herbal medicines. It is an approach developed to create and strengthen a mutually beneficial relationship between herbs and humans.

As well as focusing on plants, Sensory Herbalism is also all about understanding the human body. This involves understanding how the elemental forces – wind, fire, earth, water and spirit – pervade all of life and are expressed in varying degrees in plants, in the seasons and in people as holistic organisms.

Even systems within the body have affinity for one or more of the elements. Sensory Herbalism associates each of these body systems with water, fire, air, earth or spirit. This helps to understand the energy and function of each system, as well as why disease arises in these regions and what it could mean.

Sensory Herbalism follows a seasonal journey that differs from the practice of

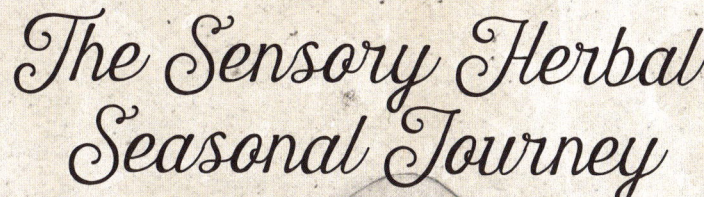

The Sensory Herbal
Seasonal Journey

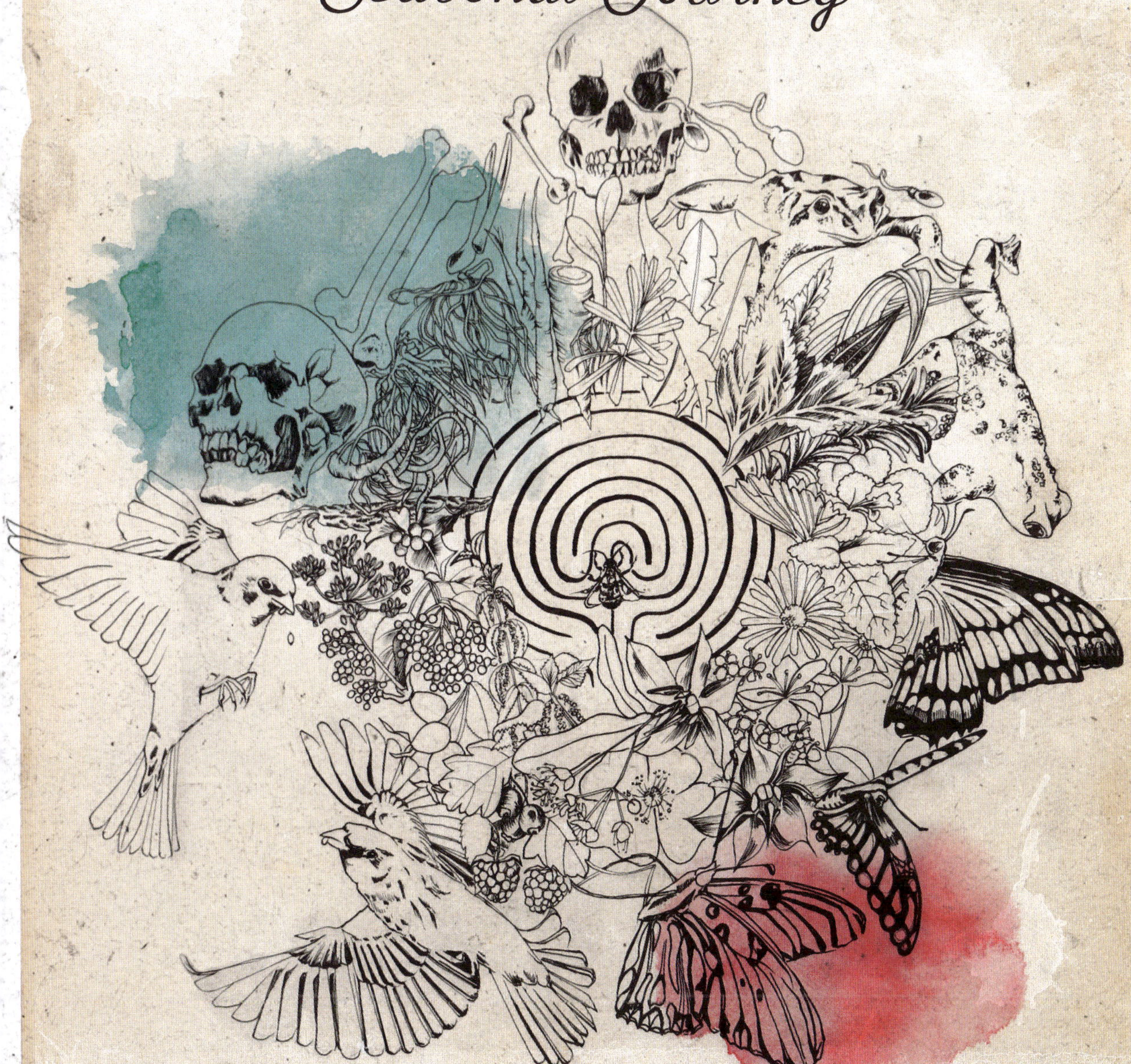

Western Herbal Medicine in focusing on how plants experience the seasons, rather than on how we as people experience the seasons.

Modern Western Herbal Medicine uses often large doses of herbs to push the body into a perceived place that it "needs to go", whereas in Sensory Herbalism sensory drop doses gently encourage a shift toward health.

Sensory Herbalism draws on ideas and theories from many medical models of the past as well as from modern medicine and research. It draws on Western allopathic medicine, Western astrology and Chinese and Ayurvedic medical models. It is, however, unique in its techniques for understanding and getting to know plants themselves and also in its detailed understanding of how the elements affect the body, emotions, seasons and the plants themselves.

In Sensory Herbalism, it's important to begin by getting to grips with the idea of "meeting" a plant or herb. This provides a foundation of confidence for an elemental journey through the cycle of the year, working with herbs as they appear. The word "sensory" is used to describe the way we work with the plants, getting to know them using all our senses. An important tool is observation, which includes using our senses to understand a plant's nature and the way it could interact with us, bringing us food, medicine and deeper messages about how we might protect ourselves and the planet.

Other tools of Sensory Herbalism include intuition, interpretation, characterization and plant dream creation. These connect us with the plants and allow us to understand their language, ultimately enabling us to take lessons from nature and use plants to reshape our social norms.

As you explore Sensory Herbalism further, you will connect the elements of water, fire, air, earth and spirit to the seasons and look at how these elements are expressed by the plants themselves, as well as in the human body – physically, emotionally and spiritually. Sensory Herbalism follows the elements on their dance through the year. Water, fire, air and earth correspond to each of the four seasons, and to specific parts of the plants. Spirit or ether, the fifth element, exerts influence throughout the year. Spirit informs our ritual practices with plant medicines, and drives our connectivity.

Sensory Herbalism is designed to aid people on their journey to health. It is a unique style of healing that encompasses many art forms. There is a strong focus on physical movement, meditation, art and ritual in the practice, but it is always centred around the herbs. Practising Sensory Herbalism will open up your intuition and as you start to interpret colours, forms, tastes and scents, you will open your heart to nature – and nature will extend life in all its beauty back to you.

HOW THE SEED SISTAS BEGAN

We are a collective of eco-proactivists with a mission to reconnect us all to the often overlooked power of plant medicine. We do this through creating community medicine gardens and inspiring others to do the same, teaching, and initiating arts projects. We are herbalists, educators, writers, mothers, artists and rebels.

The Seed Sistas began when the two of us, Kaz and Fiona, bonded over a love of the natural world when we were studying together for a Bachelor of Science degree in herbal medicine. Immersed in nature from childhood, we both had developed a deep love of this beautiful green planet. Our questioning natures and rebellious spirits led us to develop our own system of medicine, carving out a new path for ourselves and for others who choose to resist the status quo. We learned to trust our intuition, to trust ourselves, to go against the grain. Be free, be wild and let individual creativity shine is the call of Sensory Herbalism!

DAISY MAGIC

Daisy (*Bellis perennis*) was the first herb that taught us to pay close attention to our intuition, and also revealed that understanding the language of plants does not have to be complicated or mystical. Once a staple of

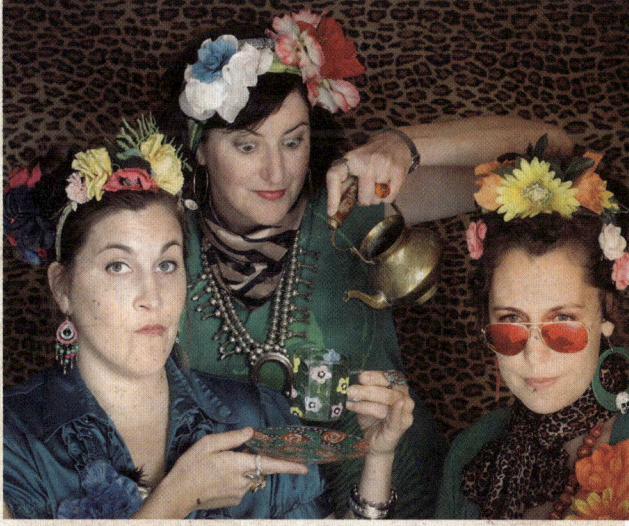

Seed Sistas Fiona and Kaz (in front), with artist Belle (behind)

herbal medicine (its common name was bruisewort, indicating just one of its many healing gifts), daisy had fallen out of fashion by the time we were training to be herbalists, so we were not taught anything about this incredibly common little flower, considered a garden weed. Noticing these delicate blooms everywhere, we decided to gather a harvest, create a syrup and see what this wild medicine had to offer us.

We set out with our baskets one blazing sunny day and soon became absorbed in the

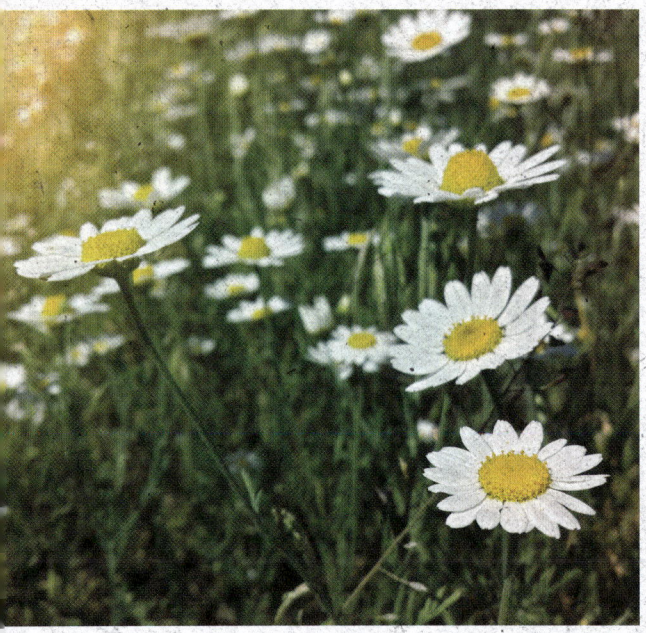

Daisy inspires our inner child to play and be joyful.

pop, pop, pop of the white-and-yellow flower heads as we plucked them from their hairy stems. Sheer delight compelled us to pick another and another, knowing that daisies regenerate quickly and our copious harvesting wouldn't damage them. When we considered our impulse to keep going, it dawned on us that daisy might be useful for supporting those with compulsive behaviour patterns.

We tasted a few flower heads, using this sense to detect possible actions that this herb might have; sweet, metallic, soapy, bitter, were some of the flavours that greeted our taste buds. We knew then that these precious daisies had many medicinal virtues. For example, the soapy flavour indicated saponins, plant constituents with an expectorant action, helping to clear the lungs.

We made gallons of daisy syrup that year. We researched the use of *Bellis perennis* in the work of Dr Edward Bach on flower essences, and found that it is indeed used when repeated patterns of behaviour become problematic. Daisy itself had taught us one of its medicinal applications simply by our becoming aware of how we felt while harvesting it. This first sensory, intuitive experience was gifted to us by daisy. Having our intuitions corroborated by Bach's research encouraged us to delve deeper into the joys of the plant world, and to open ourselves up to being led by the herbs.

Daisy's message was that it was needed in today's society. One of its abilities is to revive our inner child; it is here to help address the manic work ethic, worry and anxiety that are prevalent in this modern age. Daisy doesn't snap or crush when stood on. It bounces back and can often be seen still in flower on freshly mowed lawns. With its messages of "play and be joyful", "don't take life too seriously" and "bounce back from emotional bruising", it became integral to our own herbal blends. We created Drops of Courage and Passion Potion, and set about giving drops to as many folk as we could at festivals and other events.

The feedback was astonishing. People loved the herbs; they were experiencing positive shifts and wanted to know more. The Daisy Revolution had begun.

Our plant knowledge deepened as we travelled over Europe, exploring the natural environments of native European plants. We developed ever more herb preparations to support a plethora of emotional, physical and spiritual imbalances, from needing more courage or self-nurture to seeking more passion, from thinking more clearly to recovering after a bout of illness.

Our voyage to understand nature has taught us to listen closely to our intuition and to listen to our souls. We spent years observing how plants grow and interact with people. Both our intuition and these observations led us to discover and translate the language of plants in our own way.

We called our dream, to connect folk with herbs and continue our adventure with plants, Sensory Solutions Herbal Evolution. Acquiring a 1960s American Airstream caravan, our silver bullet, we toured the UK, running workshops and providing our Sensory Herbal drops to those who wanted them. To demystify using herbs as medicine, we showed photos of herbs at various stages of growing, harvesting and remedy production. Over many years of midsummer heather quests in the mountains, riverside peppermint bounties, autumnal horseradish digging and hedgerow foraging for hips and haws, we laid out the principles of practice for Sensory Herbalism, informed by lessons we learned from nature. Everything that's needed to learn the ways of the plants is inside each of us, and, with a little guidance, nature can truly open up to reveal its magic.

It has been an incredible journey, and we have met some of the most inspiring and wonderful people on their own journeys, promoting positive change through writing, education, growing projects, arts activism and creating collectives. We have watched lives transform through the work that we have done and feel privileged to have worked with people from all walks of life, from HIV support groups and domestic abuse hostels to homeless young people. We have run workshops, organized walks, created gardens and initiated art and creativity – and noticed that working in this way with herbs has provided a place to explore ourselves.

Together, we have dedicated our lives to finding creative ways to give as many people as possible access to knowledge about the medicine of plants.

The Seed Sistas were later joined by Belle, an accomplished artist and early graduate of the Sensory Herb Apprenticeship. An activist, herbalist and artist, she is the brilliant illustrator of the plant drawings, prints and sketchbooks featured throughout this book.

WHY PLANTS MATTER

Humans and plants have evolved together. This is demonstrated by the interaction of plant compounds with receptors in the human body, compounds that can be almost identical to hormones or neurotransmitters. We are in essence made of the same stuff.

Plants and people have lived together side by side from the very beginning. We share a rich, colourful history. We are intertwined.

There are around 300,000 plant species on our planet. They are the only life forms that can produce their own energy source from sunlight. Through photosynthesis and transpiration, they create an environment suitable for us and other animals to live in, regulating our planet's water and air supply.

Herbal medicine is an art and, in more modern times, a science. Plant healing has ensured our survival, allowing us to cure ourselves and thrive as a species. Every community has utilized its native plants for medicine. According to the World Health Organization, 80 percent of people in Africa still rely on traditional herbal medicines as their main healthcare, often conducted with a sacred connection to the plants.

How did our ancestors discover the medicinal potential of plants? We can only speculate. Most likely they observed the plant and animal kingdoms, and used their instinct to discover the wonderful healing qualities of plants, knowledge that was then passed down through the generations. It's fascinating to observe this inherent knowledge in animals. Horses will self-medicate when they're sick, naturally foraging for nettles if given access to them. These nettles can provide a horse with essential minerals, can help reduce the inflammation of laminitis, treat kidney complaints, help with allergies and support lactation issues, among other ailments. Similarly, a horse will naturally avoid ragwort if there are plenty of other food sources (a yellow-flowering plant in the daisy family, ragwort commonly grows in fields but is toxic to horses).

FOOD

Almost everything that we ingest comes directly or indirectly from plants. Throughout human history approximately 7,000 different plant species have been used as food. Wheat is thought to have been the first plant cultivated, in the Middle East *c.* 8000 BCE.

CLOTHING

Cotton, flax, hemp, nettle and bamboo are among the plants generously giving us their harvest to make fabrics. The use of plastics in fabrics is contributing to our current environmental crisis; when washed, these fabrics shed plastic microfibres into the water system. We need ecologically friendly fabrics – the awesomely strong fibre of stinging nettles is an excellent choice. Nettles have hollow fibres that are filled with air, creating natural insulation. In fact the use of nettles in clothing dates back some two millennia; it was only with the arrival of cotton in the 16th century that this useful plant fell from favour. In World War I, when cotton ran short in Germany, nettles were used to make army uniforms.

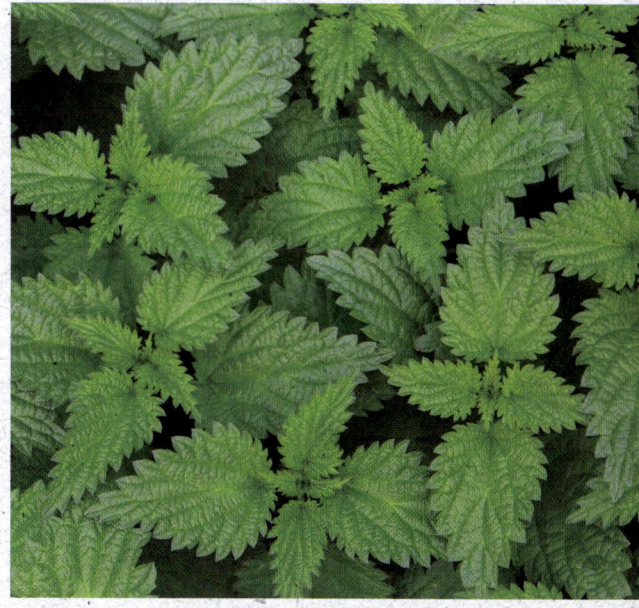

Nettles: a fabulous source of food and clothing

MEDICINE AND RITUAL

Plants have long been used for medicinal purposes. Ancient Chinese and Egyptian papyrus writings describe medicinal uses for plants as early as 3000 BCE. In cultures where practices have remained relatively unchanged for millennia, herbs are still used in healing rituals. Traditional medical systems that involve prolific use of herbs, such as Ayurveda in India and Traditional Chinese Medicine, are so embedded in the culture of their country that they are still part of more mainstream medicine today, with herbs administered within hospital systems.

In many places across the globe, there is fantastic diversity in native and naturalized plants and a rich ancestral history of plant medicine that is still being uncovered. Herbal medicine has evolved over time with cross-pollination between many cultures. Scientific models are now being applied to some of the oldest texts available. For example, research has been carried out on the recipes and herbal actions in the *Leech Book of Bald*, written in Saxon times. Science is confirming the wisdom that has been known for centuries.

Animism – the belief that there is God or spirit in all things – can be found in many ancient Earth-based wisdom traditions. Each plant has its own sacred spirit, which makes it more than just its physical substance. This is synergy, meaning the combined effect of the parts is greater than the sum of the separate parts. It indicates that when compounds work together their effects are enhanced. This sacred or ethereal aspect has been utilized in rituals for purification, consecration, protection and community cohesion.

When altering consciousness for religious ceremonies, art and personal exploration, humans have used psychotropic plants and fungi to celebrate and connect with spirit for millennia. There are theories that the religious experience was initiated in humans originally through mushroom intoxication. Could it even be that psychedelic experiences played a part in the evolution of the human brain?

PAPER

From the Bible to Harry Potter, literature is filled with references to our plant allies. The very paper on which books are printed comes from the plants, too. The word "paper" derives from the Latin *papyrus*, which is the name for a plant once abundant in Egypt and used by the ancient Egyptians, Greeks and Romans to produce a thick sheet-like material for writing and painting.

FOLKLORE

A multitude of stories have been told about the folklore of plants, their characters and spirits. Several botanical names of plants derive from Greek and Roman myths. For example, the Roman goddess Diana was the huntress. In Greek, her name is Artemis, the moon goddess, and many species of plants with her namesake, Artemisia, cast a silvery moon-glow from their leaves. The protector of small children, she helped her mother to birth her twin brother Apollo immediately

---

Pharmaceutical Drugs

The modern pharmaceutical industry still relies heavily on plants; a quarter of all prescription drugs come directly from, or are derivatives of, plants. Some of the more famous ones are:

✴ Quinine, which is used to treat malaria and is synthesized from cinchona bark.

✴ Digoxin, which is used to treat heart conditions and is derived from foxglove.

✴ Diacetylmorphine, which is better known by its trade name "heroin" and was originally sold, incorrectly, as a non-addictive substitute for the naturally occurring morphine in poppy plants.

✴ Aspirin, also known as acetylsalicylic acid, which is an artificial reproduction of salicin, found in willow bark and meadowsweet.

✴ Taxol, which is an anti-tumour drug derived from the bark of the Pacific yew.

✴ Artemisinin, derived from a cousin of the mugwort plant, *Artemisa annua*, is a potent anti-malarial medicine discovered in 1972.

after she had been born. Artemisia species such as mugwort are used in labour to help bring down the baby. There is a long tradition in Chinese medicine of using Moxa sticks, which contain charcoal and mugwort, during and just before the birth process. Mugwort stimulates oxytocin, the hormone that is released during birth (and also in orgasm).

Yarrow, or *Achillea millefolium*, is named after Achilles the warrior. It is said that Achilles used the plant to staunch the wounds of his fellow soldiers, and indeed it is known as a styptic, staunching the flow of blood.

DISCONNECTION

People have always lived interdependently with plants and yet we no longer value them, no longer treat them as sacred. Mass agriculture has changed our outlook. Our wild spaces are getting smaller and smaller. We are still hugely dependent on plants but we no longer recognize this. Now the corporations are chemical producers and we are the lab rats. As herbalists, we see untold damage done to many people by prescription medications. Drugs have side effects. What's the solution? Take another pill. This reliance on pharmaceutical drugs plays a big part in the ill-health of our planet and our physical, emotional and spiritual disconnection from the plant world around us.

People in much of the Western world have lost touch with the medicine of the Earth,

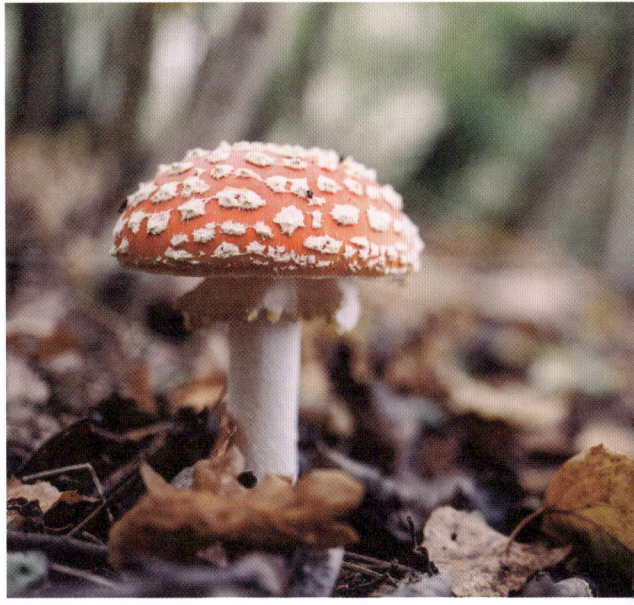

The iconic fungus fly agaric, also known as Soma, the divine mushroom of immortality

and have consequently forgotten how to care for her. Herbalism is a nearly forgotten art in many places, seen as antiquated "folk" or "old wives'" medicine. The skills of our great-grandparents to treat simple complaints are no longer deemed relevant and much of the herbal knowledge of the past has died out.

POLITICS AND PLANTS

The medical profession and politics have always been intertwined. The focus of healthcare in any given country is determined, in part, by the ideals of the political party in power. With the rise in influence of drug companies in recent decades, the medical profession is often at their mercy. Much medical research is conducted with a specific goal in mind, determining how and where money is spent in the healthcare system. Power is often removed from the doctors, and access to medicine is determined by the pricing of drugs and alliances between the government and the pharmaceutical companies.

Our aim is to protect the Earth from greed and violence by linking people with their local medicinal plants. If people can recognize and harvest medicinal herbs, a reconnection with nature develops. On the foundations of self-empowerment, respect for the Earth and knowledge of the past, a whole new system of healing can be built, creating greater community cohesion, autonomy in healthcare and participation in grass-roots activism.

Seed politics is of paramount importance. This refers to the freedom to grow, harvest and then save seeds without interference from large corporations who want to monopolize the production and management of seeds. If we reduce crop strains, we risk creating huge issues around disease and food shortage. We are inspired by the work of activists such as Dr Vandana Shiva who called seed saving a political act. She has worked tirelessly to change farming practices where "terminator"

seeds produced by massive agro-farming companies have destroyed livelihoods through their inability to produce future generations of crops.

Seed politics and seed saving are inextricably linked to herbal medicine. As the Seed Sistas, we spread the word about the importance of seed saving. We campaign for the ideal of a medicine garden in every community – a dedicated growing space filled with abundant medicinal herbs, accompanied by educational signs to support everybody's learning and connection with the plants.

MOVING FORWARD

Access to herbal medicine and information is vital if we are to shift toward a more responsible society. It's often forgotten that we have the power as individuals to make choices. Getting to know how our bodies work, and making changes for our emotional and spiritual wellbeing, promotes happier, healthier societies. Connecting people to plants strengthens the bonds of protection and love for Mother Earth.

There are many benefits to modern allopathic medicine, but also costs in terms of wellbeing and finance. Today, individual plant compounds are extracted, then refined for use as allopathic drugs to treat particular conditions. While this has certainly led to faster treatment of certain conditions, these drugs also have side effects. A whole plant containing a multitude of chemical constituents has a very different action on the physical body, because all those phytochemicals work synergistically. For example, the herb meadowsweet contains the compound salicylic acid, the constituent that aspirin is derived from. Aspirin's side effects include corroding the stomach lining and causing ulcers. Conversely, meadowsweet is actually indicated for stomach ulcers in herbal medicine, because of other constituents that it contains in addition to salicylic acid, all working in synergy.

Today, laws specify that some plants are illegal to grow and possess. Others are seen as colossal cash crops to be taxed and exploited. Governments dictate how we can and cannot distribute herbal medicines, yet often these governments themselves have little knowledge about plant medicine.

Herbal medicine, in contrast, is alchemy, the creative power to transform a plant into a potion for positive change. Traditional pharmacy taught that herbal preparations should be presented in a beautiful way, and this was part of the healing. And right up until the middle of the 20th century, the presentation and packaging of all medicine was indeed beautiful. Have you ever seen old glass medicine bottles? They are usually made from hand-blown, coloured glass, decorated with pattens and logos. Presenting the medicine attractively honours the life force of the plant and draws the recipient toward a cure. Belief in the medicine and appreciation of its beauty inspires healing.

The core intention of Sensory Herbalism is to encourage as many folk as possible to connect with the Earth, to protect her from greed and violence and place the power of plant medicine back where it belongs, in the hands of the people. Our Earth needs as many secret heroes as possible. Knowledge about the plant world and its medicinal powers makes secret heroes of us all, working together toward a better future.

We are committed to developing projects that will spread through all parts of society, in order to achieve a massive shift in consciousness, toward thinking more holistically about health, wellbeing, education and community. Thankfully, today people are becoming interested in herbal medicine again. They are taking notice of the green spaces around them and wondering what marvels these can offer in terms of food and herbal medicines. Our children should be brought up with knowledge about the medicinal plants that grow around them, and learn to cultivate and nurture them in order to make simple herbal preparations. We hope this book will inspire people to work with plants in a creative way – that it will inspire greater self-awareness and a desire for knowledge that can be passed down to the teachers of the future, our children.

HOW TO USE THIS BOOK

This book is designed to give you more confidence in connecting with and embracing herbs in your everyday life, to improve health and wellbeing. Whether you are brand new to the way of herbs, have always felt you had a calling as a herbalist but never knew where to start, or are a qualified herbalist who wants to incorporate Sensory Herbalism into your practice, this book will guide you step by step as you connect with plants, your own health and the seasons that support us in our dance through life.

As you work through this book, consider creating a herbal journal in which you note down anything that comes up emotionally or that you would like to know more about or question. Researching plants, and creating food and medicines from them, gives you the space to explore your own physical and emotional responses. Allow the plants to lead you on your own journey.

This is a guide to Sensory Herbalism, looking first at the theory underpinning the approach, then offering a practical guide to learning the language of plants, and finally taking you on a seasonal journey through the elements of water, fire, earth, air and spirit. It is an elemental guide to understanding your own health through the seasons of the year with the plants at the helm.

PART 2: THE FOUNDATIONS OF SENSORY HERBALISM lays out the theories behind Sensory Herbalism. We will look at the systems that have been drawn upon and integrated in the development of Sensory Herbalism, and how we can begin to trust our own senses to understand the workings of plants. Read the whole section and then look back when you find reference to certain theories or practices later in the book.

PART 3: THE TOOLS OF SENSORY HERBALISM is a practical section to help you start experimenting with Sensory Herbalism. It suggests exercises to do with the plants that grow around you so that you can start to learn their language and interpret their medicinal value. You will be encouraged to unleash your creativity, to immerse yourself in your reflective nature and to create your own sensory herbal – a log or journal recording your experiences with plants.

PART 4: THE SEASONAL JOURNEY explores the elemental cycle, the changing seasons of the year and their associated plants. Each element – water, fire, air, earth and spirit – is reflected in our body's physical and emotional health. Awareness of this can bring greater understanding of how to utilize plants for health and wellbeing. Read through the whole of this section, looking at each element, season and plant part, to glean an overall understanding. Then dip back in throughout the year to the relevant section, working with each of the plants, the rituals and the recipes as they appear in that season.

In each season you will be encouraged to reflect on how you express yourself physically and emotionally through the element. You will be asked to consider your own health and wellbeing to understand how you can guide yourself toward a state of true balance. As you work through the book, you will find:

* Theory, influences and the history of Sensory Herbalism.
* The Sensory Herbalism tools – a guide to connecting with the herbs, designed for you to experiment with each of the tools individually so that you can deepen your understanding of particular plants.
* Poems and art to encourage the unleashing of your own creative flow.
* Exercises to help you understand how your own health and wellbeing relate to the elements.
* Rituals to truly connect you to the year and the lunar cycles as they ebb and flow. Rituals can be used to empower us to become still, to play, to be reverent or irreverent and to connect with others in our friendship groups and communities.

* Fifteen of our dearest plant friends for you to make lasting friendships with. You will start to understand how to harness their plant medicine, when best to harvest them and how to prepare each herb. You will find the herbs located in the season in which they are harvested but you will also learn of their unique elemental association according to how they interact with their environment and the human body.
* Recipes to inspire cooking with seasonal vegetables, herbs and spices.

We are privileged to be able to share our journey and our life's work with you in this guide to Sensory Herbalism. Our intention is that you will gain confidence in working with and identifying plants and learn more about the power of their medicine. This guide is for you to learn about yourself and how to live in accordance with nature as she carries on her merry dance through the turning year.

We hope that you will approach the exercises in this book with an open heart and open mind and are receptive to any flutters of knowledge that wish to land on you as you work through the pages of this guide.

Ultimately, we hope that you will be inspired to work further with plants, and join the quest to improve their habitats and treat plants with the same awareness and sense of nurturing that we accord to our fellow humans and animal friends.

FOUNDATIONS OF SENSORY HERBALISM

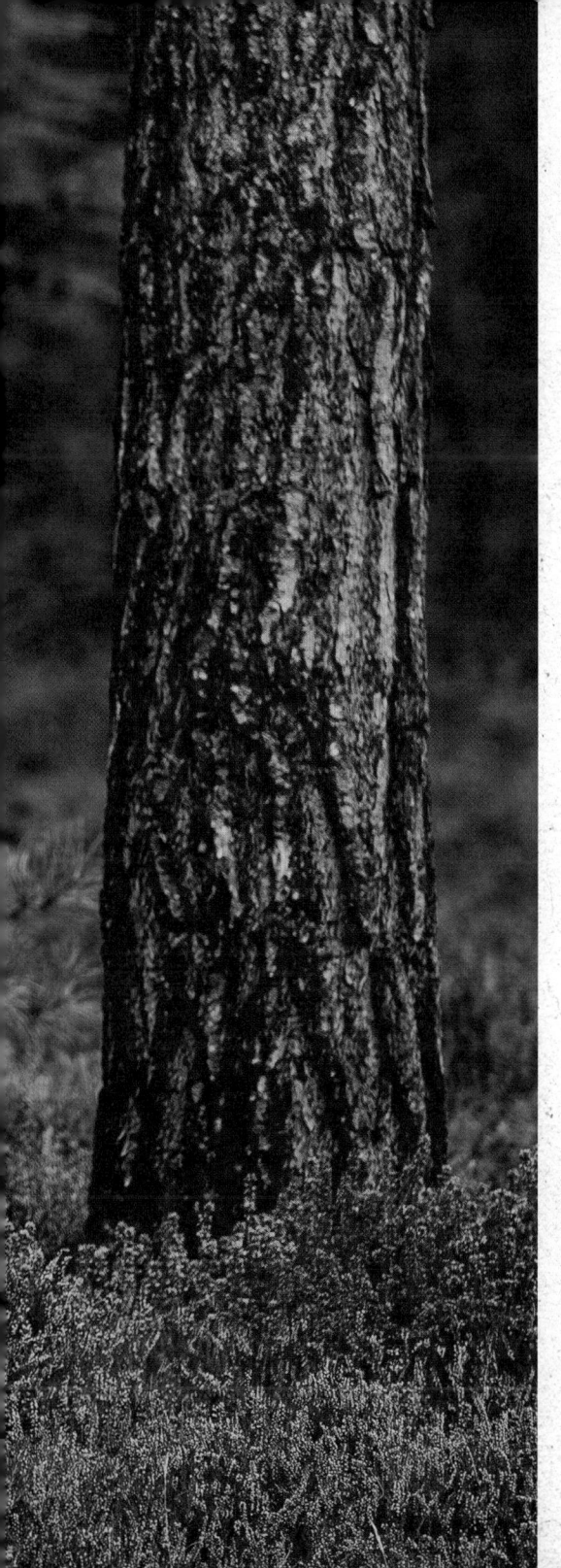

Sensory Herbalism draws inspiration
from many different medical and
spiritual theories and practices. In this
section we will take a look at some
of these foundations of Sensory
Herbalism, such as astrological
herbalism, planetary correspondence,
the chakra system and elemental
medicine – including Ayurveda and
Traditional Chinese Medicine. We
will look at how these traditions have
shaped Sensory Herbalism into a unique
system to support health.

ASTROLOGICAL HERBALISM

Found in many cultures across the globe, astrological herbalism is an ancient system that can help us to understand plants and how they interact with the body and the mind. For example, the sign of Gemini is ruled by the planet Mercury. The lungs and nervous system are under the domain of Mercury and therefore herbs of Mercury include many that are beneficial for the lungs, such as liquorice and mullein. Those with Gemini prominent in their chart may find their lungs and nervous system are areas of weakness. In Sensory Herbalism we draw on this ancient system, using intuition and logic to decipher where each herb fits within it and exploring astrological associations to gain deeper understanding of the plants' qualities and effects. However, we do this through the perspective of modern research into phytochemistry and the action of plants on receptors within the body.

Astrology was more highly respected in the past. It was the Babylonians who applied stories to the star constellations and first described the 12 signs of the zodiac (meaning "circle of animals"). Societies hunted, planted and migrated with the stars. Although today there is much scepticism about astrology, there has been a long history of considering the influence of celestial bodies over health and life. For example, an epic poem of 8,000 verses from the first century CE entitled *Astronomica* associates the signs of the zodiac with parts of the body as follows:

ARIES ♈ – head, face, brain, eyes

TAURUS ♉ – throat, neck, thyroid gland, vocal tract

GEMINI ♊ – arms, lungs, shoulders, hands, nervous system, brain

CANCER ♋ – chest, breasts, stomach, alimentary canal

LEO ♌ – heart, chest, spine, spinal column, upper back

VIRGO ♍ – digestive system, intestines, spleen, nervous system

LIBRA ♎ – kidneys, skin, lumbar region, buttocks

SCORPIO ♏ – reproductive system, sexual organs, bowels, excretory system

SAGITTARIUS ♐ – hips, thighs, liver, sciatic nerve

CAPRICORN – knees, joints, skeletal system

AQUARIUS ♒ – ankles, circulatory system

PISCES ♓ – feet, toes, lymphatic system, adipose tissue.

NICHOLAS CULPEPER

The English apothecary and physician Nicholas Culpeper (1616–1654) was also a political radical who wrote pamphlets against the king, priests, lawyers and licensed physicians. Dedicating himself to serving the sick, the poor and the powerless, he was one of the first to translate medical texts into the layperson's language – English. Until this point Western medical literature was written in Latin and therefore only accessible to an elite few. In doing this, Culpeper not only made medical information more accessible, but also threatened the monopolies of university-trained physicians.

Culpeper popularized the practice of attributing qualities to herbs, and making planetary associations with them. His *Complete Herbal* is still the text we use to discover the relationship between astrology and the uses and qualities of plants. He worked with plants in an experiential way, observing how they acted directly on people who were ill.

INFLUENCE OF THE PLANETS

Until the invention of the telescope in 1608, humans had only witnessed the night sky through the naked eye. The days of the week were associated with the five nearest planets, the moon and the sun, which were visible without a telescope. If we look at some of the European languages of Latin origin, we can see how the days' names clearly relate to these visible celestial bodies: Monday is linked to the moon (in French, Spanish and Italian *lundi*, *lunes* and *lunedi*); Tuesday is linked to Mars (*mardi*, *martes* and *martedi*); Wednesday is linked to Mercury (*mercredi*, *miércoles* and *mercoledi*); Thursday is linked to Jupiter (*jeudi*, *jueves* and *giovedi*); Friday is linked to Venus (*vendredi*, *viernes* and *viernes*); and Saturday is linked to Saturn: *samedi*, *sábado* and *sabato*. Sunday, however, was known outside Germanic languages

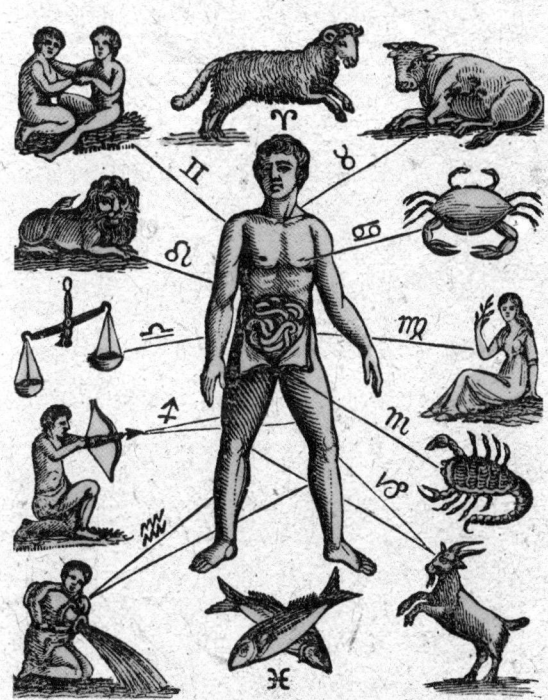

Zodiac man, from a 1923 astrological almanac

as the day of god, from the Latin *dominica* (*dimanche*, *domingo* and *domenica*).

It is interesting to regard the energetics of each planet as being stronger on the day of the week to which it has ties. For example, harvest rosemary, a solar herb, on a Sunday; cleavers, a lunar herb, on a Monday; nettle, a herb of Mars, on a Tuesday; fennel, a Mercurial herb, on a Wednesday; dandelion, a herb of Jupiter, on a Thursday; rose, a herb of Venus, on a Friday; and plantain, a herb of Saturn on a Saturday. Our own observations have led us to believe that plants harvested with greater awareness and intention produce more potent tinctures.

ZODIAC ASSOCIATIONS

Each celestial body has its own qualities, assigned by astrologers. Based on their observations, the planets were given names relating to gods that best fit with the qualities they appeared to exude and the influence they had over people and plants on Earth. Were they solid like the Earth or made of gas like Jupiter? How quickly did they orbit the sun? Mercury, for example, does this in only 88 days and was therefore associated with the quick-witted and fast-paced god Mercury.

These qualities align with the workings of the human body. Mercury, a planet made of gas, has the qualities of speed and quickness, and therefore rules over the nervous system and communication. Venus, the sensual

goddess, rules over the reproductive organs. It was believed that the body at birth is an expression of cosmic energy, characterized by the planetary alignments at that time.

According to legend, Jupiter, as the god of light, rain and lightning, infuses vitality into the universe, and promotes health and strength. In medieval times, it was believed that this planet exercised great influence on people's health. A tradition of writing the ancient Roman symbol of Jupiter – Rx – started among physicians, to convey good wishes and the hope that Jupiter may initiate speedy recovery. "Rx" is still used nowadays almost universally on prescriptions, a remnant of ancient practice still existing in modern allopathic medicine and a tiny recognition of the magical beliefs of old!

The summary in the tables opposite and on the following two pages of the qualities of the planets and their alignment with the human body and herbs is based on our reading of Culpeper and other traditional herbals combined with years of experience in practising Sensory Herbalism.

Another consideration is which phase the moon is in, whether it is waxing or waning, full or new. This directly affects the constituents within the plants. As the moon becomes full, constituents are drawn up into the aerial, or above-ground, parts. The ideal timing of the harvest will depend on which part of the plant you need. A waxing or a full moon is an optimum time for harvesting leaves and flowers. A new moon is ideal for harvesting roots. (See page 72 for more on the moon.)

THE DOCTRINE OF SIGNATURES

According to the Doctrine of Signatures, which dates back to ancient Greece, herbs resembling various parts of the body can be used to treat ailments of those body parts. It was said that God (or spirit) shaped plants so that we might recognize the body system, organ or fluid that the plant has an affinity for. For example, daisy's open flower head, with its white petals and yellow centre, watches the sun as it transits the sky. It is the eye of the day, the day's eye – daisy. It closes at the end of the day. The plant's appearance and behaviour are thus reflected in daisy's traditional use to heal eye problems.

In Sensory Herbalism, you are asked to observe a herb's appearance and manner of growth. The Doctrine of Signatures can help us to interpret this information. It is not a set dogma but rather one that requires creativity and intuition to ascertain what a herb may be communicating. You will notice how the connections you make just by observing a plant are backed up by its known medicinal actions when you turn to herbals to gain further information.

Effect of Celestial Bodies on the Human Body

ASTROLOGICAL BODY	NOTES	HERBS IN THIS BOOK
Moon ☾	**QUALITIES:** Maternal, provides nurture and protection, is cooling in nature **BODILY EFFECTS:** Affects water in the body, alleviates hot symptoms, relates to emotions, influences lymph, relates directly to the womb and ovaries, governs and affects sleep **ASSOCIATIONS:** Artemis, Diana **ASTROLOGICAL SIGN:** Cancer **HERBS:** Plants living by the water (e.g. watercress), cooling plants (e.g. chickweed)	Cleavers Mugwort Poppy

ASTROLOGICAL BODY	NOTES	HERBS IN THIS BOOK
Mars ♂	**QUALITIES:** Hot, fiery, assertive, direct, pioneering and combative, passion, penetration **BODILY EFFECTS:** Influences muscular system, adrenals/kidneys, red blood cells **ASSOCIATIONS:** Mars, Roman god of war **ASTROLOGICAL SIGN:** Aries, Scorpio **HERBS:** Plants growing under adversity (e.g. blackberry), plants with thorns or prickles (e.g. hawthorn, nettle), plants generally heating in nature (e.g. horseradish)	Horseradish
Mercury ☿	**QUALITIES:** Encourages movement, promotes clear communication, air, represents the bright intelligence and the free flow of nervous energy **BODILY EFFECTS:** Governs nervous and respiratory systems, involved in matters of conscious perception **ASSOCIATIONS:** Mercury the winged messenger and a god of trade, thieves and travel **ASTROLOGICAL SIGNS:** Gemini, Virgo **HERBS:** Plants with hairy, fuzzy leaves (e.g. mullein), plants that have finely divided leaves like the bronchi of lungs (e.g. dill, fennel) or vines that grow on trees (e.g. honeysuckle), plants relating to the nervous system (e.g. skullcap, lavender, valerian)	Fennel Yarrow Valerian
Jupiter ♃	**QUALITIES:** Expansive, encourages bile production and flow, power and status, optimistic, aspirational **BODILY EFFECTS:** Relates to blood, liver, arteries **ASSOCIATIONS:** Jupiter or Jove is the king of the gods and the god of sky and thunder **ASTROLOGICAL SIGNS:** Sagittarius, Pisces **HERBS:** Herbs that promote a positive frame of mind (e.g. dandelion), large edible plants, representing expansiveness (e.g. burdock, centaury)	Dandelion

ASTROLOGICAL BODY	NOTES	HERBS IN THIS BOOK
Venus ♀	**QUALITIES:** Attraction, sensuality, warmth, grounding **BODILY EFFECTS:** Associated with the womb, kidneys, venous system **ASSOCIATIONS:** Venus, Roman goddess of love, beauty and fertility **ASTROLOGICAL SIGNS:** Taurus, Libra **HERBS:** Plants with lots of mucilage (e.g. marshmallow), plants with beautiful flowers (e.g. rose, vervain, violet), plants with red fruits (e.g. raspberry, rosehips), herbs that calm overindulgence in food (e.g. sage)	Daisy Elderberry Heather Rosehips
Saturn ♄	**QUALITIES:** Constriction, contraction, encourages boundaries **BODILY EFFECTS:** Support for mucous membranes, support and reinforcement for bones, joints and connective tissue **ASSOCIATIONS:** Saturn, Roman god of time **ASTROLOGICAL SIGNS:** Capricorn, Aquarius **HERBS:** Plants that remedy swollen joints (e.g. comfrey), perennials with long leaves (e.g. plantain), plants with annual rings or woody plants, often poisonous plants (as linked with death, e.g. datura, aconite, belladonna)	Datura Plantain
Sun ☉	**QUALITIES:** Positive, lively, warming, vital, light, paternal figure, associated with pride and the ego **BODILY EFFECTS:** Influences the heart, thymus gland **ASSOCIATIONS:** Apollo, worshipped for growth of harvest **ASTROLOGICAL SIGN:** Leo **HERBS:** Plants beneficial to the heart and circulation (e.g. rosemary, ginger), plants that lift the spirits (e.g. hypericum, motherwort)	Daisy Rosemary

COLOUR AND THE CHAKRA SYSTEM

The chakra system is a fantastic example of how a system of medicine can change as differing interpretations are added in layers through the ages. Chakra theory stems from ancient Vedic scriptures, but in recent decades this concept has been taken up by the New Age movement in the West, along with many other yogic principles.

Through meditation and yogic practice, energy centres known as chakras were

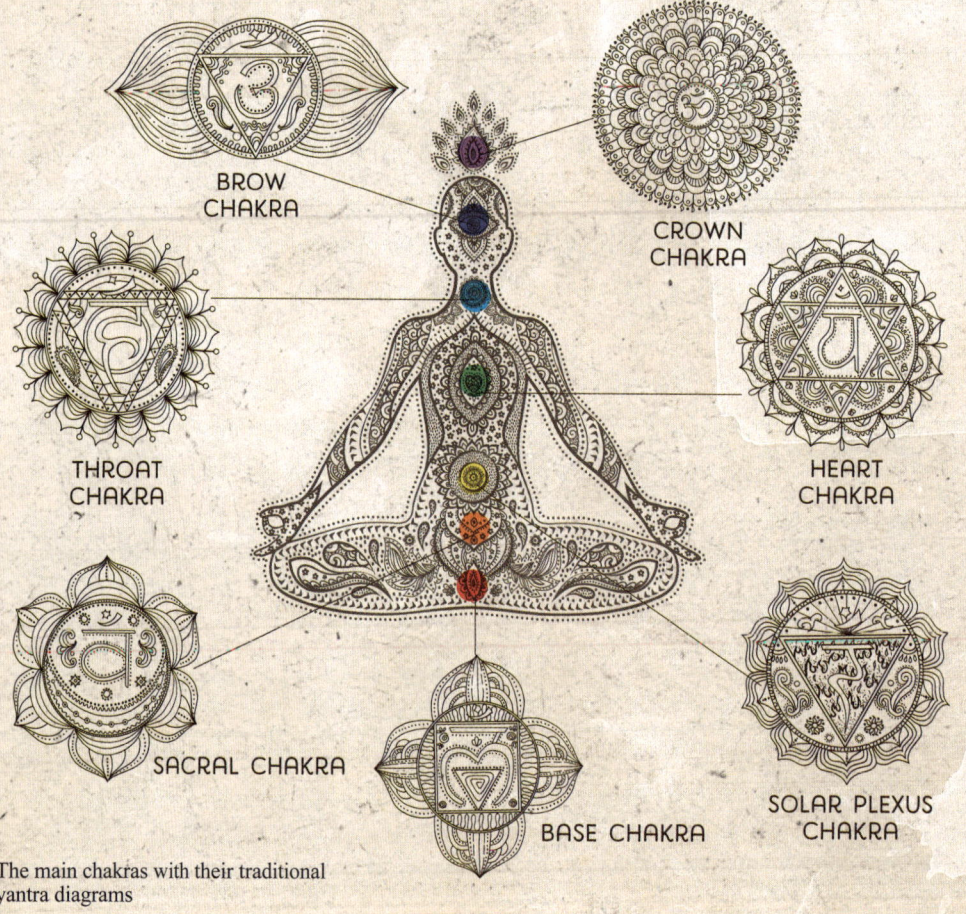

BROW CHAKRA

CROWN CHAKRA

THROAT CHAKRA

HEART CHAKRA

SACRAL CHAKRA

BASE CHAKRA

SOLAR PLEXUS CHAKRA

The main chakras with their traditional yantra diagrams

visualized as being located through the body. These areas were intuited as power points, each one representing a different energy. The seven main chakras (described on the next two pages) were thought to align with the spine, and each one was associated with one of the seven spectrum colours of red, orange, yellow, green, blue, indigo and violet, the energy of each chakra resonating with the energy of its colour. The chakras were thought to develop from birth through to adulthood, starting with the base chakra.

Although these power points or energy centres were identified thousands of years ago, it can now be observed that they correspond to the location of hormone glands within the body. There is often also a nerve plexus, where there is condensed amounts of nerve activity, located at the exact areas the chakras are located. Hormonal release and response, coupled with nerve energy could be part of the explanation for the condensed activity and the location of the chakras.

Each area is affected by correlating emotions and experiences that can increase or decrease energy output and density at the specific locations. This is beautifully illustrated by the connection between the thymus gland and the heart chakra. We know that after shock or trauma we feel more vulnerable, and may describe ourselves as having "a broken heart" or "heartache". Because the thymus gland is found to be

tiny in autopsy, it was once thought to be active only until teenage years, after which it starts to decrease in size. However, it is now known that the thymus gland can shrink by 50 percent in just one day from illness, stress or shock. Its function of excreting growth hormones drops off after puberty, but it carries on producing immune cells throughout life. When shock or trauma has occurred, there is a decreased output of immune T-cells and a person becomes prone to infection. The whole area shuts down, which will be seen as markedly reduced energy flowing through the heart chakra.

Sensory Herbalism draws on chakra theory as another tool for understanding the body and emotions in more depth. For example, the liver is located in the solar plexus chakra region. The solar plexus is linked with a sense of self and purpose in the world. If there is an issue with the liver (a sign of this might be a floating poo in the toilet, which can indicate poorly digested fats), this could stem from issues around sense of self.

Ask yourself what are the problem areas in your body, then consult the tables on the following pages to see which chakra they relate to and assess if any of the emotional issues that may knock that chakra out of balance are applicable to you.

The Chakras with Associations and Imbalances

CHAKRA/ ENERGY CENTRE	ASSOCIATED COLOUR	ASSOCIATED THEME	CHAKRA IMBALANCES
Base	Red	Adrenal glands, tribe, fight or flight, immune system	Excessive negativity, cynicism, eating disorders, greed, avarice, illusion, excessive feeling of insecurity, living constantly in survival mode, feeling alone, sciatica, hypertension, impotence, colitis, eating disorders, prostate issues in men, constipation, circulatory issues
Sacral	Orange	Ovaries, testes, relationships	Dependency, co-dependency with other people or a substance that grants you easy access to pleasure
Solar plexus	Yellow	Pancreas, the ego, sense of self in the wider community	Low self-esteem, lack of boundaries, addiction, procrastination, inability to make decisions, depression or anxiety, co-dependency, poor digestion, lung difficulties relating to diaphragm, liver and/or kidney involvement, nerve pain, arthritis
Heart	Green	Thymus, nurture, give–take balance	Loneliness, social anxiety, self-criticism, judgemental, inability to let go, difficulty giving and receiving, suspicion and fear, especially in friendships and romantic relationships, poor circulation, lung problems

The Chakras with Associations and Imbalances

CHAKRA/ ENERGY CENTRE	ASSOCIATED COLOUR	ASSOCIATED THEME	CHAKRA IMBALANCES
Throat	Blue	Thyroid, communication, honesty	Never feeling settled, inability to relax, fear of speaking out, feeling judged or pressured to not speak your truth, being unable to accept a situation, possibly emotional trauma, not believing in yourself, disconnection from your true nature/ individuality, neck pain or chronic headaches, dental pain, chronic sore throat, inability to listen
Brow (sometimes referred to as the third eye)	Indigo	Pituitary gland, control centre, intuition	Controlling over small things, obsessiveness, inability to let go of the past, living in the past, insomnia, delusions, depression, anxiety, paranoia, migraines, sinusitis, poor vision
Crown	Violet	Pineal gland, spiritual connection, dreaming	Ungrounded, airy-fairy, possible God complex, obsessive thoughts, lacking purpose, clumsy or poor balance, forgetfulness, neurological conditions (such as Parkinsons, dementia, muscular disease), sensitivity to light and certain sounds

THE PAGAN WHEEL OF THE YEAR

The wheel of the year, or the Pagan calendar, marks specific moments in time. The winter solstice occurs when the Earth's axis is tilted at the furthest point away from the sun, giving us the longest night. The summer solstice, in contrast, is when the Earth's axis is tilted toward the sun, giving us the most daylight hours. Halfway between these two points are the equinoxes, when day and night are of equal length. There are also midway points between each solstice and equinox.

These, too, are recognized as celebrations in the wheel of the year, and therefore there are eight celebrations each year.

The table below shows the names of the eight modern pagan festivals and the span of dates during which they are celebrated in the northern hemisphere.

For farming and foraging, these pivotal points are significant, marking the cycle of the seasons. Crops and wild plants respond to the seasonal changes in energy, influenced

Pagan Festivals Through the Year

DATE	ENGLISH NAME	CELTIC NAME	HERBS FOR HARVESTING
31 October	Halloween (All Hallows Eve)	Samhain	Horseradish, valerian
19–22 December	Winter Solstice	Yule	Mistletoe
1 February	Candlemas	Imbolc	Plantain, dandelion root, nettle
19–22 March	Spring Equinox	Ostara	Plantain, dandelion leaf, cleavers, daisy
1 May	May Day	Beltane	Elderflowers
19–22 June	Summer Solstice	Litha	Rosemary
1 August	Harvest Festival	Lughnasadh	Milk thistle, mugwort
19–22 September	Autumn Equinox	Mabon	Elderberries, rosehips

by variations in the amount of light and the atmospheric temperature. The more you work with the Earth's cycles, the more you will naturally recognize the shift in the seasons.

Although these specific dates mark the seasonal turning points, in practice the timing of celebrations in days gone by often depended on the weather and harvest. If there was a crop to bring in and the first fair weather for weeks, folk would be out harvesting, not yet in celebration. Similarly, farming communities would have celebrated at different times from fishing communities. The roots of paganism – or the worship of the seasons, spirits and deities of the land – are intertwined with the physical reality of harvesting food and medicine.

As part of your Sensory Herbalism practice you will start to follow the cycle of the seasons through the year. Each season will begin to hold deeper significance, the more time you spend on the land, foraging and harvesting. Harvesting gives a grounding and practical side to a spiritual practice, putting you in tune with the changing seasons and the ever-changing tilt of the Earth's axis. Spring brings a bounce to your step with the excitement of the arrival of fresh, green, leafy medicine. Summer warmth and light bring fertility and passion. Autumn is a time of bountiful harvests – hips, haws, berries and fruit practically spill out the door as you struggle to find surfaces on which to

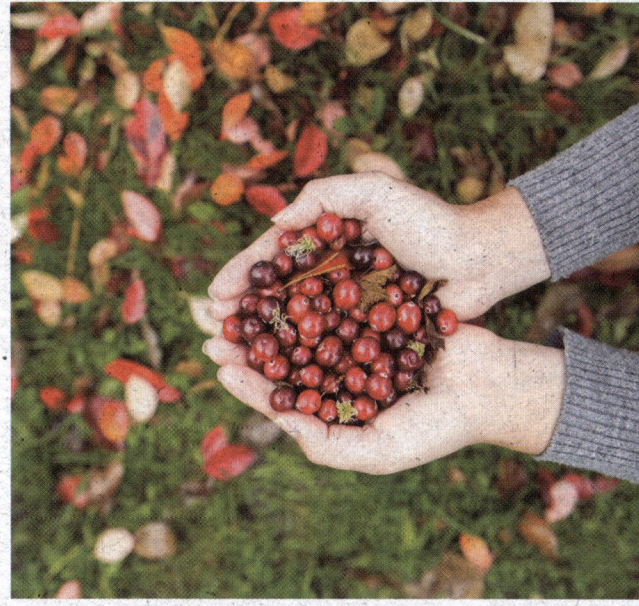

In autumn, nature provides a bountiful harvest of berries, hips, haws and fruit.

process them! And winter allows time for planning and preparing for the next cycle. It is important to observe your surroundings and learn when the medicines that grow around your home are ready.

Following the pagan wheel of the year gives eight significant points through the year that can be celebrated communally. If these festivals resonate with you, you could start to organize get-togethers, have a fire, share seasonal food and invite like-minded folk to join you. It's a wonderful way to start creating and nourishing community.

ELEMENTAL MEDICINE ACROSS THE WORLD

Ancient systems of philosophy and medicine have always drawn on elemental theory to describe the world of nature and matter around them. In Sensory Herbalism, we also draw on the five basic elements of the ancient world – water, fire, air, earth and spirit – to inform our whole system of medicine.

It is important to highlight some of the models that have influenced us and taught us much over the years. Without the systems that have gone before we wouldn't have been inspired to create an alternative perspective.

In all of the ancient systems – Ayurveda, Chinese Medicine, Western Medicine, and in Sensory Herbalism, too – good health or an individual's chi or vital force is dependent on all the elements being in balance within the body. In the case of excess damp or water, a person may be prone to conditions that are opportunistic in such an environment. These could include lung conditions presenting with excess phlegm or digestive conditions with harmful bacterial overgrowth such as *Candida albicans*. An excess of water or damp in the system could also leave someone hyper-emotional and unable to rationalize.

When you look at each individual, you will see that they will be more naturally aligned with one element, with influences of the others. Someone may naturally be more fiery and passionate, another person more solid and steadfast. This does not mean that they are out of balance but rather they present in a certain way that, if everything is in balance for them, means they are healthy and vital. They have a strong vital force. The difficulties arise when an element starts to take over that is not in their natural state, or they become overly hot or overly stuck in the earth element. "Dis-ease" will start to arise.

This fine balance is affected by a complex web of influences. What these influences are varies according to the system of medicine. The next pages explore some of the systems that we have studied over the years and that have influenced Sensory Herbalism.

AYURVEDA

Developed thousands of years ago, Ayurveda (meaning "the science of life") is the predominant medicine in India. It looks at balancing body, mind and spirit for good health. People are characterized into three different "doshas", or energetic types, in order to build a picture of what may be beneficial for them in terms of food, weather and types

Elements in Ayurveda

SEASON	ELEMENTS	ENERGETICS	DOSHAS
Late winter Early spring	Water and earth	Oily, cool, heavy, sticky, sluggish, smooth, dull	Kapha
Late spring Summer	Fire and water	Oily, hot, light, intense, fluid, soft, spreading	Pitta
Autumn Early winter	Air and space	Dry, cold, light, erratic, mobile, rough, irregular	Vata

of exercise. When you are born, one dosha is usually more prominent in your "prakruti", or specific make-up or presentation, and this stays with you for life. Similarly, in the Sensory Herbalism model one element may be more naturally ascendant or influential. The table above shows how, in Ayurveda, the doshas are associated with the seasons, just as the elements are in Sensory Herbalism.

CHINESE MEDICINE

Chinese medicine views the five elements as phases of the year (see the table on page 38). The idea of one element being present in each season suggests something fixed, whereas in reality a ten-day crossover of each season called "doyin" allows for movement rather than stasis. At that time, any of the four seasons' weather might appear. This explains why snow may appear in April, for example.

Chinese medicine incorporates a complex array of theory applied to acupuncture and Traditional Chinese Medicine (TCM). Even the time of day is taken into account in TCM. If someone wakes at a specific time each night, this could be indicative of issues with a certain organ. For example, 1–3 a.m. is related to the liver, while 3–5 a.m. is related to the lungs.

The five elements in Chinese Medicine – wood, fire, earth, metal and water – are categorized into seasons, organs, tastes, colours … the list goes on. We have been influenced by the form of Chinese medicine rather than the particulars. We have embraced some organ and element associations, such as the link of the stomach with the earth element and the view of systems or organs as an expression of an element rather than just functional equipment in the human body.

Elements in Chinese Medicine

ELEMENT	SEASON	ORGAN	ENERGETICS
Wood (Mu)	Spring	Liver, gall bladder	Wind
Fire (Huo)	Summer	Heart, small intestine	Heat
Earth (Tu)	Late summer	Spleen, stomach	Dampness
Metal (Jin)	Autumn	Lungs, large intestine	Dryness
Water (Shui)	Winter	Kidney, bladder	Cold

WESTERN MEDICINE – THE FOUR HUMOURS

Humoral theory, also known as humourism or the theory of the four humours, was a model for the workings of the human body that was systemized in ancient Greece, although its origins may go back further still. The theory was central to the teachings of Hippocrates, the father of modern medicine (*c*. 400 BCE), and Galen, a prominent Greek physician and philosopher (*c*. 170 CE). The dominant medical theory in Europe for many centuries, it remained a major influence on practice and teaching until well into the 1800s.

In this theory, humours exist as liquids within the body and are identified as blood, yellow bile, black bile and phlegm. The health of a person depends on the balance of these fluids in the body. These fluids are in turn associated with the fundamental elements of air, fire, earth and water respectively. This traditional scheme is still adopted by many modern herbalists. It is

Elements in Western Medicine

ELEMENT	SEASON	ORGAN	ENERGETICS
Air	Spring	Liver	Warm and moist
Fire	Summer	Spleen	Warm and dry
Earth	Autumn	Gall bladder	Cold and dry
Water	Winter	Brain/lungs	Cold and moist

very focused on the bodily fluids, whereas in Sensory Herbalism, we consider how the elements present within the body and emotions. Inevitably, however, our practice echoes this system, as we were taught within the Western tradition of herbal medicine.

Marcos Patchett, a contemporary medical herbalist whose practice is still rooted in the tradition of humourism, sums up humoural medicine as this: "Heat generates life and cold removes it. Dryness disperses and desiccates leading to infertility and moisture collects and generates producing fertility. Heat eventually destroys moisture, then disperses itself, producing cold. Cold gradually collects moisture, which eventually collects and generates heat."

He goes on to explain how this is reflected in the turning cycle of the seasons (or a day), each with its own qualities, from the hot, sanguine youth of spring (or early morning) to the cold, phlegmatic old age of winter (or the hours between midnight and dawn).

SENSORY HERBALISM AND THE ELEMENTS

Sensory Herbalism links the elements to the seasons according to how the plants show themselves most prevalently at that time. It follows the plants on their journey through the year and sees the elements reflected in the plant part that is most readily available in each given season. This differs from some of the ancient systems of medicine. Let's take winter for example. In Traditional Chinese Medicine and the humours of Western medicine, winter correlates to the element of water. The earth is seen as water-logged and damp-related disease becomes more prevalent. In Sensory Herbalism, we see winter as the time when all of the energy of growth retreats into the roots to revive ready for spring. Early winter or just before spring is therefore the time when we harvest most of our roots, when they are full of earth energy. We equate winter with the grounding element of earth, as a time to take stock, retreat and restore. Come spring, the plants draw up water from the earth and start to produce verdant, water-filled leaves. Spring is a time for cleansing and remineralizing, flushing the system and cleansing the emotions. Spring, in Sensory Herbalism, is therefore equated with water.

Sensory Herbalism focuses on the plants themselves, on how they reflect the elements and therefore on how we humans interact with the plants at each given season. In our years of practising and teaching in this way, this approach has provided a simple structure for people to connect with the seasons and for the harvesting of medicinal plants. You will see in the Seasonal Journey how, as with traditional systems, we also correlate systems within the body with elements according to the energetic function of those systems.

For example, the digestive system processes food, bringing us back to earth if we are in shock or having a blood sugar crash. A person with a malfunctioning digestive system will often present as floaty and hard to pin down, thoughts are challenging to grasp and they may loose their trail of thought or speak about things that seem irrelevant. The digestive system in its proper functioning will provide grounding, an earth element.

It might be seen as reinventing the wheel to take a traditional system apart and rebuild it in a new way. In truth this is how medicine has grown and developed over the centuries; people question the current paradigm and add their own interpretations. Ancient Greek medicine was developed from Egyptian medicine. Each and every system before Sensory Herbalism has been developed by somebody else as a result of his or her observations of nature and the human body. Incidentally, what has been recorded and therefore developed into the accepted paradigm is mainly written by male scholars. This gives us a one-sided view of the world and maybe it is time for a rethink.

The four basic elements – water, fire, air and earth – form the foundation of life itself. They are expressed in us through the way our bodies function. They are expressed through our emotions. They are expressed in plants and in the seasons. Sensory Herbalism follows the elements through the cycle of the year by observing how they are expressed most fully in each season and expressed in the plants as they grow and develop through each season. It looks at the expression of the elements in the human body – emotionally, physically, spiritually.

Water correlates with spring

When the rivers are in spate from the melting snow, the showers come more frequently, rejuvenating the earth, and dormant nature sprouts into action. Lush leaves start to form, full of hydration.

Fire correlates with summer

The energy of fire is in abundance when the sun is at its highest and reproduction in nature occurs most readily.

Air correlates with autumn/fall

Autumnal winds create diaspora by blowing the seeds to pastures new to regenerate once again, come the right time and conditions.

Earth correlates with winter

Earth is embodied fully in the winter months, when energy drops down into the ground. Growth above ground stills and plant roots hold nourishment for the following year.

Spirit pervades throughout the year

Throughout the 13-moon yearly cycle, spirit initiates magic in the natural world.

ELEMENTS IN THE EMOTIONAL OR ENERGETIC BODY

It is common to classify people "elementally" without even being aware that you're doing it. Someone may be described as wet or slippery, fiery or hot, airy-fairy or grounded and practical. Even when thinking of a person as wise or spiritual, we evoke the spirit or ethereal element. What words do others use to describe you? What words might you choose to describe yourself? Are you aware of how you feel or present elementally? For those of you interested in astrology, you may already have a story or idea in your mind according to which signs the planets were in at your birth.

As we've discussed earlier, one element is usually more dominant in an individual's make-up. This doesn't mean that there is an imbalance and can often be explained through the astrological birth chart. This astrological chart determines the position of certain planets in the zodiac at birth, and can create a sort of blueprint as to how you may move through life. It can be astonishingly accurate and has been used for centuries across the globe. The blueprint does not affect your free will, or your capacity to shift from predetermined traits.

The table on page 42 explores how expressing one element more than others can still be harmonious. It also shows how excess or deficiency of an element may present in an individual. It is important to remember that this is not a definitive guide. Interpretation is important and takes practice. For example, a lack of the element of air making an

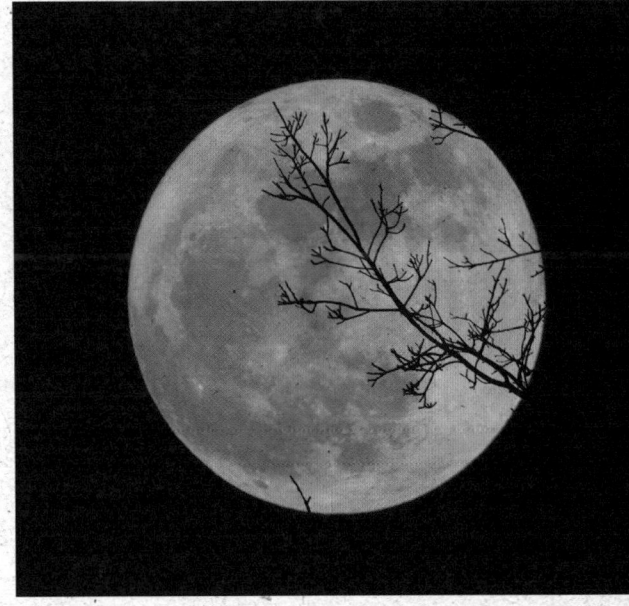

The moon brings the element of spirit into nature throughout the 13 moons of a year.

individual appear static, uninspired and heavy could look similar to an excess of the element of earth, which could present as stubbornness or seeming unmoved emotionally.

Considering the emotions as map to the physical body helps to build a picture of the internal environment as expressed in an emotional way. For example, heat in an over-taxed liver could be expressed as anger; an excess of the element of fire.

As an example of how to use the table on page 42 to assess others, an artist came to us who was a fairly sociable, communicative type. He was always the heart and soul of a party, up for fun and a laugh. He was also extremely organized and practical, naturally an air type with aspects of earth. But he was feeling uninspired. The ideas had run out, he was dead to his creative flow and finding social situations challenging, as he felt he had nothing to talk about. He wanted to get back to his natural state of creative flow and harmony. His experience of a lack of

Elements in Balance/Excess in Sensory Herbalism

ELEMENT	ELEMENT IN BALANCE	ELEMENT IN EXCESS	DEFICIENCY OF ELEMENT	ASTROLOGY	HERB
Water	Compassionate	Pushover, wet, histrionic (needs fire to push out the damp)	Rigid, brittle	Cancer Scorpio Pisces	Cleavers
Fire	Passionate	Jealous (needs to be cooled with water element)	Apathetic	Aries Leo Sagittarius	Daisy
Air	Communicative, inspired	Ungrounded, flighty (needs to be grounded with earth element)	Unimaginative	Libra Aquarius Gemini	Fennel seed
Earth	Pragmatic, practical, organized	Stubborn (needs relaxation of boundaries)	Lacking in will	Capricorn Taurus Virgo	Dandelion root

imagination suggested that he had a lack of the air element. Fennel is a prime example of an air herb whose plant part (the seed) also expresses the air element. This made fennel the perfect match. He was given drops to take with an affirmation: "I am open to receiving inspirations." He felt that the focus on the affirmation and the regular zingy taste of the fennel rebalanced him and inspiration started to flow again.

In this case, we can see that the artist was experiencing a lack of air. In the case of an excess of an element, it needs to be opposed. This is a very simplistic system and when you get into more complex health treatment, the approach needs to be holistic, taking into account physical presentation of symptoms, which organs are linked, what this could mean emotionally, and so on. However, it is nice to experiment simply with drop doses of a herb, with specific intentions to shift the elemental emotional presentation.

From the table opposite, we can see that an excess of air will benefit from being grounded with the earth element. Dandelion root provides grounding root energy. In the case of an air excess, dandelion, taken in conjuction with an affirmation, could be used to bring earthly grounding. You may want to think of other herbs that express predominantly one element and start to build up an elemental herbal tool kit.

Elements, Seasons and Systems in Sensory Herbalism

ELEMENT	SEASON	BODY SYSTEM
Water	Spring	Lymphatic system Urinary system
Fire	Summer	Heart Circulatory system
Air	Autumn	Nervous system Lungs
Earth	Winter	Bones Skin Digestive system
Spirit	13 moons	Reproductive system

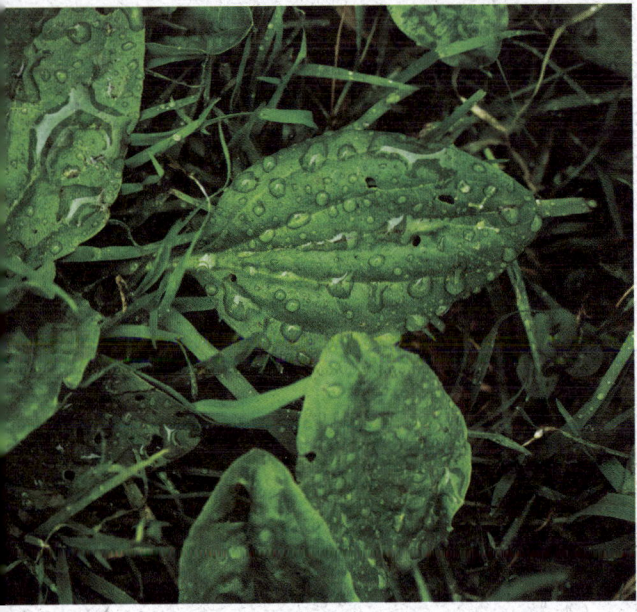

Leafy plantain protects the boundaries of the body.

ELEMENTS EXPRESSED IN THE PHYSICAL BODY

In Sensory Herbalism, the elements correlate to different systems in the body where the energy of that element is most represented. **Water** can easily be seen in the kidneys and bladder – the urinary system. The lymphatic system is heavily dependent on good hydration for efficient functioning, so we have also linked lymph with water. **Fire** correlates with the heart and circulation and the energy needed to move the blood around the body.

Air is linked with the nervous system, shaky and impulsive in character. The lungs or respiratory system provide a physical interface with the air around us. **Earth** is associated with bones, which hold us steady, and with skin which holds us in. Earth is connected to the digestive system where we process food grown in the earth; here we ground and nourish ourselves. We have linked **Spirit** to the male and female reproductive systems and with the womb, where we all begin our evolutionary cycle.

ELEMENTS EXPRESSED SPIRITUALLY

There are a multitude of ways to connect with the divine to come to acceptance and unity, from prayer, meditation, yoga or tai chi, to practical ritual such as methodical preparation of wood for the fire, to the ingestion of perception-altering plants. Spirit is present in all beings and is accessible in different ways. It may be expressed as deep knowledge, as championing causes, as inspiring social change and justice, or as psychic abilities, magic or intuition. Spirit informs our ritual practices with plant medicines, and drives our connectivity.

ELEMENTS EXPRESSED IN THE HERBS

In Sensory Herbalism, the plants predominantly express one of the five elements and this in part relates to their astrological associations. So, for example, plantain is ruled by the planet Saturn, linked with the earth element … warm, grounding, generous. Plantain is therefore seen as a plant representing the earth element. Plantain as a mucous membrane restorative improves the stability of our own physical boundaries. Mucous membranes are a boundary between the outside and inner worlds, preventing pathogens or allergens from penetrating the system and into the bloodstream. Boundaries, the skin and mucous membranes are seen in Sensory Herbalism as part of the earth element of grounding and structure.

In addition, we generally use the leaf of plantain as the medicinal part of this plant. In Sensory Herbalism, leaves represent the succulence of the water element. Plantain leaves are harvested in the spring, which is associated with the water element. So plantain leaf becomes the earth element of water. They carry the mineral-rich energy of the spring soil.

The more you get to know the plants, the more this will become clear. In the table of the emotional expression of the elements on page 42, we have chosen plants in which the element is represented by both the plant and the plant part. So cleavers is a water herb of the moon and we use the leaf, also the water element. Daisy is associated with the sun (as well as Venus) and is a flower associated with the fire element. Fennel is a Mercurial air plant and we use the seeds for medicine. The autumnal seeds are linked with air and the nervous system and lungs. Dandelion, however, is a law unto itself, each part of the plant expressing a different element. Although it is ruled by Jupiter, the planet of expansion, the yellow, sun-like flowers can be seen as fire of fire, the urinary system-associated leaves are water of water, the digestive system-related roots are earth of earth and those air-borne dandelion clock seeds are air of air. Dandelion is an anomaly. Generally the whole of a plant will be more expressive of one element and its plant parts then bring in the energy of that element.

ELEMENTS EXPRESSED IN THE PLANT PARTS

The seasons correlate to the part of the plant most prevalent and generally most medicinally valuable at that time. Spirit can be found throughout the plant and at every stage of its development and reproduction. As with people, different parts of a plant express more of one element or another. We have linked the leaves, flowers, seed and roots of the plants to the five elements:

WATER = SPRING = LEAF
FIRE = SUMMER = FLOWER
AIR = AUTUMN = SEED
EARTH = WINTER = ROOT
SPIRIT = 13 MOONS = ALL

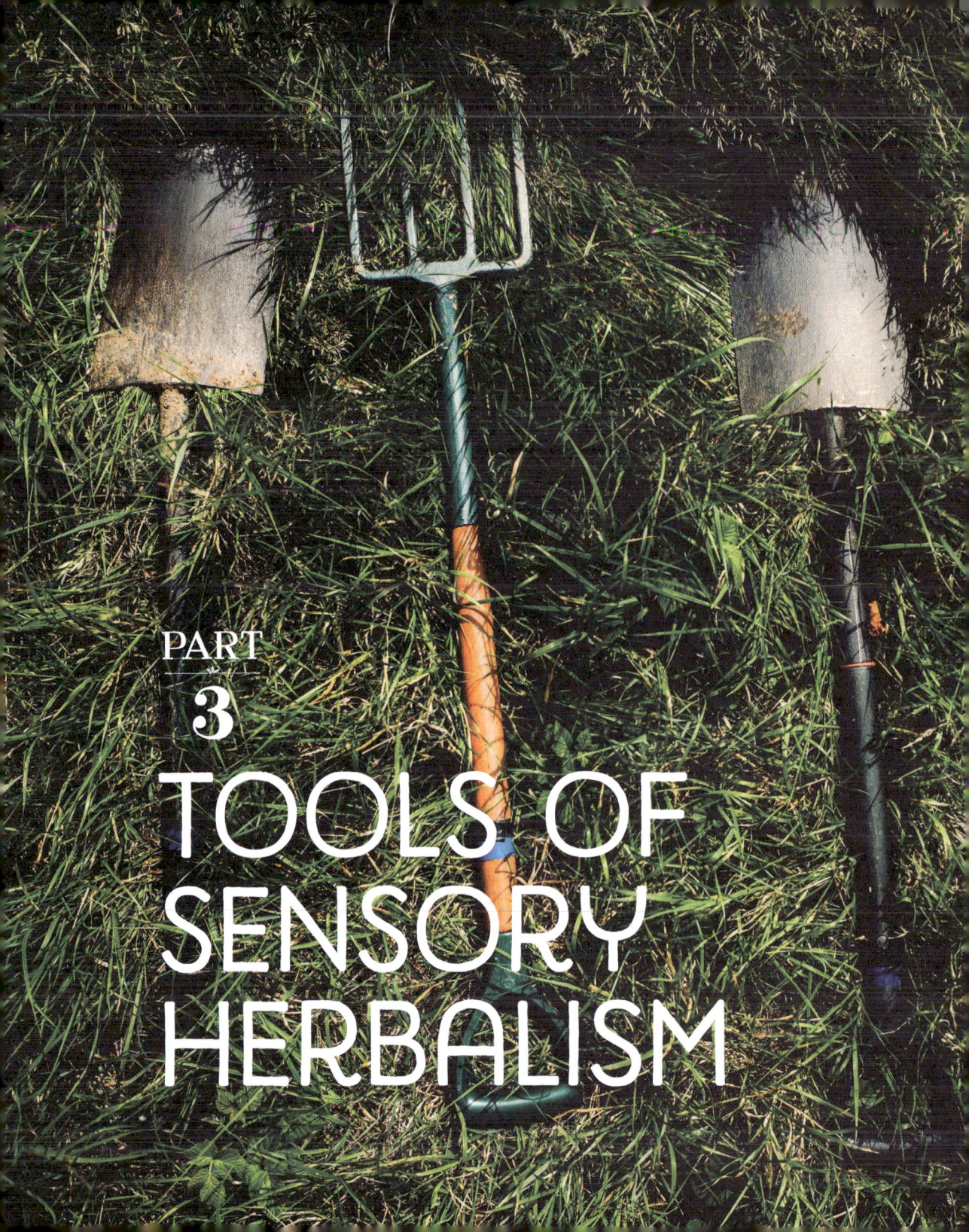

TOOLS OF SENSORY HERBALISM

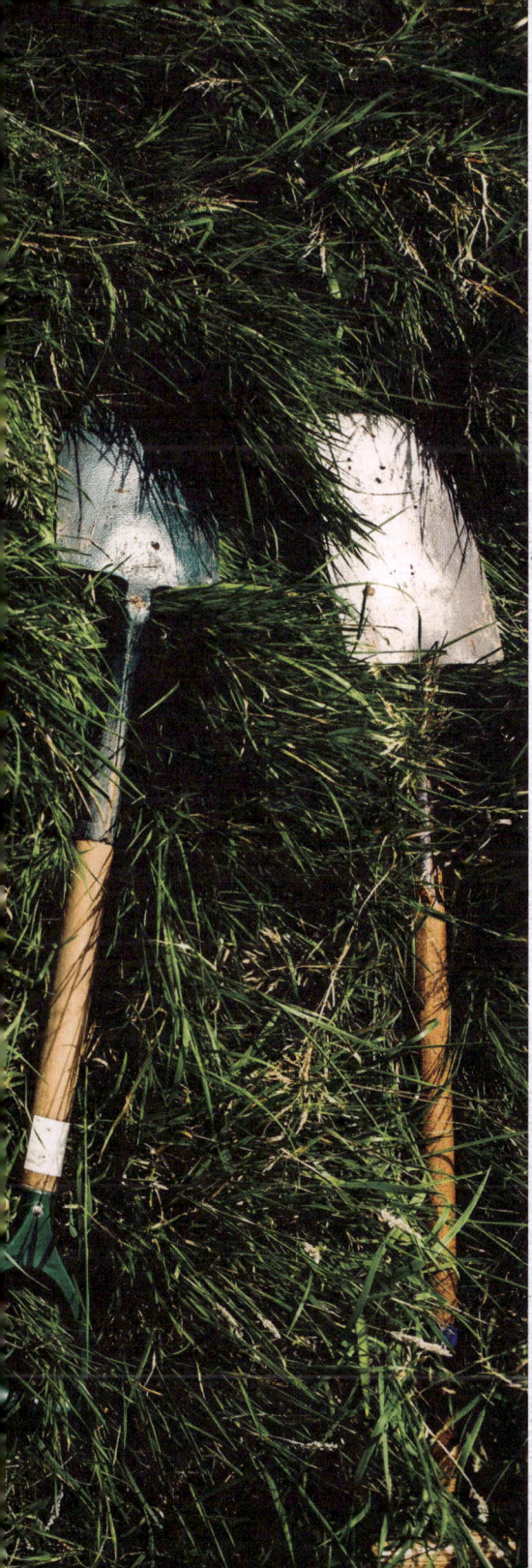

Plant compounds elicit responses from us by interacting with receptors in cells and nerve endings. We are composed of much the same substances as our plant cousins; we have grown and developed together over millennia. We can speak the same language if we just give ourselves the chance to do so. Taste a bitter lettuce or a sweet apple and the conversation begins. The way a plant tastes gives us clues to its physical actions. Plants also communicate with us through their visual appearance, their scent, the way they feel to the touch and the energy they emit. Taking time to stop and breathe, to sense and experience, brings us an awareness of how each plant forms a relationship with us. The more we experiment, explore and practise speaking to plants in this way, the deeper our relationship goes. Sensory Herbalism offers simple techniques for tuning into, and learning to trust, your own senses, translating the language of the plants.

FIVE TOOLS OF SENSORY HERBALISM

Sensory Herbalism reveals our own inherent plant knowledge through observation, intuition and interpretation, as we watch, taste, touch, smell and draw to connect deeply with herbs. Meditation, creative writing and discussion also help us decode the language of the plants, while creating characters and folklore for the herbs breathes new life into ancient legends.

Working with plants for the first time can be daunting. The tools of Sensory Herbalism will give you a structure to work with as you move through the cycle of the year, meeting the plants that flourish, and produce the parts you need, in each season. If you use these tools, you will gain a deep and lasting understanding of the plants. As with any new friend, the more time we spend getting to know the plants in different ways, the deeper and more profound the friendship becomes.

The five Sensory Herbalism tools that guide you as you meet the plants are:
1. OBSERVATION
2. INTUITION
3. INTERPRETATION
4. CHARACTERIZATION
5. PLANT DREAM CREATION

As we consider each tool, we will use rosemary as an example of how to apply it.

CREATE YOUR OWN SENSORY HERBAL

To truly immerse yourself in Sensory Herbalism, we recommend that you fill a sketchbook with the information you discover from each plant you work with. You could have a section for each herb, with drawings as well as all your observations, thoughts, feelings and stories. This will become your own sensory herbal, a reminder of your discoveries and a useful reference, as well as a beautiful object to treasure.

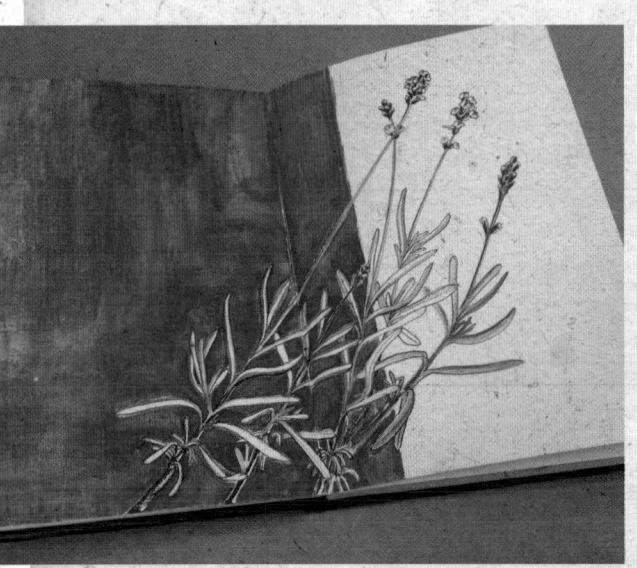

Lavender lovingly depicted in a sensory herbal

OBSERVATION

The more familiar you become with the way a plant looks, smells, tastes or feels, the more you begin to notice similarities with other herbs. Then, plants that are new to you might seem recognizable, reminding you of a more familiar plant ally, just as we sometimes make an instant connection with a stranger who reminds us of a close friend or relative.

We recommend you start with a plant whose identity you are sure of. Clear your mind of any preconceived ideas about that plant and try the exercise below.

SIGHT

Let's use the herb rosemary as an example. Find a rosemary plant, perhaps in a garden or a garden centre. First, have a look at the overall structure of this evergreen bush from a few metres away. What colour is it? How dense is it? What shape is it? Take a cutting and sketch a loose outline of this. Then try drawing something much more intricate; you may like to examine the individual leaves with a magnifying glass for a detailed image. Don't worry about your drawing skills; this exercise is about your powers of observation.

SMELL AND TASTE

Smell and taste are particularly vital in the observation tool kit. They can give an indication of compounds contained within a plant. Every plant part (roots, leaves, seeds, flowers) contains a host of different phytochemicals that serve different functions within the plant and each of these constituents will affect the human body in its own way. It may seem a somewhat reductionist way of looking at the wonder of plants, but linking tastes and smells with these constituents gives us an indication of a plant's potential medicinal actions. For example, plants that taste soapy and make saliva frothy when chewed contain the phytochemical compounds called saponins. These have an expectorant action on the lungs. Therefore, a plant that creates frothy saliva may be useful for phlegmy coughs. Recognizing individual tastes or sensations in the mouth helps to simplify the complex presentation of flavours found within one plant. Indeed, the same plant can have a different taste in its roots compared to its leaves, and the compounds will differ, too. Leaves that grow nearer to the ground may differ slightly in constituents from those located higher up the stem. The multiple constituents of each plant work in a synergistic way in which the overall effects are beyond the measure of individual compounds. However, as with any new language, simplifying helps us to learn it.

Notes on Observation

TOOL	NOTES
Sight	Make detailed notes of the plant, observing: What is the colour/shape/structure? How is it growing? What is the soil like (chalky, rich, wasteground)? Is it in a shady or sunny spot? Make a detailed drawing including as many botanical observations as you can. Look at the leaf edge and veins, how the leaves grow from the stem and where the flowers grow. Make a pressing (either in a flower press or between two pieces of kitchen towel pressed inside a thick book). For larger samples we recommend at least an A4 flower press. Take photos. This can help to commit the plant to memory and to verify identification. Dissect with a thin sharp knife. This is a fascinating way to see inside the plant part, whether leaf, flower, seed or root. You can start to list the botanical parts you notice.
Touch	How does it feel? Waxy, soft, prickly, irritating, stinging, wet, dry, smooth, rough?
Hearing	When rubbed or picked or torn, how does it sound?
Smell	If you rub the plant, what scents can you identify? Freshly mown grass, floral, pungent, medicinal, fruity, honey-like? What is your reaction to the smell? Is it repugnant, heady, enjoyable? Does the smell remind you of anything else? This might be another plant but equally might be something seemingly random. Everything is worth noting down.

TOOL	NOTES
Taste	Start with a little of the plant and place it on the end of your tongue and then chew (be certain of the plant's identification and safety before embarking on tasting it). Become aware of any tastes – there are often many. Is it acrid, green (yes, often used to describe the flavour!), bitter, fruity, mushroomy, sour, cereal-like, malty, salty, sweet, nutty, metallic, hot/spicy, pungent? How does it feel in the mouth? Are there any reactions? Slimy, drying, refrigerant, tingly, numbing, frothy saliva, drying/astringent/puckering, burning/acrid coating, oily? Where exactly can you feel it on the tongue?
Harvesting	Is it easy or a challenge to pick? At what height does the herb grow? Do you need a ladder to reach it? Is it growing in water? Is it easy to dig up? Consider the amount of herb that is possible to harvest. Is it growing in abundance? Is it hard to find? What tools are needed (e.g. gloves, knife, trowel, basket)? Observe your own reactions to harvesting. Is it compulsive, enjoyable, tough, etc?
Processing	Processing a herb may involve: stripping from a central stem crushing up leaves straining the herbs from oil or alcohol noting if the herb is challenging or easy to process.

PLANT CONSTITUENTS AND WHAT THEY MEAN

It helps to know a little more about plant constituents in order to build up a detailed picture when you are observing, tasting and smelling a herb. For example, it is helpful to know that richly coloured berries are often high in flavonoids (see page 52). Like all life forms, the complex plant compounds contain carbon atoms, which bind with other

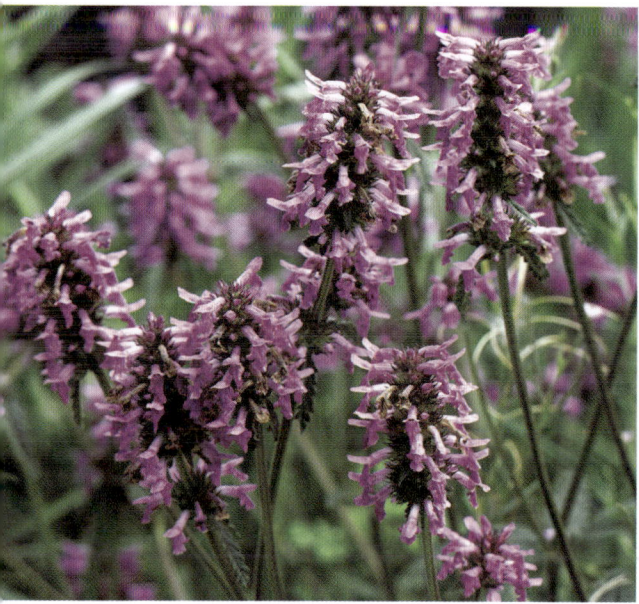

Wood betony, known for easing stress headaches

substances to give them a specific structure or form. Their composition determines how they will interact with the human body. The tables on the next three pages summarize some attributes associated with particular plant tastes and sensations.

AROMATIC VOLATILE OR ESSENTIAL OILS mostly possess antiseptic properties, but some are more specifically antifungal or antiviral. They are the aromatic scents that are notably released from a plant part when crushed. Essential oils are located in tiny secretory structures in various parts of plants, such as thyme leaves, lavender flowers or juniper berries.

IRIDOIDS are characterized by a bitter taste. They are produced by the plant as a defence mechanism. Aucubin is one of the most common iridoids and is bitter but also mushroomy in flavour. Its presence indicates a relaxing quality; herbs containing aucubin affect the nervous system, helping one to become more chilled out. It is present in herbs such as skullcap, which is famous for cooling a hot-headed state, or wood betony, a herb fabulous for helping with a headache caused by nervous tension.

FLAVONOIDS are widely distributed in plants. The name flavonoid comes from the Latin *flavus*, "yellow". They (and carotenoids) are mainly responsible for the colouration of flowers, fruits and vegetables. They attract pollinators or ward off predatory herbivores with their bright pigments. Flavonoid compounds have been associated with lots of health benefits, including protection of the skin, improving blood sugar regulation, and anti-inflammatory and antioxidant effects. They have been linked with anti-cancer diets and associated with boosting the immune system. As they are mainly found in fruit and vegetables, a diet high in flavonoids would naturally be packed full of other nutrients and minerals too.

TANNINS are found in many species of plants. They protect against physical

Tastes, Sensations and Associated Actions of Herbs

TASTE/ SENSATION	ELEMENT ASSOCIATED IN SENSORY HERBALISM	ASSOCIATED CHEMICAL CONSTITUENTS	INDICATION	HERBS IN THIS BOOK
Sweet	Earth	Carbohydrate, fat and protein (predominantly found in roots and seeds)	Tonic, demulcent (relieves inflammation), soft, soothing, cooling	Dandelion root
Sour	Water and earth	Acids	Digestive stimulant, increases bile, gently stimulating to whole system	Rosehips Elderberry
Salty	Earth, fire and water	Minerals	Stimulates appetite, nourishing to the nervous system	Cleavers
Spicy	Fire and air	Terpenes and iridoids	Heating, invigorates blood flow, encourages sweating, stimulates metabolism	Cleavers Horseradish Valerian
Perfumed	Air	Aromatic volatile oils (high in mint family)	Supports lung function	Mint Rosemary Lavender Lemon balm

TASTE/ SENSATION	ELEMENT ASSOCIATED IN SENSORY HERBALISM	ASSOCIATED CHEMICAL CONSTITUENTS	INDICATION	HERBS IN THIS BOOK
Bitter	Air and earth	Many compounds, including: iridoids alkaloids (often most toxic compounds) flavonoids	Toning to mucosa of the gastro- intestinal tract, increases digestive secretions, anti- inflammatory, anti-bacterial, anti-pyretic (fever), promotes peristalsis and urination, reduces itching, swelling, oozing on the skin	Dandelion root Horse- radish Mugwort Rosemary Valerian Yarrow
Astringent	Fire and air	Tannins (high in rose family)	Drying, repairs wounds, neutralizes bacteria, reduces leakage of bodily fluids (e.g. sweating, bleeding, diarrhoea)	Heather Rosehip
Metallic	Air	Trace metals	Encourages transformation, self-reflection	Daisy
Mucilaginous, slimy	Water	Polysaccharides	Soothes irritated mucous membranes	Dandelion root
Frothy saliva	Water and air	Saponins	A soapy quality that indicates expectorant action	Daisy
Tingly, numbing, cooling	Water and air	Volatile oils	Anodyne when in contact with mucous membranes or applied topically	Poppy Fennel

TASTE/ SENSATION	ELEMENT ASSOCIATED IN SENSORY HERBALISM	ASSOCIATED CHEMICAL CONSTITUENTS	INDICATION	HERBS IN THIS BOOK
Oily	Water and earth	Lipids (including fatty acids)	Important for healthy functioning of cells and membranes	Fennel Mugwort Yarrow Rosemary
Sticky, coating, fragrant	Earth	Resins	Anti-microbial	Rosemary Yarrow

predators and act as pesticides. They also regulate plant growth. The astringency from tannins causes a dry and puckering feeling in the mouth. Tannins are also mildly antiseptic.

POLYSACCHARIDES are long chains of sugars, including starch, glycogen, cellulose and inulin. Starch and glycogen serve as short-term energy stores. Cellulose is used to build cell wall structure. Inulin compounds have many medicinal benefits including hypoglycaemic properties for blood sugar regulation. They may add a sweetness or a subtle, almost nourishing sensation.

SAPONINS serve to protect the plant against microbes and fungi. They derive their name from the soapwort plant. They taste soapy and create frothy saliva. They are poisonous to fish, and therefore plants high in saponins have been used in river fishing: large amounts of saponins washed into a river stun the fish, making them easier to catch but without making them toxic to humans. Saponins break down red blood cells, so are not used on open wounds. They irritate mucous membranes in the gut. By reflex action via the nervous system, more specifically the vagus nerve, they cause the lungs to expectorate phlegm.

PHYSICAL ACTIONS
The physical actions a plant has on the body are also a key to the more emotional or spiritual attributes of each herb. Rosemary is high in essential or volatile oils produced as protection from pathogens. Rosemary protects us on a physical level against microbes and also provides emotional and spiritual protection. It is carried to ward off negative influences or is traditionally planted outside the home to protect from robbers.

INTUITION

People often stop in their tracks to wonder at a particular plant or tree that they pass. They may feel compelled to stroke the leaves, smell the flower or take a photo. Some of the braver ones may take a nibble. What is this calling? Our primordial instinct may be telling us this plant needs to be in our lives.

How does our intuition work? How can we harness and hone this incredible ability? By turning our attention to our heart space and opening ourselves up (for example through breathing techniques or meditation), we become aligned with and more receptive to the callings of the natural world.

This part of Sensory Herbalism is both exciting and creative. With intuitive knowledge there is no right or wrong way.

It is about connecting to what you sense when you focus inside yourself. How do you feel? What sounds are you compelled to make? What pictures or words come to you? Intuition is informed by our own experiences and by something that seems to come from deep within, an instinctive understanding.

Tapping into the spirit of the plant and going on a journey of exploration can take many forms. Whatever ideas surface, however random they may seem, they are important to note. If while you are working with a plant your mind wanders, ask yourself what you are thinking about. What memories are evoked through working with the plant? Note the conversations you have if you are out harvesting with friends. It's all useful.

Connecting with Horseradish

An overall feeling and experience can be translated into useful information about how and when to use a plant. When interacting with the horseradish plant, for example, most people first feel familiarity when they employ their sense of smell. The pungent heady odour "hits" the nostrils and provokes some sort of vocal reaction in most people. Then their eyes begin to stream as the volatile oils react with the cornea. The taste of the fresh root is so intense it provokes a flurry of sneezing, coughing and spluttering. This is notably a heating, pushy, circulatory plant. After taking this powerful herb, it is hard not to notice our airways opening, enabling us to breath more fully and deeply. This experience translates into educating us that horseradish is extremely useful for sinus infections, as an intensely warming circulatory remedy, brilliant for clearing the respiratory system when suffering from a cold or the flu.

Once, while gathering lady's mantle, our conversation turned to the relationships we have with our mothers and grandmothers. We connected our conversation with our other observations (see box, below) and since then we have used lady's mantle with great success to help people release unhelpful patterns of health and behaviour passed down through the maternal ancestral line. Lady's mantle has an affinity with the female reproductive system and is used in a plethora of conditions, including optimizing fertility. Consider the fact that female babies develop in utero with all their eggs in place. The egg that created half of our genetic make-up was already in our mother's womb when she was growing in our grandmother's ovaries.

CONNECTING WITH A PLANT

When the body is completely relaxed there are tools that can be utilized to help connect

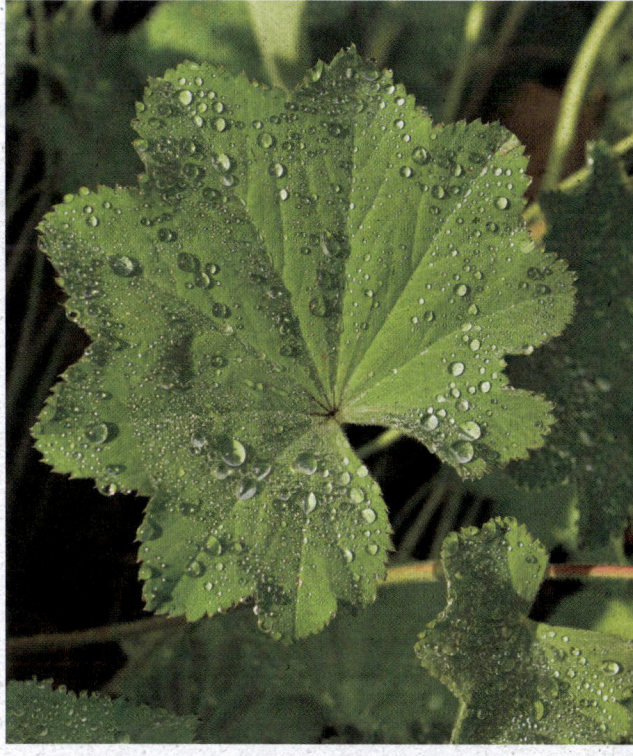

Lady's mantle, supporting matriarchal understanding and connection

---

Observing Lady's Mantle

When we initially observed lady's mantle, it reminded us of an upside-down family tree. Our interactions took us on a journey through time, noticing patterns of behaviour that might be remnants from our ancestors, passed down through the generations. This plant is a sort of visionary scaffolding, supporting us as we explore places that might not feel so comfortable to visit but benefit us in the long term. Its long association with Mary Magdalene and alchemy (Latin name *Alchemilla vulgaris*) adds credence to its reputation for transforming stuck and unhelpful patterns, particularly those affecting the female line.

in different ways with a plant, energetically and imaginatively. Once the body and mind are calm and relaxed, you can choose to sit with the plant, observing how you feel in its presence to gain insight into its overall feel or energy. You could try a guided meditation or going on an internal journey to meet the plant, allowing your thoughts to unleash an internal experience by setting an intention to meet the spirit or guide associated with the plant. This can be done not only in the presence of the plant, but also by holding the image of it in your mind's eye. Altered states of consciousness can be achieved in the presence of rhythmic sound. This imagination practice often takes time and effort.

MEDITATION

Try this guided meditation to get to know a plant better. You can create clarity before you start by setting your intention. In the case of our rosemary plant, the intention of a guided meditation could be "to get to know it better and understand the medicine more deeply". Draw any colours and pictures that come to mind, write thoughts and feelings down.

* Close your eyes, take three deep breaths in and out through your nose; make them full and down into your belly. Place your hands on your belly and feel them move as the air is expanding inside yourself.
* Centre yourself, feel as though rootlets are coming out from all parts of your body that are touching the floor, grounding you and connecting you to the earth.
* Take all your attention to the crown of your head and visualize the night sky and the large, luminous full moon and all its craters, feel the cooling, energizing rays.
* Move down to your third eye, the space between your eyebrows, see the clouds moving through the sky, make out their shapes, see their textures.
* Draw your attention down to your neck area, imagine the wind in the treetops, hear the sound of the trees rustling.
* Draw your attention down to your heart, feel your heart beat and the blood moving around your body, imagine a spring day with the birth of new life.
* Draw your attention down to your solar plexus, a couple of inches above your navel. Breathing into this area, imagine yourself lying on a warm, flat stone in the heat of the sun, basking like a snake.
* Move your attention down to your pelvic region, the sacral area. Imagine flowers opening and bees collecting sweet nectar and pollen.
* Take your breath down to your base and imagine roots travelling down into the warm, rich, moist soil of the earth, moving down deeper and deeper.
* Relax here for a moment, enjoying your breath flowing freely through your body and the feelings of both invigoration

and relaxation that can be felt by having explored your energy centres.

* Imagine a rosemary plant that you know that grows or imagine a place you think it might grow.
* Walk toward the rosemary in your mind's eye and reach out your hand and brush it across the plant, releasing its scent into the air.
* Ask the plant if it has a message for you and be with it a while to see if any emotions or feelings occur; maybe a character will appear with a message or maybe just being with the plant is enough.
* Give yourself a few minutes and notice anything that occurs in this time.
* Bring your attention back to your root.
* Draw your inhalation up from the root through the pelvic region, the solar plexus, heart, throat, third eye and out through your crown.
* Allow your breath to return to normal, gentle exhalations and inhalations, allowing the breath to move as it pleases.
* Rub your fingers against your thumbs.
* And when you're ready and in your own time, open your eyes.

QUESTIONS TO CONSIDER

When you are working intuitively with a plant, keep the following questions in mind:

* Are you reminded of anything as you work with this plant?
* What emotions or feelings are conjured up by your interaction with this plant?
* Are there any particular words that pop into your head?
* What do you notice about your breathing?
* What stories come when you let go of mental constraints and open your imagination to the spirit world of the plants?

Posing these questions leads to useful information that can then be interpreted to indicate how best to utilize the herb medicinally.

Let's take rosemary as an example again and apply it to intuition.

All through the observation exercise, note anything at all that you are feeling. For example, if the rosemary triggers joy or grief, note these emotions down. As you study the section of the plant and draw it, make a note of any images or ideas that pop into your mind. Remember that everything is important to the process. Perhaps your intuitive experience is that rosemary could support grief. You will then discover that rosemary has traditionally been used in remembrance. Scientific research also tells us that rosemary improves circulation to the head and may aid in neural links and improved memory. This could be a helpful action in the grief process, remembering a deceased or lost loved one and experiences that were shared.

INTERPRETATION

The interpretation of information is the real grounding element of Sensory Herbalism. What does it all mean? And how can it be applied? We can have a wonderful time playing with plants, and this might be enough for some people, but if we want to be able to apply the information we have acquired for medicine, interpretation is key.

Observations and intuitions need to be interpreted in a useful way to determine how best to use a herb for medicine in a physical, emotional and spiritual way. Ask yourself: What do the observations I noticed mean to me? What indications are there of the actions of the plant? Try to make sense of your intuitive exploration of the herbs. Are there any clues within your own experiences?

To support your interpretation, research what others say about the plant and cross-reference this with the things you have discovered. Prepare to be amazed at how accurate your interpretations are. As you develop this practice, your trust in your observational and intuitive skills will grow.

If we take all the observations and intuitions we have about rosemary and try to make sense of them, our notes might say:
* vibrant and erect with upward movement
* stem snaps off with a cracking sound
* breaks away easily
* stem feels dry
* smells very strong
* smells uplifting and energetic
* clears my head
* tastes super-strong
* tastes perfumed, oily, slightly bitter and is coating my teeth
* makes breathing deeper and fuller
* upward-moving energy
* feeling my heart and movement in my body
* reminds me of a funeral when I wore a sprig (rosemary for memory)
* intuitively I feel happy and full of life with rosemary
* feels protective and lucky.

These notes now need to be interpreted and this is where you can reference research found in books and other sources. There is a sense of intense energy and excitement when you cross-reference your findings with factual information and find that the perfumed smell and taste indicates the aromatic/essential oils, the bitter quality denotes digestive actions, the coating shows the plant is high in resins and the movement felt in the body connects to the herb's circulatory action. Intuition highlighted the protective nature of those essential oils in keeping pathogens away.

CHARACTERIZATION

Another Sensory Herbalism tool is the creation of plant characters to personify and represent the qualities of each herb. It is a useful and effective method for remembering the information studied.

By using observation, intuition and interpretation, we allow the plants to reveal themselves as individuals – and they often become our close friends. The deeper the friendship, the more familiar their character becomes and the more their individual medicine is revealed and understood. It may be that different herbs speak to you more clearly at different times in your life.

Developing plant characters is a way of weaving the stories of the plants together and is the origin of herbal folklore. In this book, you will meet characters for each of the 15 featured plants.

By personifying the plants and giving them recognizable characteristics, it is easier to remember aspects of the herbs more clearly. These characters help you form relationships with your plant friends. Like people, plants each have their own individual personality traits. Some you like, some you don't; some you absolutely fall in love with and some you fear. Exploring our emotional responses, we can draw parallels with our friends and family members and start to see how certain types of people resemble certain types of plants. As with people, the plants can reveal different parts of themselves to us as individuals, just as different friends might see different aspects of us depending on the relationship and connection we have with them. Interestingly, years of exploring this in workshops has revealed that there is usually a common plant personality that comes through for most people. For example, nettle is always a little hard to handle! Plants speak to different people in different ways; there is a common message but how it is picked up or interpreted depends on the individual experiences of the person meeting the plant. A walk outside is never lonely, not with all of those steadfast, rooted friends to meet, each with their own secrets and personalities.

STORYTELLING

Many traditional folk tales, myths and legends contain references to plants, or deities and archetypes that represent them. Creating our own tales about plant characters can embed their image and characteristics deep in our imagination, so that we remember the essence of the herbs as we hear them. Through stories and poems, the wisdom of the herbs can be more easily absorbed and knowledge passed on to future generations.

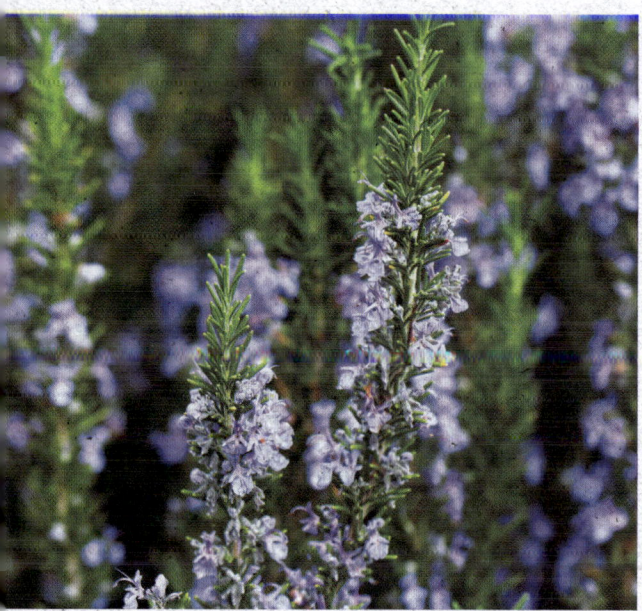

Protective, uplifting rosemary blooming beautifully

Storytelling is one of humanity's oldest art forms. Storytellers are entertainers, teachers and healers, maintaining a spiritual tradition. Stimulating the imagination and building a sense of community between teller and listener, herbal folklore carries with it the gifts of nature in a beautiful medium.

CHARACTERIZATION – WHO IS ROSEMARY?

Spend some time now being playful as you let your pen flow over the paper and jot down some ideas about the character of rosemary. This initial character creation is the starting point of creating folklore and stories to tell, a way of sharing the knowledge you've gained and helping you to unleash some creativity.

The box below describes Rose-Marie Seashore. Her characteristics are linked to the medicinal gifts of rosemary in order to make them more memorable. What characteristics can you give to rosemary, or another herb, to cement in your mind the knowledge you have gained and in the minds of others you share the story with?

ROSE-MARIE SEASHORE ...

is a hot-blooded, passionate reader of cards; she lives in Andalucía next to the Mediterranean Sea. She always dresses in sharp threads, really funky clothes, and when she walks into any room all eyes are on her. She rarely sits down and loves to dance. She is strikingly beautiful and never seems to age. A fabulous cook, whatever she serves you to eat is healthy and nourishing, full of flavour. She has an incredible memory, never forgetting anyone's birthday. She is the sort of person you need in a crisis, guaranteed to give a practical, clear response, never losing her head.

PLANT DREAM CREATION

Plant dreams are a product of all the information gathered from the murmurs of plants themselves. Using this final tool, every bit of knowledge – all the observations, intuitions, interpretations and characterizations – are woven into a poem that encapsulates the spirit of the plant for you. The dream language of each plant is represented by the written word.

A plant dream is often ethereal in nature and encompasses everything you have gained through your observations, intuition, interpretation and characterization. It can include some of the folklore of the past, snippets of your observations during the drawing process, feelings or visions you have experienced or feel about the plant. It gives a real sense of the energy of the plant. These poems and stories are lovely tools to read before you go into meditation on the plant. You can even record them and play them back to yourself.

PLANT DREAM BASED ON FINDINGS OF ROSEMARY

Here is a poem that highlights the medicine and magic of rosemary, a pushy, circulatory stimulant that is always there if you need a bit of psychic or physical protection. This plant dream describes the folklore, medicine and messages that we have gleaned from working with the plant.

I AM ROSMARINUS

Evergreen rose of the sea
Purple-blooming femininity
Straight-lined sprigs of strength
Gifting crystal memory
Solar surge
Tactility offering stimulant scent
Aromatic circulatory

Holding amulet protection
Gypsy-lore luck
On waves of adventure
Merge with inside energy
Creating synergy
Courage on a cliff edge

I am rosemary

You will find plant dreams for the 15 featured herbs in this book, included to inspire you as you create your own. The plant dreams on the two following pages are the work of two of our Sensory Herbalism apprentices. Each year, we are blown away by the creativity and magic our apprentices express.

ODE TO COMFREY
by Tracey

On the bank by the river, grows the much-
loved comfrey
Queen Symphytum officinale, server of plants
Great wound healer, cell proliferator and
knitter of bones
She is altruistic, a magnanimous humanitarian
A dynamic nutrient accumulator, she feeds
the soil with her deep root system
Pulling minerals from the belly of the warm,
moist worm earth to feed her abundant leaf
system beneficial insect attractor
She feeds and heals the animals
A benevolent beauty, she gives generously and
is loved by all
In fact you will find her now standing by the
river bank reading her love letters from the
creatures who love her:

I have a number of reasons to tell you why
I love you
I cannot live without you
I am bewildered by the magnificence
of your beauty
and wish to see you
with a hundred eyes
I am charmed
Your humble servant, Fly

You are the finest, loveliest, tenderest and most
beautiful plant I have ever known and even
that is an understatement
Yours forever
Your very devoted, Horse

Your magical, magnificent splendour
Is beautiful my all-seeing giant
Ever yours my love, Ant

Hello darling
Come over tomorrow please,
We don't need to go out we don't even need to
wear pants
Let's lie around and eat food
A thousand kisses
Butterfly

I have loved you for a thousand years, I will
love you for a thousand more
Yours with fondest and deepest love, Bee

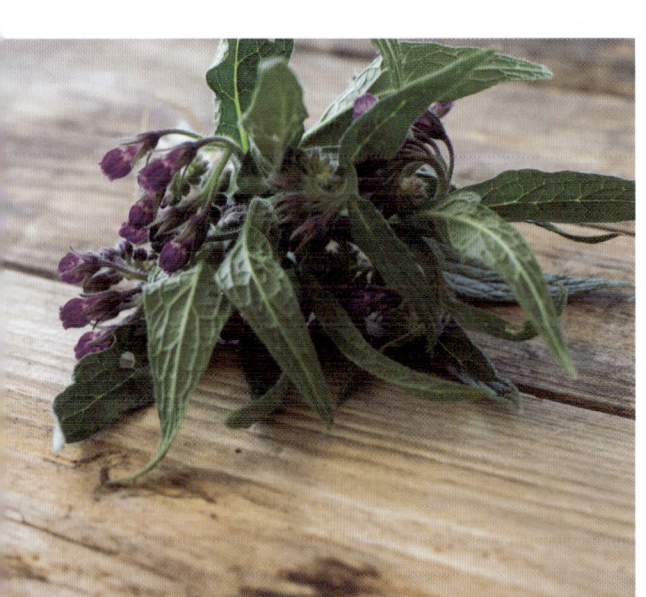

Comfrey (*Symphytum officinale*)

VIVA LA MENTHA!
by Alice

Viva la Mentha!
Vivid and tough.
Rough
Round the edges.
Zigzag leaves look gnarly and protective
But mint, your kind and inventive
Ways – of both calming and bringing zing
You are the thing

That tingles me, excites me and wakes me up
Mint, I want you in my cup
Come and relax my digestive tract!
Stands strong and gardens it permeates. Sweet
  strength brings clarity and creates space.
For the new.
For the new.
Refresh the spirits and deep breathe the air.
Refresh the spirits and deep breathe the
  cool air.
Viva la Mentha!

Sensory Herbalism Tool Recap	
OBSERVATION	Observe through drawing, tasting, harvesting and processing. Make links with tastes and possible constituents and actions of the plant.
INTUITION	Ask questions about what you intuitively sense from each plant and make notes.
INTERPRETATION	Interpret all the information you have gathered and see if you can make any useful sense of how the plant might be used for medicine. Cross-reference your ideas and interpretations with what others have said about the plant, gradually building up a picture of the qualities of the plant.
CHARACTERIZATION	Use all you know about the plant, from where it grows and the plants that grow nearby, to its taste, energetics and medicinal values to create a plant character.
PLANT DREAM CREATION	Finally, when you feel you really know the plant, you can let your creative juices flow and see which words come to you in your own plant dream. In essence, allow the plant to talk through you.

OTHER KEY TOOLS

AFFIRMATIONS AND MANTRAS

Modern medicine is delving into new realms to discover how mental attitudes can determine health and, more importantly, how we have the potential to transform our bodies through the power of thought.

We have found ourselves that when we harvest herbs for medicine and create a remedy, having a specific person in mind makes the remedy more potent. Unlike in most modern Western Herbal Medicine, Sensory Herbalism uses very small doses, sometimes just a few drops, of a medicine to elicit powerful change. All our medicines are created with incantations (affirmations or mantras repeated out loud) while harvesting. They are also administered in conjunction with a written affirmation, which can be displayed to be seen and repeated regularly.

An affirmation is a tool that allows you to guide your thoughts in a conscious way. Repeating these short, powerful statements, or just listening to them, has profound effects and can help create positive change. Using language in this way connects you with your conscious thoughts by declaring something firmly and asserting something to be true. Affirmations are powerful when set in the present tense, making the statement true right now.

It has been suggested that we have between 45,000 and 51,000 thoughts a day. That is up to 35 thoughts a minute. But there is the difficulty of defining what a single thought is. Where does one thought end and another begin? It has been postulated that up to 80 percent of the thoughts we have are negative, so mind training, learning how to master our thoughts, is an important tool.

THOSE WHO WANT TO KNOW THE TRUTH OF THE UNIVERSE SHOULD PRACTISE THE FOUR CARDINAL VIRTUES. THE FIRST IS REVERENCE FOR ALL OF LIFE. THIS MANIFESTS AS UNCONDITIONAL LOVE AND RESPECT FOR ONESELF AND ALL OTHER BEINGS. THE SECOND IS NATURAL SINCERITY. THIS MANIFESTS AS HONESTY, SIMPLICITY AND FAITHFULNESS. THE THIRD IS GENTLENESS, WHICH MANIFESTS AS KINDNESS, CONSIDERATION FOR OTHERS AND SENSITIVITY TO SPIRITUAL TRUTH. THE FOURTH IS SUPPORTIVENESS. THIS MANIFESTS AS SERVICE TO OTHERS WITHOUT EXPECTATION OF REWARD.

– Lao Tzu –

When you say, think or even hear positive mantras, they can become your conscious thoughts and subsequently inform your reality. "I am happy, I feel healthy, I feel ecstatic." Conversely, negative mantras can also become self-fulfilling prophecies. When we have used mantras to put our intentions into practice, we have seen them create magic. Synchronicities start to occur more and more often, which in turn affirm life.

Forms of magic, such as spells and incantations, draw on the power of words and how they resonate in our consciousness. The technique of using affirmations can be traced back thousands of years. "Mantra" is a Sanskrit word meaning literally "instrument of thought" and referring to a sacred sound, word or group of words believed to have psychological and spiritual power. Sanskrit has sets of sounds that represent earth, air, fire, water and ether. By utilizing these sounds in different ways through chants or mantras, different energetic vibrations are raised, the words and their sounds being specifically chosen for the intention of the mantra. Words carry a vibration, not just in their meaning but also in the way that they sound. Think of the difference between "hack" and "hush".

You are probably familiar with the classic mantra "Om", which refers to the original sound of the universe, the first vibration, representing birth, death and rebirth.

Chanting the sound "Om" is said to bring us into harmonic resonance with the universe. Some yogic mantras are much longer, even pages long, and are sung as bhajans or kirtans (devotional songs and chants).

MASARU EMOTO

Perhaps some of the most profound evidence to support the power of affirmations is found in Masaru Emoto's work with water crystals. Emoto, who died in 2014, was a Japanese researcher whose work demonstrated how human consciousness can influence the structure of water. He showed that water changes shape to reflect a mood consciously projected onto it; so it alters when music is played nearby, when the written word is held up or placed under it, and even when mental visualizations are projected onto it. Emoto's photographs show that crystals from water frozen after being exposed to a positive affirmation were far more beautiful than those not exposed.

We know that we comprise approximately 60 percent water. So if we can change the structure of the water within our body by repeating positive affirmations about ourselves, we are on to a winning formula. Repeating positive statements enhances not just patients' lives, but also the potency of the herbs harvested and thus the medicines created from them. Aligning with Emoto's ideas, reciting an affirmation when harvesting herbs potentially enhances their potency by altering the water structure within the plant.

Dr Edward Bach is well known for his intuitive work with plants, and for categorizing specific characteristics that present in a person, giving an indication of which remedy they may need. His system was created through sitting and working with the plants, tapping into their energy and sensing their vibrational medicine. We are all capable of this. The American herbalist Stephen Harrod Buhner writes eloquently about perceiving the energy of plants through the electromagnetic field of the heart. He describes how to tune in to plants and discover their interaction with our physical and emotional bodies. Plants effect subtle shifts in human beings on an energetic level. The support of plants enhances the potency of affirmations and vice versa.

SEASONAL NUTRITION

Consuming plants as food is another important aspect of Sensory Herbalism. With different plant parts in abundance at different times of the year, we maximize the nutritional benefit of the plants by using produce fresh from nature, which improves wellness, prevents illness in the future, and nurtures a sense of daily connection to nature through food.

Nutrition and diet can be a minefield, with body dysmorphia and eating disorders now causing a great deal of suffering. There are thousands of different diets and nutritional theories out there, from cabbage soup to banana diets to calorie counting. Also in the mix are choices driven by health necessity or ethical or political reasons such as gluten-free, dairy-free, veganism, GMO-free diets, acid/alkaline, palaeolithic, organic only … the list goes on. Baffling, to say the least.

The father of medicine, Hippocrates, is renowned for saying "let thy food be thy medicine." Fresh, seasonal fare is exactly what our bodies assimilate the best. There has been a recent revival for growing your own foods and medicines, and for foraging wild foods. Fantastic community growing projects have sprung up all over the place, so do go and look up your local orchard, allotments or community gardens to connect with others. Get outside and get your hands dirty, walk in the wilds and connect with what you are eating as much as possible. One cause of ill health is the fracture of the connection between people and the origins of their food. We recognize hundreds, maybe thousands, of corporate logos but many of us cannot tell what medicinal weeds are growing in the garden or which berries are safe to eat. It is time to reclaim our connection to nature.

In the Seasonal Journey, each season closes with a section on nutrition, examining how we can use that season's key plant part (leaves, flowers, seeds or roots) in our food.

Drops of Courage – *"Courage to move through"*

When we create a sensory potion it always has an accompanying affirmation that sums up the resultant effects of the herb blend. We specifically developed Drops of Courage to give the "courage to move through", offering support when stress and strain is starting to take over.

INGREDIENTS:
Dandelion root, borage flower, daisy

DANDELION ROOT *(Taraxacum officinale)*

Dandelion root shifts stuck energy through its bitter stimulating action on the digestion. It grounds with its super-tenacious tap root reaching down into the earth, strengthening the emotional body and giving a clearer sense of self. It directly supports the liver and helps to dissolve confusing, "irrational" feelings. As we dig these roots we chant "Keep us rooted, grounded and clear."

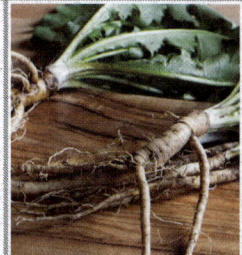

BORAGE FLOWER *(Borago officinalis)*

Both borage and dandelion are ruled by the giant planet Jupiter which has a creative, expansive energy. Borage's beautiful, purple star-shaped flowers are traditionally used for courage. They support the adrenal glands, making all of life's challenges easier to face and giving us quiet strength in our convictions. As we pick the delicate flowers, we use the words "Walk with us and bring us the courage to face all challenges with grace."

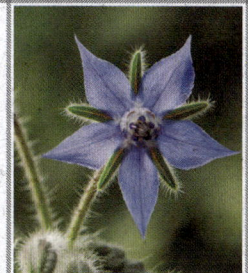

DAISY FLOWERS *(Bellis perennis)*

Daisy brings joy to those who take it. As a herb of the sun, it cleanses and lightens. These little flowers are constantly being trodden and mown down, but amazingly, bounce back up to face the sunlight. They also can be used to support the lymphatic system, clearing the skin and encouraging immunity. As we pick the blooms we often sing, "Joy, light, resilience."

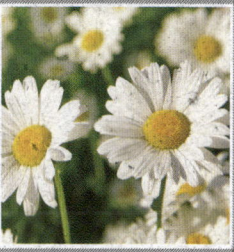

These three herbs are mixed in equal parts for the potion: 10ml dandelion root tincture / 10ml borage flower tincture / 10ml daisy flower syrup.
The words "courage to move through" are written on each bottle.

SAFETY

Plant medicine is an ancient mode of healing with countless systems and theories and can be daunting to the novice. Approaches to holistic health are diverse and complex and a comprehensive understanding of our physical, emotional and spiritual bodies is essential in supporting the body's healing process.

Managing optimum health as a day-to-day endeavour, adding herbs to meals, drinking daily herbal teas and reaching for specific herbs when you notice illnesses approaching, can give a sense of wellbeing and empowerment, optimizing health in a way that is uncomplicated, inspiring and fun. The need to take herbs as medicine can be decreased by incorporating them in daily life, using berries and flowers as cordials and jams, making herb vinegars for salads and using seeds and petals in bread and cakes. Following what is seasonally available avoids cumulative toxicity or potential adverse health risks of long-term use of any one herb.

This book offers pointers for starting to connect with herbs, understanding them and improving your general health and wellbeing. It is not intended as a manual for treating yourself and others for complex health issues. For deep-seated health issues we recommend that you find someone local to you who can support and guide you in

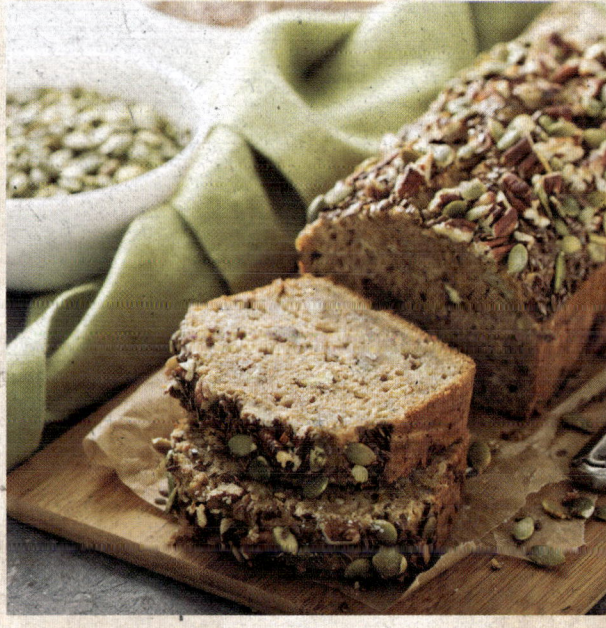

Seeds and nuts bring a little Sensory Herbal magic to your daily bread.

treating ailments that might come up on your health journey. Practitioners such as body workers, psychodynamic practitioners, nutritionists and herbalists can all work together in an integrated fashion with the correct communication strategy. General practitioners within the allopathic medical model are required for specific diagnosis and signposting to other disciplines of medicine. If you see a doctor for a health complaint, try to gain as much information as possible about what they have found, what they think the issue is and any test results. That way, you are still empowered with knowledge about your body and its workings and in a much better position to choose your treatment strategy.

During pregnancy, we recommend you work with someone well versed in the world of herbs. Many herbs are contraindicated in pregnancy so you need to be careful. Women who are pregnant often have a greater desire to care for and nurture themselves, so they may turn to "alternative" medicine, yoga and health techniques during this time. Acquiring a support network of practitioners in pregnancy will lay the foundation for continuing after the baby is born.

HOW MUCH DO I TAKE?

Recommended medicinal daily doses vary from herb to herb but there is still a crude gauge of how much is a "medicinal" dose. For a tea, a heaped teaspoon of herbs per cup is a good rule of thumb. In Sensory Herbalism, we work with drop doses of tinctures of herbs to create subtle shifts in the body, encouraging innate healing rather than forcing the body to heal.

Herbs can be extremely effective and fast acting in children (brought up on herbal teas, our own children accept a wide range of tastes). It is important to work with children alongside a qualified herbalist, so that you can feel confident that you are making the right decisions and combinations of herbs.

It's a good idea to attend herbalist workshops or courses to learn about the potency and effects of medicinal plants. To become more confident in identification, look out for herb walks and other events in your local area, join wildlife groups, horticultural and herb societies and visit local nature reserves. Nothing beats taking someone a little more knowledgeable on a forage!

Small Doses, Big Effects

In herbal medicine it is routine to take relatively large doses of herbs. However, the subtle vibrational and physical effects of a herb or herb combination can also work powerfully in very small doses. Drop dosing of herbal tinctures reflects the premise that less is more. Using small doses of plants can elicit powerful effects by stimulating the subtle energy patterns of the mind, body and spirit. Physiological responses are initiated, encouraging physical and emotional balance. Even through the sight and smell of a plant, subtle shifts occur within the body as it responds through the nervous and endocrine systems or electromagnetic energy exchange. You can start to experience the medicine of plants before imbibing them simply by being with them and experiencing them through the tools of Sensory Herbalism.

HARVESTING HERBS

Learning to harvest herbs (as well as prepare, dry and store them, see pages 74–8) is important if you want to use a herb beyond its leafing, flowering, fruiting or rooting season. When harvesting herbs to make home remedies, it is imperative to recognize the shifting seasons in order to catch the spring greens, the summer flowers, the autumn berries or the winter roots for your medicinal cabinet, before they pass you by until the following year. The seasons are an ever-turning circle of treats in our gardens, parks and wild spaces, and of preparation, birth, growth, flowering, fruiting and harvesting.

Confidence in identification is also key. Even when you think you know a plant, there are some that can be tricksters. We have had apprentices return to us with buddleia instead of heather, self-heal instead of ground ivy … the list goes on. So you need to make absolutely sure you know how to recognize the plant you are setting out to harvest. Even the familiar stinging nettle can be mistaken for the dead nettle if you are not careful and many plants purposefully mimic each other.

The safest way to build your confidence in working with plants is to stick to what is in some way familiar already. Please make sure you confirm the identity of any herbs that you have even the vaguest doubt about before moving on to harvesting and using them. When you're starting to harvest, we

Influence of the Moon

The moon has a powerful influence over all life, including the plants. She governs the water on our blue planet, causing the tides of the oceans. Regulation of the flow of water within our bodies and within plants are also under the domain of the lunar enchantress. As the moon waxes from new to full, providing more light in the night sky and greater gravitational pull, the plants' constituents are drawn upward into their aerial parts. This makes a waxing or a full moon an optimum time for harvesting leaves and flowers.

At the new moon, energy is drawn down into the earth, with less light in the sky. We like to harvest roots at the new (or dark) moon. This is a general rule of thumb, and if the weather and the herbs allow it, gathering plants in harmony with the phases of the moon can enhance your harvest. We also note which astrological sign the moon is in when we harvest. For example, a label might read, "Daisy flowers picked on a waxing Leo moon". The more attention and energy you put into harvesting herbs, the more potent your remedies will be.

recommend that you begin with a plant you know well.

The best ingredients for creating herbal remedies are fresh good-quality herbs that you've picked yourself. Nature is intelligent and there is a theory that all the medicine that we need grows around us. We like to think that this is true and that everything necessary to aid the body to find balance in health can be gathered within walking distance from your home.

Harvesting gives you an opportunity to focus intently on your actions. It can be used as a form of meditative practice. We like to approach each harvest as a ritual and we use the common mugwort as part of this. Mugwort is a gateway plant, opening portals to alternative realms. Connected to the dream state, this herb enables you to slip gently and safely into a liminal state of consciousness. We make a strong brew of mugwort tea: one heaped teaspoon of the dried herb in a pot of freshly boiled water, infused for 13 minutes.

Drink the tea while taking a few deep breaths to settle your mind, then go out and start to observe everything about the herb that you have chosen to work with:

* Where is it growing?
* What is it growing with?
* Does it look healthy and vibrant?
* And is there enough of it that it will still flourish after you have gone?

Think about sustainability. Leave some healthy plants to keep growing and producing seed, and only take plants from areas where they are prolific. Always leave enough of the flowers or berries to continue the reproductive cycle.

Other aspects to consider when harvesting are the weather and the phase of the moon (see box, opposite). Aerial plant parts (anything growing above ground) are best harvested on a dry, sunny day around the waxing and full moon, after the morning dew has evaporated. The perfect time to harvest roots is when the moon is waning or new, so there is less light and the plant constituents are concentrated in the roots.

Sensory Herbalism considers the astrology of each herb. If this appeals, you can harvest on the day that corresponds to a plant's planetary alignment; for example, nettle is a herb of Mars and Tuesday is the day named for Mars (see page 25).

HARVESTING CHECKLIST
* Be 100 percent sure of a plant's identity.
* Look for healthy, vibrant plants growing away from sprayed fields or busy roads.
* Choose a sunny day.
* Consider the phase of the moon.
* Harvest with care and awareness.
* Harvest where the plant is abundant.
* Always leave enough plant behind for it to keep growing and produce seeds.

PRESERVING AND PREPARING HERBS

The following pages give guidelines on preserving herbs and preparing them for use.

DRYING

There are loads of different ways to try drying herbs.

* To dry herbs quickly, put them in the oven on a very low heat. Leave the door open so moisture can escape. Great for herbs with a high moisture content, such as comfrey.
* A dehydrator is a really effective way of drying herbs, as it maintains a constant temperature and dries the herbs quickly.
* A super-easy method is to dry the herbs in a basket somewhere warm and dry like an airing cupboard, shaking them every day.
* Tie the herbs in bunches and hang them to dry. This is especially good for plants with long stems, such as mugwort.
* Spread the herb out on newspaper.

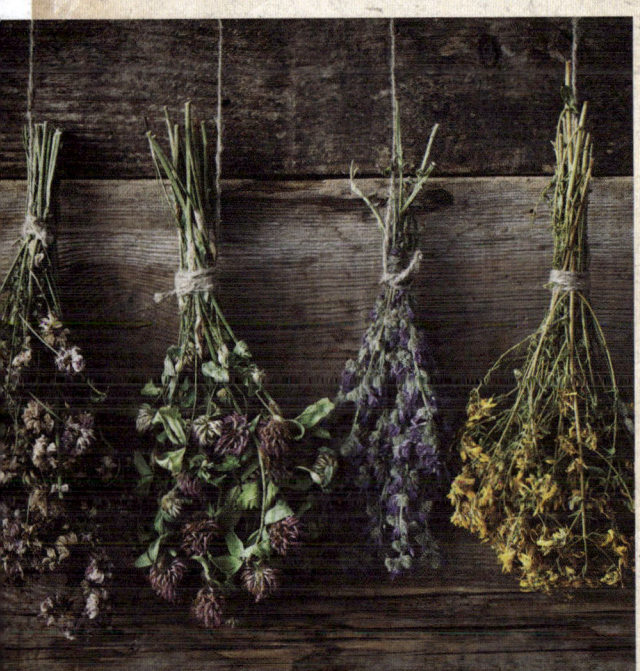

Herbs tied in bunches and hung for drying

With all these methods, it is key to put the herbs somewhere warm, dry and where air can get to them – but keep them away from the sun. The more efficiently your herbs dry, the more herbal goodness will be preserved. Direct sunlight will bleach them.

As a general rule leaves will crunch when they are dried. Note also that roots should be chopped before drying as they become very hard. When your herbs are dry, which could take anything from a few days up to a month depending on their moisture content and where you're drying them, store them in an airtight container. We prefer glass to plastic because some plastics have the potential to transfer chemicals to your herbs. Again, store your jars away from direct sunlight because bleaching drains herbs of their potency. It is good practice to label your jars, as it is super easy to confuse one jar of green herbs with another! Label them with the herb name, and the location and date of the harvest. You can add other information if you wish, such as the lunar phase in which the herb was harvested.

INFUSIONS/DECOCTIONS

You can use fresh or dried herbs (leaves, flowers, bark, fruit, roots or seeds) to make a herbal tea. An infusion is where boiling water is poured over the herb in a drinking vessel or teapot. A decoction is where tougher material, such as roots or fruits, may need simmering in water for a period of time to draw out the medicinal compounds. To decoct actually refers to reducing the liquid but is in effect a way of creating a potent tea from the parts of herbs that are harder to extract from.

To make an infusion, as a general rule place one teaspoon of dried herb per cup of water into a teapot. Pour boiling water over the top and infuse for 5–10 minutes. Strain and drink. We love to do this as a ritual, repeating a loving affirmation as you prepare the herb and pour the water. You can then sit calmly while you enjoy the tea, experiencing the flavours and sensations.

A decoction is generally made in a stainless steel, copper or enameled pan (avoid aluminium or non-stick Teflon). We usually decoct roots, seeds and fruits, placing one teaspoon per cup of water into a pan. Pour the water over the top, bring to boiling point and then simmer for approximately 10 minutes or until the liquid has the desired depth of colour. Use a lid to prevent all the liquid evaporating.

TINCTURES

Tinctures are alcoholic extracts of herbs made using a variety of different alcohols. The more care and energy you put into producing them, the more potent the final product. After harvesting, the fresh herbs are chopped up and macerated in alcohol. Some people believe that using a fresh herb makes a weaker tincture due to the water content diluting the final medicine, but in our experience this is not the case. There is something of the original essence of the plant captured in a fresh herb tincture; it also tastes more alive. Once the herbs are fully macerated the tinctures need to be strained.

The finished tinctures are then stored and can be used in combination with other herbs to produce situation-specific remedies. We always anticipate the first taste of a new tincture with relish to see what properties we can experience.

INFUSED OILS

Infusing herbs in oil can create remedies such as medicinal creams, ointments, rubs, lip balms, ear drops and skin oils. Balms and oils can be used for lots of ailments including eczema, cuts, scrapes, ear infections, cold sores, chapped lips, aching muscles, arthritis, nappy rash and many more.

To make an infused oil, gather the herbs on a sunny day, then dry them to remove any excess moisture before infusing them in oil, usually organic almond oil. We infuse the oils in the earth or in the sunlight depending on which herb we are using. Burial of earthenware is a traditional method of herb oil maceration – the cooling properties of the earth's energies are imparted into the oils.

We have experimented with the earth-maceration method and had great results. We collect the plants for maceration at full moon and dry them out for two weeks until the next new moon. They are added to an oil in the earthenware and then the sealed bottles are buried in the earth. At the time of the new moon the earth's energy has retreated underground. In burying the oils at this time the plants become energized with the strong, grounding earth element.

The infusions are left buried for at least one lunar cycle, then dug up and strained. We have buried them next to a fig tree in our allotment, leaving a stone spiral to mark the spot.

The expansive, warm, creative sun energy, however, suits the maceration of some plants better. These herbs, such as St John's wort, are harvested around the summer solstice (when solar power is at its strongest) and macerated in oil on 21 June. The infused herbs are left to macerate in sunlight (for example, on a sunny window-sill) to gather the rays for a further three months, or even longer; we had some St John's wort infusing in oil for over a year, during which time we watched it turn a darker and darker red.

SYRUPS

Preserving with sugar is a traditional way to work with many herbs. Over the past few years, sugar has been much maligned and many substitutes are now available. We have experimented with fructose, coconut sugar, honey and apple juice concentrate.

To make each syrup we place the flowers, berries or leaves in a pan, cover with water and gently bring to the boil. Then, we either turn off the heat and leave it to infuse (for flowers) or simmer gently for 10–20 minutes (for roots). Sticking to traditional recipes, we then add organic fair-trade cane sugar and natural flavours such as vanilla pods or star anise, and simmer gently until the sugar has completely dissolved.

VINEGARS

This is a wonderful way of preserving herbal medicines without alcohol, the vinegar capturing their nourishing goodness. Apple cider vinegar has been used as a health-giving agent for centuries. Hippocrates, the father of medicine, is said to have used only two remedies: honey and vinegar.

There are many healing powers attributed to cider vinegar, including helping to lower cholesterol, improving skin tone, moderating high blood pressure, preventing or countering osteoporosis, and improving metabolic function. When vinegar is combined with mineral-rich herbs, it can be more wholesome than mineral supplements.

Herbs and vinegar are a superb combination: the healing and nutritional properties of vinegar married to the aromatic and health-protective effects of mineral-rich green herbs (adding a splash of vinegar to cooked greens is a classic trick).

Minerals are important for the health and proper functioning of our bones, our heart and blood vessels, our nerves, our brain (especially memory), our immune system, and our hormonal glands. Adding vinegar to your food actually helps build bones because it frees up minerals from the vegetables you eat.

Vinegar extracts (aceta) are weaker than alcohol-based tinctures, so the required dose is higher. And, while vinegar won't draw out all the same phytochemicals that alcohol will, it does excel at drawing minerals and vitamins from a plant.

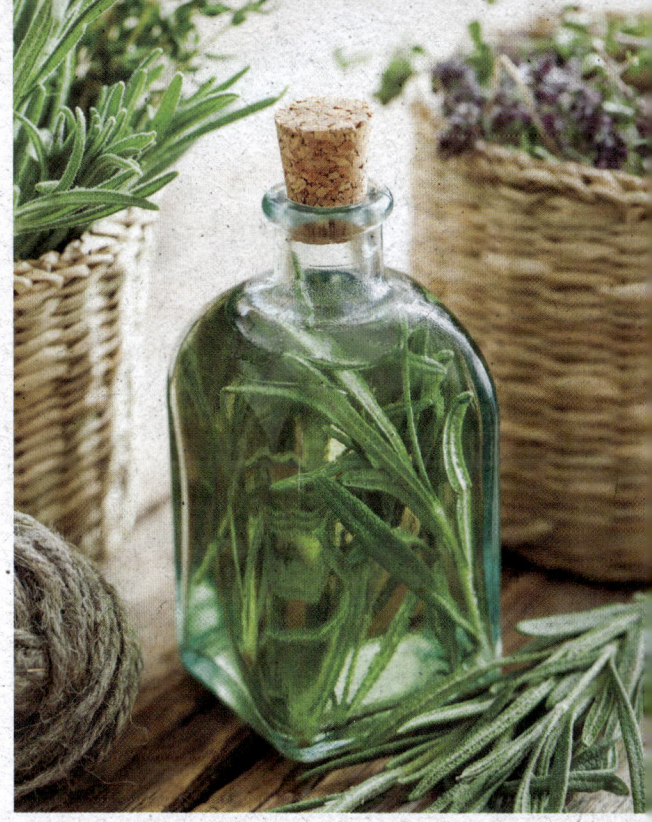

Rosemary vinegar

MAKING HERBAL VINEGARS

* Fill any size jar with freshly harvested and coarsely chopped aromatic herbs: leaves, stalks, flowers, fruits, roots, or even nuts. For best results and highest mineral content, be sure the jar is well filled and the herbs well chopped.
* Pour room-temperature vinegar into the jar until it is full.
* Cover or seal the jar: a screw-on lid, several layers of plastic or wax paper held on with a rubber band or a cork are best. Avoid metal lids – or protect them

well with plastic – as vinegar will corrode them.

* Label the jar with the name of the herb(s) and the date.
* Store away from direct sunlight.
* Strain after a maximum of two weeks.

USING HERBAL VINEGARS

Herbal vinegars taste so good, you'll want to use them frequently. Regular use boosts the nutrient level of your diet with very little effort and virtually no expense.

* Pour a spoonful or more on beans and grains as a condiment.
* Use them in salad dressings.
* Add them to cooked greens.
* Season stir-fries with them.
* Use herbal vinegar instead of plain vinegar in any recipe.
* Add a big spoonful to a glass of water.
* Use rosemary or lavender vinegar as a hair rinse.

OXYMELS

The word "oxymel" comes from the Latin *oxymeli* meaning "acid and honey". Oxymels are preparations using both vinegar and honey. These mixtures have a long history of use in herbalism, dating as far back as the ancient Greeks.

Hippocrates spoke highly of oxymels for coughs but cautioned against their use for people with a cold and dry constitution (these people are commonly always the coldest in the room, wearing sweaters when others have T-shirts on, and may have dry skin, dry eyes, etc.). He also suggested heating these mixtures gently when they are being consumed during cold weather.

William Cook, a physiomedicalist of the 1800s, preferred vinegar as a solvent when treating issues of the respiratory system. He felt that it concentrated the herb's actions on the respiratory system.

Honey offers us a wide range of benefits for coughs and sore throats. It's anti-microbial, inhibiting the growth of pathogens as well as being slightly expectorant.

To make an oxymel, combine a herb-infused vinegar with a herb-infused honey. Play with ratios to suit your own tastes.

MAKING HERBAL HONEY

* Take a jar, fill it loosely with whatever fresh herb you're using.
* Pour the honey over your herbs.
* Make sure the honey settles and all of the air bubbles come to the top.
* Add more honey as needed.
* Seal your jar and once or twice a day turn the jar on its head to "stir" the mixture.
* Strain after two weeks.

All the above preparations have their benefits for different situations and are generally chosen according to the season or herb.

USING HERBS AS MEDICINES

If you are inspired by working with herbs, you may want to consider studying further. Understanding a picture of how disease has occurred is paramount in supporting an individual's health. The contemporary herbalist Simon Mills has laid down some fundamental principles of traditional therapeutic systems in his book *The Essentials of Herbal Medicine*. Sensory Herbalism draws on these therapeutic ideas in making sense of the way the body is functioning and how that may be affecting the holistic wellbeing of the person.

ASSIMILATION

In a consultation, we explore everything taken into the body or energy field, from energy, ancestral influence, breath and prana/chi to nutrients, experiences, sensory input and communication. What is the person eating and drinking over the course of a whole day? Do they wake up and drink a glass of water, or look at their phone? Is their environment at home calm and warm?

INTEGRATION

We also find out how they are integrating what they experience, physically and emotionally. This includes the functioning of the gut and the kidneys, the heart–brain connection, the endocrine system, and gas and cellular exchange, as well as how experiences are absorbed. Is their gut able to absorb nutrients? Are they meditating, walking, doing yoga, taking time out?

CIRCULATION

We look at how movement and transport takes place in the body, including the circulatory, lymphatic and nervous systems, as well as exercise. How are nutrients moved and transported around the body? Is this promoted by massage and exercise? Is it hindered by muscular tension?

ELIMINATION

This category covers excretion, including the functioning of the liver, kidneys, sweat glands, skin, lungs and mucous membranes. How efficiently are waste products being excreted? Are the bowels opening regularly, is the person waking to urinate at night? Is the liver under additional challenge from excessive coffee and alcohol? We also look at emotional crisis from this perspective.

These principles help build up a picture of imbalances, enabling us to support the person with advice and herbs. An individual's physical and emotional state needs to be taken into account when prescribing herbs to fit a holistic model

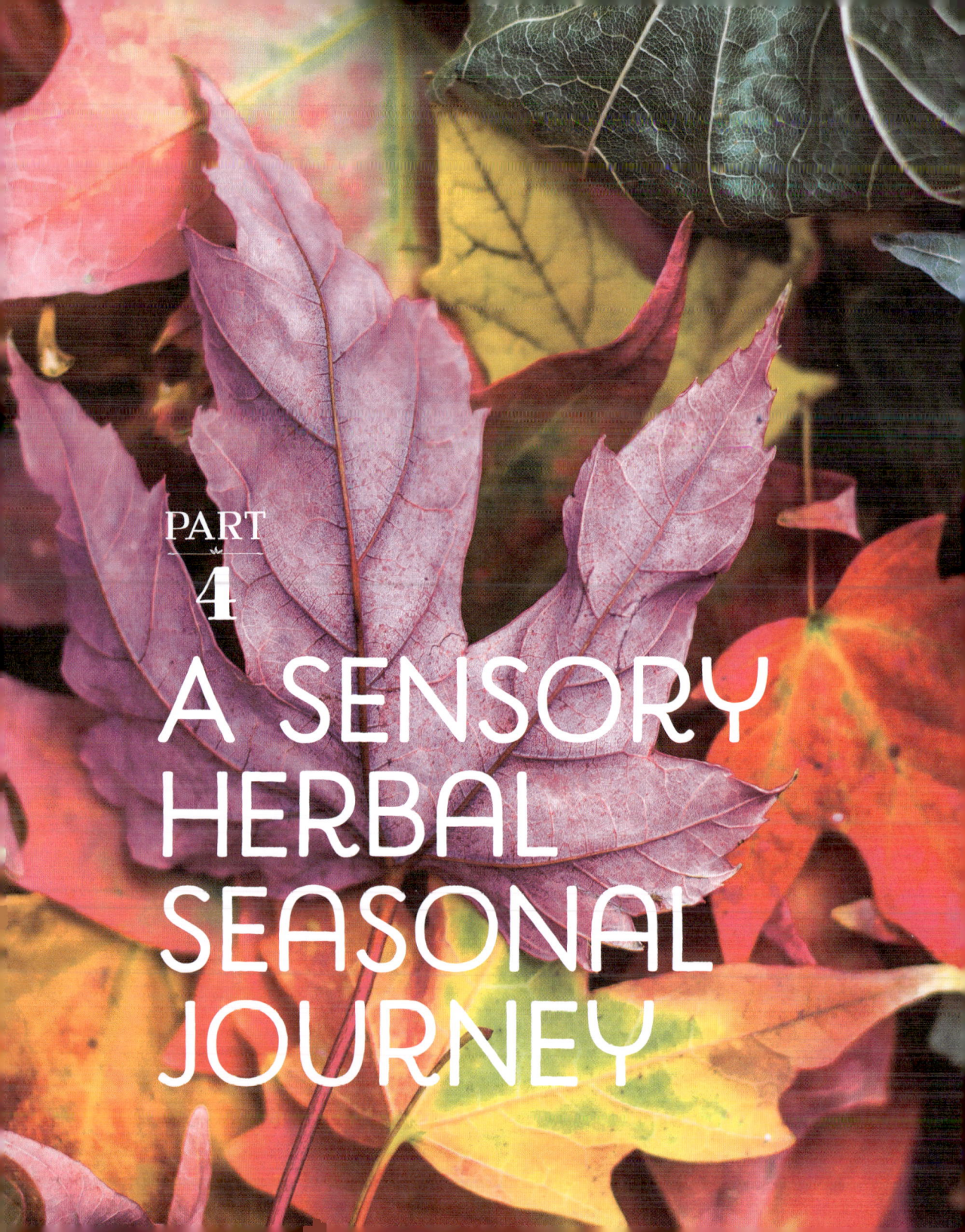

PART

4

A SENSORY HERBAL SEASONAL JOURNEY

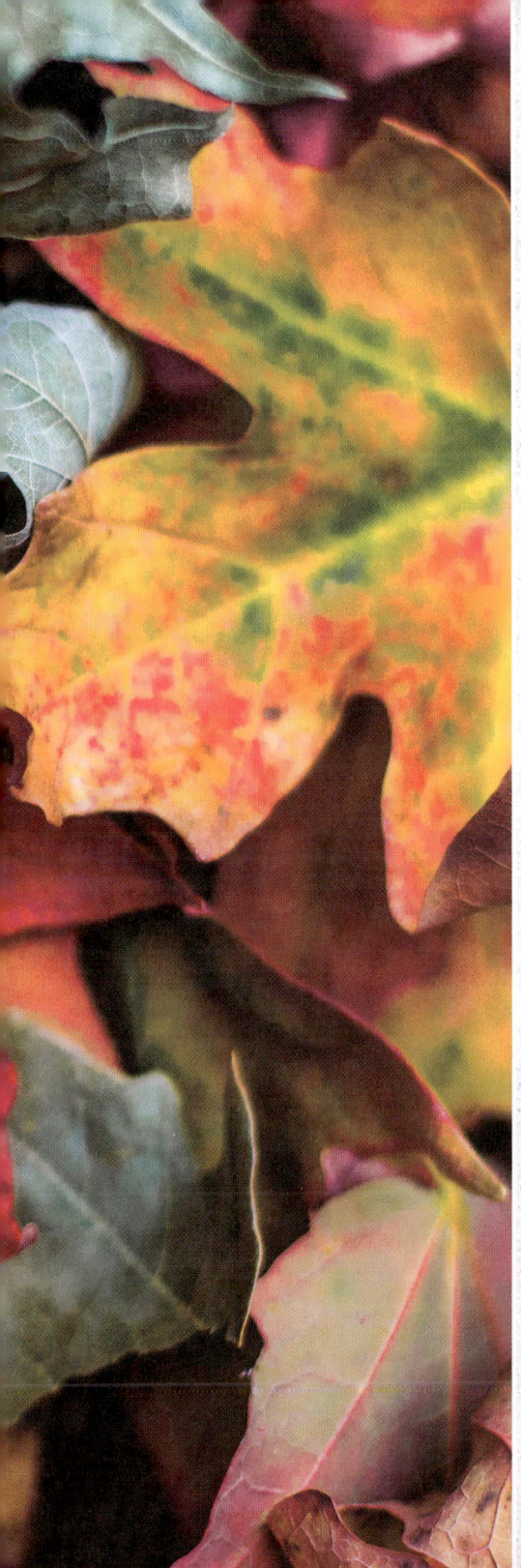

The changing seasons are our guide to the rhythm of the Earth. It is essential, therefore, when you are working with plants, to be in tune with the cycle of the seasons. Herbs need to be watched until the perfect time to harvest them; the weather and the lunar cycles are important considerations, too.

Each of the following chapters focuses on one season and on the element that most influences plants and people in that season. We also explore which part of the plant – leaf, flower, seed or root – especially reflects that element during that time. And we look at how to use each season's herbs in medicine, nutrition, rituals, art and other ways to support balance, good health and wellbeing throughout the year. This is your guidebook to a Sensory Herbal Seasonal Journey, a path to discovering and connecting with the plant world all around you.

STARTING THE SEASONAL JOURNEY

The Sensory Song

FRESH SPRING WATER
BURST FORTH LUSH LEAVES,
CLEARING, WASHING OUR EMOTIONS

SUMMER FIRE FLOWERS
IGNITE OUR PASSIONS,
ATTRACTING POSITIVE MOVEMENT AND
GROWTH

AUTUMNAL AIR
BLOW IN THE SEEDS TO INSPIRE,
FILLED WITH THE POTENTIAL ENERGIES OF
GENERATIONS TO COME

SWEET WINTER EARTH
NOURISH OUR ROOTS
CONNECTING AND HONOURING OUR
ANCESTORS

OPENING OUR HEARTS TO SPIRIT
TO GUIDE OUR FEET THROUGH THE DANCE.

Sensory Herbalism follows the elements on their dance through the year. Water, fire, air and earth correspond to each of our four seasons. Spirit or ether, is the fifth element in our system, exerting influence all year round. We become aware of how these elements are expressed in the seasons, how they're expressed in us, physically, emotionally and spiritually, and how they manifest in the plants themselves – whether in the leaves, roots, flowers or seeds. In addition, Sensory Herbalism asks us to get to know the plants themselves, to meet them at a deep level, using all our senses and intuition. By doing this, we create a profound connection with each herb and gain an understanding of its language, its nature and the way it might interact with us, as well as how to use it for health and wellbeing.

A Sensory Herbal Seasonal Journey is an exploration of the five elements. Looking at each element, we will explore the corresponding systems within the body, considering how we can influence our own health in that season by using the herbs that grow around us.

In each season (and in the 13 moons of spirit, which is a cycle that lasts the whole year round), we explore three plants that can be harvested and made into remedies to store and use throughout the year. There are also suggestions for creative and ritual activities, as well as ideas for using seasonal nutrition to support your wellbeing.

By the time you have worked through every season, you will have gained an understanding of the elemental dance that takes place through the year and within our bodies, as well as acquiring practical skills for creating medicines and knowledge of how to use them. You may want to read through the whole Seasonal Journey first, and then go back to explore each season again as it becomes relevant.

FOR EACH SEASON WE WILL LOOK AT:

* the element that appears most prevalently in the plant at that time
* how we see the element reflected energetically in people
* the body systems in which the element is expressed
* three of our favourite herbs associated with that season
* the plant part (leaves, flowers, seeds, roots) linked with the element of that particular season.

THE ELEMENTS

SPRING is when water rises, expressed in the leaf. Leaves offer chlorophyll-rich nourishment, kidney and lymphatic support through spring-time detoxification.
SUMMER is when an increase in light and warmth encourages passion, makes flowers blossom, blood flow and circulation improve.
AUTUMN produces seeds that are rich in essential fatty acids and which nourish our nervous systems. The communicative quality of air perfectly represents the nervous system. Nature's rich harvest at this time offers us inspiration for future projects as seeds are carried on the wind.
WINTER is when the energy of the plants heads down into their roots. We need time to take stock of the events of the year and prepare physically for the next cycle. The digestive system is linked to this time of processing information. A healthy digestive system brings clarity of thought and decisiveness. Without the grounding nature of a healthy gut people can become "ungrounded", unable to concentrate or focus, potentially very nervous or flighty. In Sensory Herbalism we often ascribe these symptoms to a lack of the earth element.

THE HERBS

Selecting herbs for this book was a difficult process. There are so many wonderful plants to choose from! The 15 herbs we settled on can work to treat a whole host of ailments and, in knowledgeable and loving hands, can support the healing process of practically any imbalance of the human condition.

The plants that are ready to harvest in each season often reflect the needs of people at that time, in terms of health and wellbeing. That is, the herbs that grow in a specific season will often be helpful for conditions that are commonly found, or become worse, at that time. For example, in spring, when we start to see a rise in hay fever, there are abundant nettle tips, which have

Putting It All Together for the Seasonal Journey

SEASON	ELEMENT	BODY SYSTEMS	HERBS	PLANT PART
Spring	Water	Lymphatic system Urinary system	Plantain Rosemary Cleavers	Leaf
Summer	Fire	Heart Circulatory system	Daisy Heather Yarrow	Flower
Autumn	Air	Nervous system Lungs	Fennel Rosehip Elderberry	Seed
Winter	Earth	Bones Skin	Horseradish Valerian Dandelion	Root
13 moons	Spirit	Reproductive systems	Mugwort Datura Poppy	Entirety

antihistamine action, and plantain leaves, which soothe the mucous membranes. Colds and flu that arrive in the autumn and winter require the vitamin-rich properties of rosehips and the anti-viral agents found in elderberries.

RITUALISTIC PRACTICES AND TOOLS

Spiritual expression of life needs to be grounded with practical rituals – tools that will give support through difficult and challenging times. Creativity and imagination also help to produce more potent potions. It is important to draw on creativity and imagination as you carry out rituals with plants and people. We invite you to approach these rituals with an open heart and mind. We are not ones for prescriptive ritual and magic, but rather believe you should adapt them to your own needs and situation. The power of intention can be very powerful when working with nature. You may notice shifts in yourself or your environment as you engage in the practices. You may wish to share your experiences, perhaps carrying out rituals with others. Sometimes coming together can be more powerful than working alone.

With each herb we have included at least one recipe, to give you a foundation in herbal preparation making. The recipes can often be adapted to use other herbs, too.

SEASONAL NUTRITION

At the end of each season chapter, a closing section looks at seasonal nutrition, providing suggestions for how to include herbs on a daily basis in your life. If we consume herbs regularly in our food and drink, we are approaching our health in a prophylactic way, supporting the body's systems and creating a more healthy internal environment. So try to use at least one herb every day.

While you are on your sensory herbal journey we advise that you:

* take the opportunity to be on your own healing journey
* listen to your intuition
* have awareness of where your food (and anything else you buy) comes from; consider local and organic
* connect with nature regularly and use your new-found skills through the seasons
* dedicate time to get to know plants.

The first steps of the Seasonal Journey are herb harvesting, remedy making and simply connecting with the plants. Using the sensory tools will help you to form deep, long-lasting relationships with plants. Better to know just a few well, than many hardly at all. Start by acquainting yourself with a few of the herbs from the Seasonal Journey, to give you a foundation to build on and the confidence to explore further. Together, the 15 herbs featured in the following pages will give you the basis of a *Materia medica* (healing material) medicine cabinet.

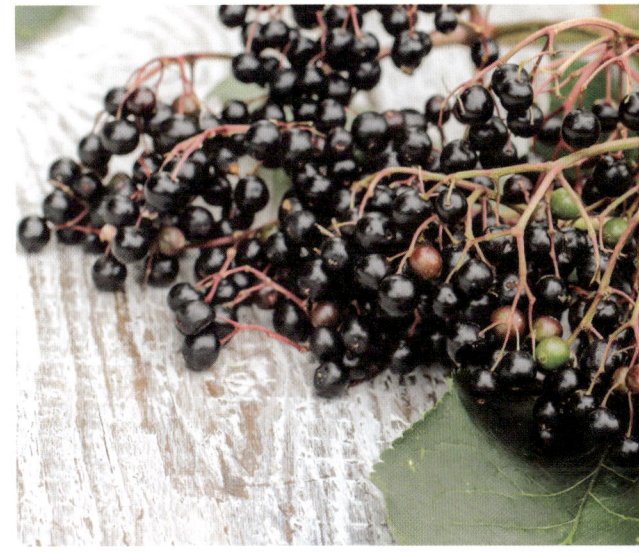

In early autumn, nature provides elderberries, rich in antioxidants to protect against colds and flu.

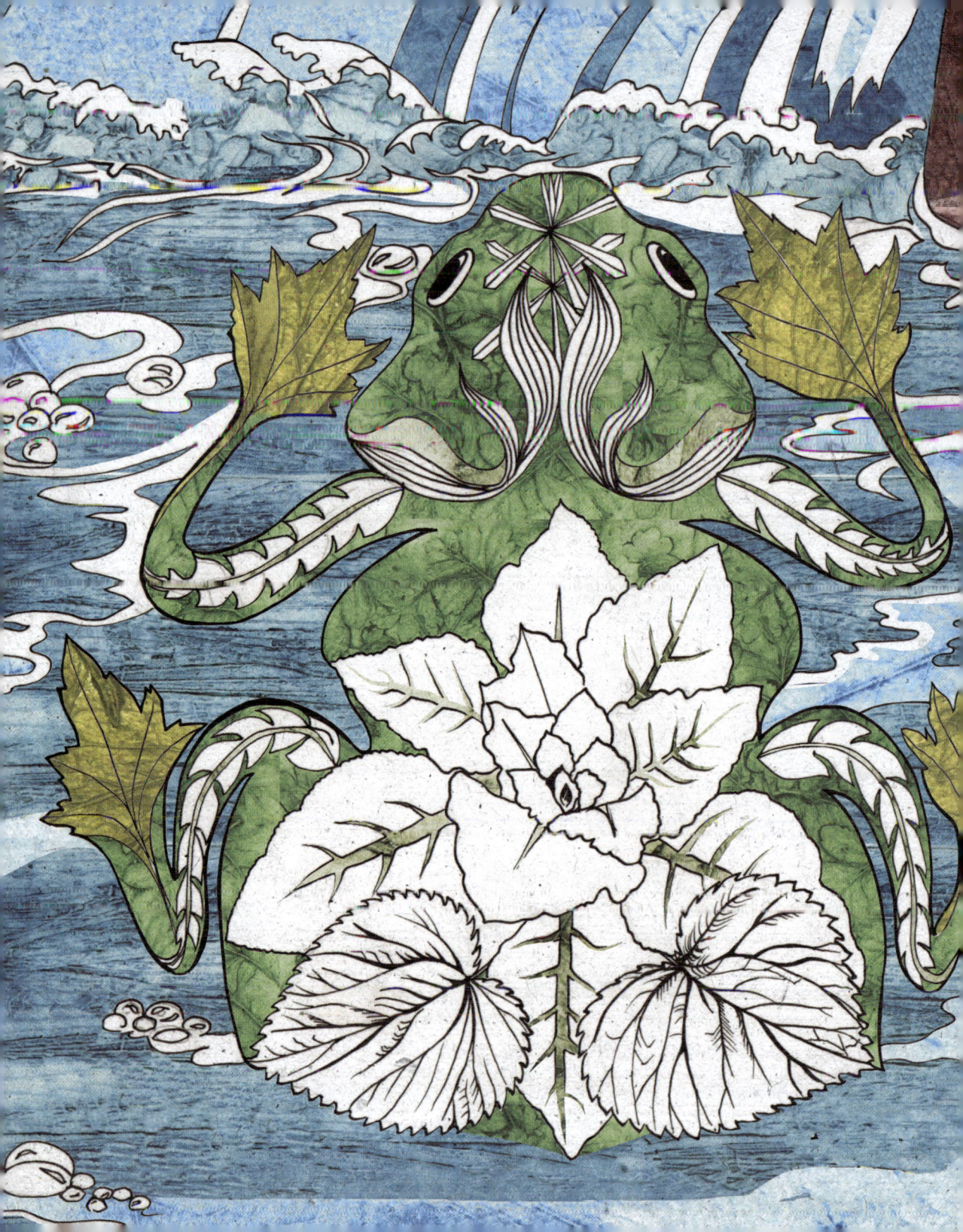

SPRING WATER LEAF

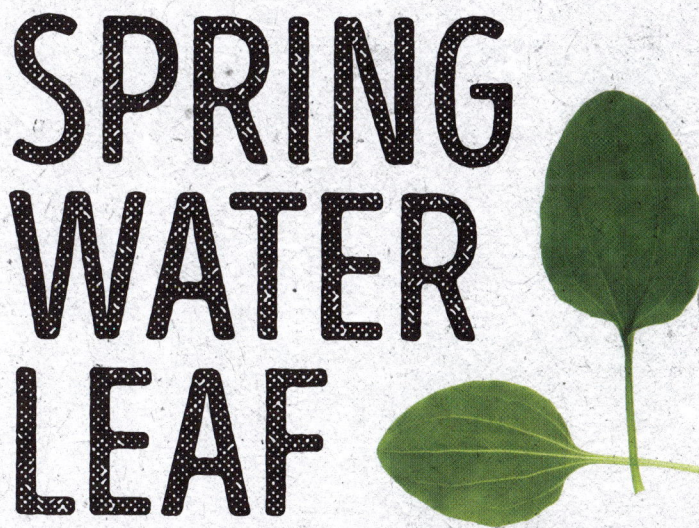

BURST FORTH LUSH LEAVES, CLEARING, WASHING OUR EMOTIONS

Spring is the dawn of life in the cycle of the year. Fresh green spring leaves emerge to offer nourishment and the promise of new life. In springtime you can see nature's gifts outside: lush mineral-rich leaves decorating the trees and plants, offering a plentiful herbal harvest.

Sensory Herbalism connects the season of spring with the element of water, the plant part leaf, the lymphatic and urinary systems and the overall theme of cleansing.

SPRING / WATER

The earth is emerging from the dark winter months, sunshine and light increasing as we approach the spring equinox, when day and night are equal. Hope, excitement and energy grow. Frustrations, too, can rise with the sap, before buds burst open into full spring — enlivening us with a spring in our step.

This is the season of juicy, green leaves, of new shoots and buds. The riverbanks and meadows are filled with delights for foraging herb lovers. Once again, after the dormancy of winter, the harvester's house becomes full of drying bundles of herbs, of jars with chopped herbs in vinegar, alcohol and oil. The creation of remedies and medicines from fresh new leaves starts once more.

Spring provides a wealth of cleansing nutrient-rich plants that are great for ridding the body of post-winter sluggishness. These greens are useful for treating the slow digestion and constipation that may arise from the excesses of the winter festivities.

WATER

Water is the liquid of life, covering 71 percent of the Earth's surface. It is cleansing and clearing, invigorating the physical, emotional and spiritual bodies   a cooling antidote to the heat of fire. Water is found in so many different forms; it can flow or provide a mirror with its stillness. Spring waters well up from deep inside the earth. Crashing salty waves, babbling brooks, waterfalls, whirlpools, lakes and stagnant puddles are all manifestations of this elemental force.

We cannot survive without the hydrating power of water. Up to 60 percent of the human adult body is water. Our brains and hearts are over 70 percent water, our lungs over 80 percent, our skin is 64 percent, our muscles and kidneys are 79 percent, and even our bones are 31 percent water! This element has numerous essential functions:

* It's vital for every cell in the body, helping to break down waste products and nutrients in the cell so that they can be filtered and moved around the body.
* It regulates our internal body temperature through sweat.
* It is required for respiration, transporting gases across the membranes in the alveoli of the lungs.
* It transports the metabolized carbohydrates and proteins that our bodies use as food in the bloodstream.
* It assists in flushing waste via urination.
* It acts as a shock absorber for the brain and spinal cord.
* It forms saliva.
* It lubricates joints.

The Water Element in Sensory Herbalism

ELEMENT IN BALANCE	ELEMENT IN DEFICIENCY	ELEMENT IN EXCESS	ASTROLOGY	EXAMPLE OF HERB
Compassionate	Rigid, brittle	Pushover, wet, histrionic	Cancer, Pisces, Scorpio	Cleavers

Good hydration is so important. If we are dehydrated, our body increases the production of cholesterol to keep cell membranes moist and pliable. This fatty thickening around the cell membrane prevents the exchange of vital nutrients and electrolytes into the cell and waste products out of the cell. In a well-hydrated person, sodium and calcium are displaced at night by magnesium and potassium, which exit the cell in the morning, leaving us feeling rejuvenated and refreshed. In the case of poor hydration, this process is not completed efficiently and traces of sodium and calcium are left in the cell at night. Then we wake up feeling sluggish and lethargic.

Dr Fereydoon Batmanghelidj observed the link between dehydration and chronic illness while he was serving a jail sentence as a political prisoner in Iran. During his imprisonment, Dr Batmanghelidj used the only medicine available to him – water – to successfully treat fellow prisoners suffering from stress-induced peptic ulcers.

WATER EXPRESSED ENERGETICALLY AND EMOTIONALLY

If water is in balance in a person, they are likely to have a good memory, be empathetic, emotionally reflective, nurturing, creative and able to deal comfortably with difficult situations. If the water element is lacking, it may be helpful to use the water-related part (the leaf) of a herb ruled by water. Cleavers is a good example. This double expression of water may help to retrieve some of water's fluidity and compassion. If someone appears to have an excess of water, you may want to consider using a plant and plant part with fiery properties, such as rosemary flowers.

WATER EXPRESSED IN THE PHYSICAL

In Sensory Herbalism the cleansing nature of spring plants is linked with the lymphatic system and the kidneys and bladder of the urinary system. These detoxification systems reflect the theme of spring cleaning.

LYMPHATIC SYSTEM

The lymphatic system is an important transport system, helping rid the body of toxins and waste. It transports lymph, a clear fluid that contains white blood cells, around the body. The lymphatic system consists primarily of vessels, similar to the circulatory system's veins and capillaries, which are connected to nodes where the lymph is filtered. In the case of infection, the lymph nodes can get overloaded and swell. Repeated or long-term infections can lead to lymph nodes becoming swollen or hardened.

COMMON SYMPTOMS OF LYMPHATIC IMBALANCE

These include: recurring sore throats, tonsil swelling, tonsillitis, pustules, spots, signs of damp in the system (such as eczema), asthma, coughs with phlegm, dysbiosis or candida overgrowth, hypersensitivity reactions (hay fever, asthma, eczema), inability to express emotions verbally, being excessively emotionally sensitive.

SUPPORTING THE LYMPHATIC SYSTEM

HERBS

* **Cleavers** is a power-packed, vibrant climber and the cardinal lymphatic herb. Cleavers is best juiced or made into fresh herb tea for medicine.
* **Marigold/calendula** gently shifts lymph stagnation and is brilliant for relieving any swollen glands. Also works as an external ointment or cream.
* **Dandelion** leaves are a diuretic and support the free flow of urine. Always

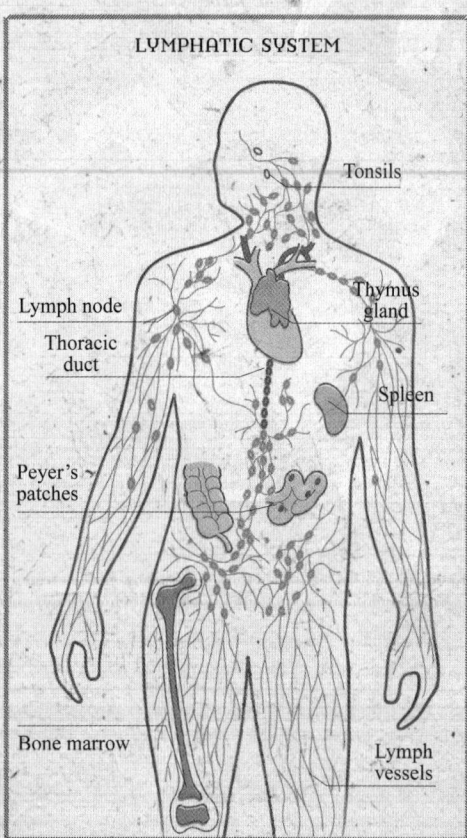

LYMPHATIC SYSTEM

Tonsils

Thymus gland

Lymph node

Thoracic duct

Spleen

Peyer's patches

Bone marrow

Lymph vessels

Lymph Conditions with Treatment Strategies for the Practising Herbalist

CAUSES	Lack of exercise, lowered immunity, infection, physical obstruction (e.g. scar tissue from injury or tense muscles)
CONDITIONS	Tonsillitis, hypersensitivity reactions (hay fever, asthma, eczema, allergic rhinitis or sinusitis), breast cancer, lymphoma
THERAPEUTICS	Improving flow and movement in the body, relaxing or stimulating tissues, supporting excretory systems such as liver and kidneys, addressing emotional reasons for stagnation
HERBAL ACTIONS CONSIDERED	Lymphatic, antibacterial, hepatic, diuretic, depurative, alterative, circulatory
OTHER TOOLS	Facial massage focusing on clearing the lymph, lymphatic drainage and massage, exercise, body brushing, increased water consumption, diet: juicing, green salads and leafy vegetables, garlic, lemon

accompany dandelion leaves with increased water intake.

* Try Detox Tea, blending cleavers, red clover, calendula, daisy and dandelion leaf.

NUTRITION
* Increase consumption of water and juices, especially green ones.
* Eat green salads, leafy veg, garlic, lemon.

LIFESTYLE
* Lymphatic drainage massage
* Meditation and yoga
* Regular exercise

Body Brushing
Try body brushing every day for at least 5 minutes before showering to get lymph moving freely through the system. Using a natural bristle brush, start at your feet and brush upward toward the heart. Similarly, when you start on your arms, begin at the hands and work upward. Use firm, small, upward strokes, or work in a circular motion. For the stomach, work in circular motion in toward the navel.

URINARY SYSTEM

KIDNEYS

The two kidneys lie to the sides of the upper part of the abdomen, behind the intestines, and either side of the spine. Each kidney is about the size of a large orange, but bean-shaped (think kidney bean!). The arteries that take blood to each kidney divide into many tiny blood vessels (capillaries) throughout the kidney. In the outer part of the kidneys, tiny blood vessels cluster together to form structures called glomeruli.

Each glomerulus is like a filter. The structure of the glomerulus allows waste products and some water and salt to pass from the blood into a tiny channel called a tubule. The liquid that remains at the end of each tubule is called urine. The urine then passes down the ureter, which connects each kidney to the bladder. Urine is stored in the bladder until it is passed down the urethra when we go to the toilet. Around 280 litres (75 gallons) of fluid passes through the kidneys for filtration daily; however, only 1–2 litres (2–4 pints) of this is excreted.

The main functions of the kidneys are:
* to filter waste products from the bloodstream, to be passed out in the urine
* to help control blood pressure – partly by the amount of water excreted as urine and partly by producing the hormone renin, involved in blood-pressure control
* to make erythropoietin, a hormone that stimulates the bone marrow to make red blood cells, needed to prevent anaemia
* to help keep various salts and chemicals in the blood at the right level.

These paired organs are governed by the flow of water. The kidneys are constantly filtering our blood and filling our bladders. The element of water is connected to the moon, the governess of our emotions, which in turn oversees the tides. The free flow of emotions can help to maintain kidney health. People who suffer from urinary problems, such as urinary tract infections, are often working through relationship issues that need resolution. There is a fine balance of the electrolytes sodium and potassium between the blood and the kidneys. It does not take much to throw this balance out, for example through dehydration, poor diet or many pharmaceutical medications. This could be comparable to the fine balance needed in relationship exchanges to maintain harmony.

In Traditional Chinese Medicine (TCM) the body is made up of meridians or channels. The kidney meridian houses our

Kidney Conditions with Treatment Strategies for the Practising Herbalist

CAUSES	Dehydration, relationship problems, unresolved ancestral issues
CONDITIONS	Kidney infection, pyelonephritis, kidney stones, cancers, acute kidney injury, renal failure (e.g. from diabetes)
THERAPEUTICS	Essential to address emotional issues alongside herbal treatment, support lymph and liver
HERBAL ACTIONS CONSIDERED	Diuretic, anti-infective, anti-inflammatory, nervine relaxants
OTHER TOOLS	Kidney band to keep them warm (cold is detrimental as it suppresses their healthy function and energy flow), increased water (with a squeeze of lemon), diet: cutting out sugar and caffeine, green salads and leafy green veg, garlic

chi, the essence given to us by our parents at conception. In utero, the kidneys go through a remarkable process known as embryonic recapitulation. They change through three different forms before settling on the final functional structure that will become the working kidneys. The first two forms echo ancestral kidneys and appear in the same order as they did during our evolution from a jawless fish-like creature into human form. This is a memory of our ancient form, so it makes perfect sense that the kidneys represent ancestry, housing the ancestral chi.

As one of the earliest organs to develop in utero, the kidneys are seen as the "root of life" in Chinese medicine. The flow of energy within the body is said to stem from the kidneys, the energy storehouse. This links with the adrenal glands, which are our driving force on a physiological level and situated on top of the kidneys. Keeping this vital energy production area warm is therefore seen as essential to good health and vitality.

The development of the kidneys is linked to that of the reproductive system. The two are often referred to together as the urogenital system. Aspects of the kidney recapitulation go on to form parts of the genitals as the kidneys move from the meso (second form) to meta (third form) phase.

In the case of chronic kidney problems, emotional work around repeated patterns of health and behaviour passed down through generations is often required.

Water has the potential to hold memory and to store and interpret information, even on a cellular level. Kidneys are the seat of power, courage and determination. When the kidney energy is vital, i.e. balanced and healthy, one is centred, fearless and clear-thinking. When the kidney energy is unbalanced, fear can prevail, often accompanied by more frequent urination.

Urinary issues such as cystitis are almost always linked with relationship challenges, usually with a significant other but occasionally with work colleagues or friends.

The emotion of fear can flow wildly and surface unexpectedly. Supporting the kidneys with herbs, nutrition and lifestyle choices can protect against the detrimental effects of this paralyzing emotion.

COMMON SYMPTOMS OF URINARY IMBALANCE

These include: kidney infections, frequent urination, repeated urinary infections, pain on urination, incontinence or urine leaking when sneezing or laughing, sense of fullness or discomfort in bladder or pelvis area, fearful emotions.

SUPPORTING THE URINARY SYSTEM

HERBS

* **Yarrow** has particular affinity with the pelvis, exerting an antimicrobial action and helping with urinary infections.
* **Marshmallow** has soothing demulcent actions and is invaluable in urinary infections, gently cooling and healing.
* **Heather** is an antimicrobial herb with specific focus on the urinary tract.
* **Nettles**, particularly the seeds, support the kidneys. The leaf is diuretic, cleansing and supporting the urinary system.
* **Cleavers** gives useful lymphatic action in urinary tract infections when extra immune help is needed.

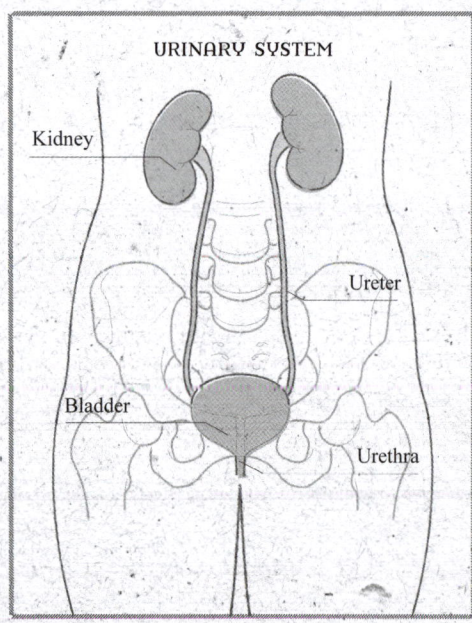

URINARY SYSTEM

Kidney

Ureter

Bladder

Urethra

Bladder Conditions with Treatment Strategies for the Practising Herbalist

CAUSES	Pharmaceutical or recreational drugs (e.g. ketamine), being "pissed off" emotionally, high-sugar diet, dehydration, infection (poor hygiene post-sex, especially in women), short urethra, sphincter weakness, obstruction (e.g. uterine fibroids or prostate hypertrophy)
CONDITIONS	Cystitis, bladder stones, irritable bladder, bladder ulcers
THERAPEUTICS	Look to soothe bladder tissues to promote healing
HERBAL ACTIONS CONSIDERED	Diuretic, anti-infective, anti-inflammatory, mucous membrane restoratives, nervine relaxants
OTHER TOOLS	Essential oils used with lower abdominal massage, hip-opening exercises, counselling, increased water (with lemon juice), diet: avoid sugar and caffeine, eat green salads and leafy green veg, garlic

* Try Piss-Ease Tea, blending heather, horsetail, marshmallow, lavender and nettle.

NUTRITION
* Cut out sugar, caffeine and alcohol.
* Eat green salads and leafy green veg.
* Use garlic – its antimicrobial actions can be helpful for conditions such as cystitis.

LIFESTYLE
* Hot water bottles on the kidneys
* Increased intake of water, with lemon juice
* Emotional work to restore balance

BLADDER
The main function of the bladder is to hold urine before excretion. In TCM it is referred to as "Minister of the Reservoir" because of its ability to manage and excrete waste products. The meridian is associated with the autonomic nervous system, so stress and tension play a key part when the bladder is overworked or its energy is depleted.

Many people suffer with recurring bladder infections and the uncomfortable burning sensation that accompanies them. It is important to stay hydrated, urinate after sex and keep caffeine and sugar to a minimum. Sugar exacerbates inflammation and feeds infection, and caffeine is a bladder irritant. The bladder also gets more irritated in those who are anxious. A healthy bladder in turn strengthens emotional flexibility.

LEAF

The energy of leaf is vital. In spring, the fertile earth once again becomes clothed in verdant vegetation. We start to feel enlivened.

The leaves that grow in spring are particularly useful for the cleansing needed in the spring months. They are bursting with the fresh energy of life, filled with minerals and various phytonutrients. Leaves picked for food and medicine at this time are rich with supporting qualities for the lymphatic and urinary systems and for remineralizing, cleansing and strengthening the body, ready for the energetic strength of summer.

Chlorophyll is the pigment that gives plants their green colour and is found in most plants and algae. Chlorophyll facilitates the process of photosynthesis, allowing energy creation from the absorption of light. Chlorophyll is green because it absorbs all the colours in the light spectrum – except green, which it reflects.

The chlorophyll molecule closely resembles haem, the pigment that combines with protein to form haemoglobin. Haemoglobin is present in the blood cells and carries oxygen to the tissues, enabling the production of energy. However, chlorophyll contains magnesium at its centre, while haem contains iron (see page 125).

THE BOTANY OF LEAVES

Leaf shape, or morphology, is an important part of recognizing plants. Start by just observing the differences in the plants around your home. How do two or three different leaf types compare and contrast?

The straight, simple vein system of the plantain leaf harks back to its prehistoric form. The simpler the structure, the less evolutionary process that has occurred. This gives an indication of plantain's straight-talking medicine. Cleavers is juicy, plump and a vibrant green. It exudes the sense that it is water-filled and as it creeps through the waysides, it seems to move like the lymph within the body. The needle-like rosemary leaves look sharper, more to the point. Rosemary has directness, and strength.

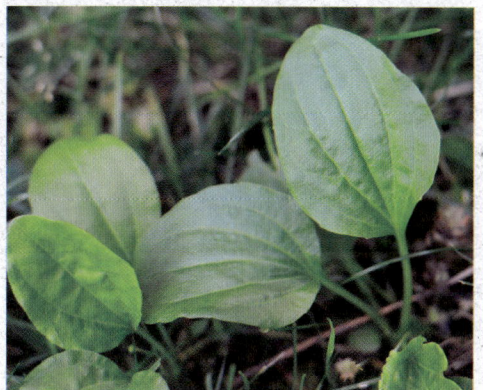

I AM LEAF

I am green
Lush, juicy green
Juicy, complex watery structure
Streaming through my venous system
Flowing responsively

Hydrated through the waxing moon

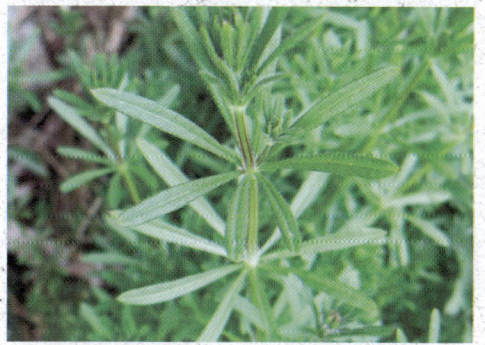

I am energy production
I am energy conversion
Trapping beams
Sunlight into sugar
Pure alchemy

Hydrated through the waxing moon

Hydrated

Prepare yourself to imbibe my pushy fluid
    mineral nourishment

I am leaf

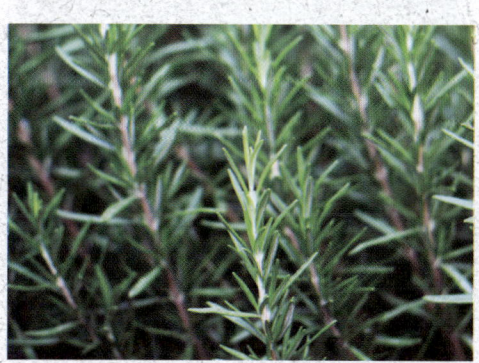

Leaf shapes of broadleaf plantain, cleavers
and rosemary

THE HERBS
THREE SPRING LEAVES: PLANTAIN, CLEAVERS, ROSEMARY

PLANTAIN

LATIN NAME:
Plantago lanceolata
FAMILY:
Plantaginaceae
ASTROLOGICAL SIGN:
Saturn
SENSORY EXPERIENCE:
Neutral green, slightly bitter
mushroomy taste

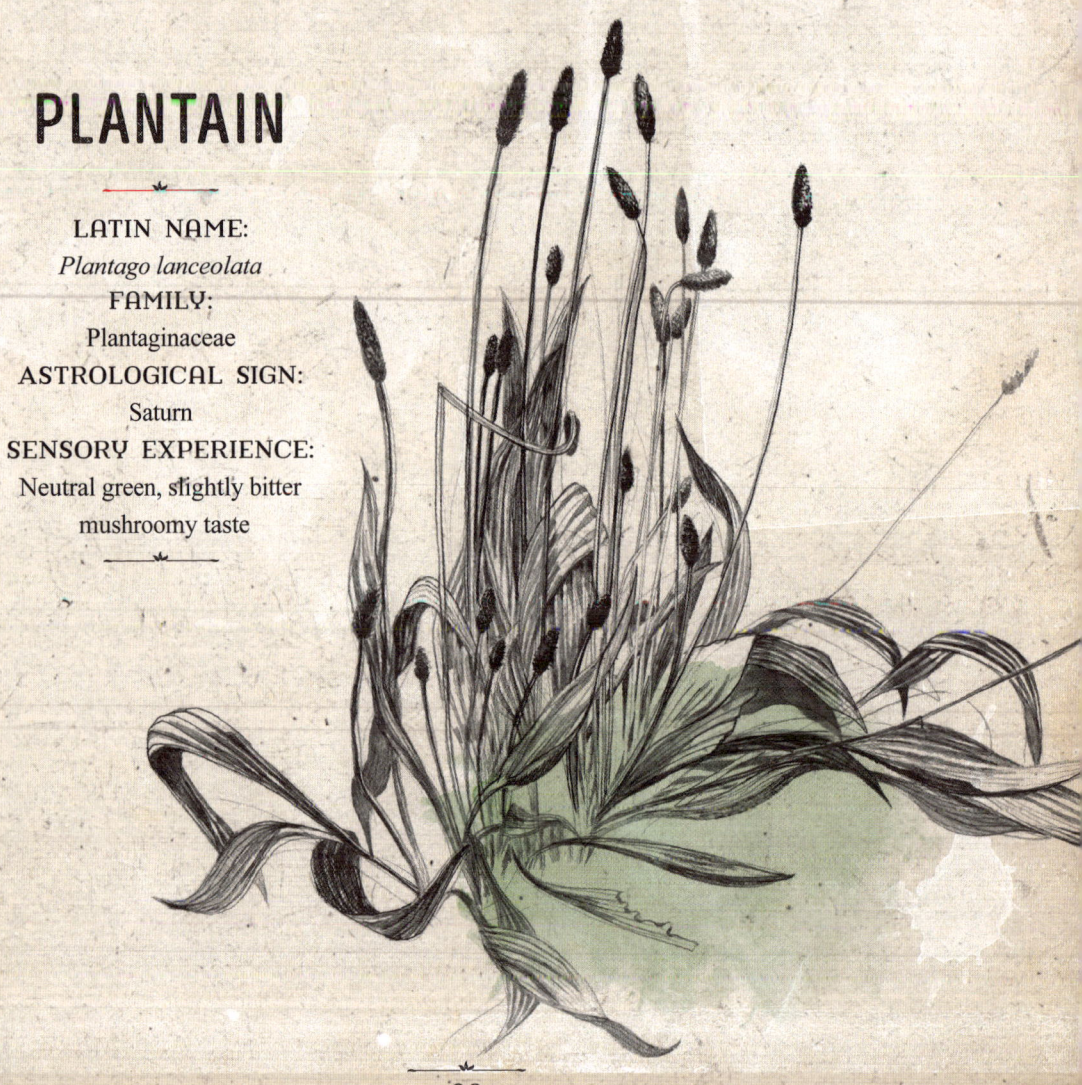

Plantain grows abundantly and can be found in almost any park, garden lawn or even waste ground. There are two distinct types of plantain: *Plantago major*, with fat, rounded leaves, and *Plantago lanceolata*, with lines of ribs stretching up its long, pointed leaves. Both types grow near to the ground, and seem to hug the earth in a beautiful floret formation. Plantain's simple design is pleasing, with long, straight lines drawing up the leaves, and its flowers rising straight and tall to meet the sun. As they blossom, a delicate crown forms around its head, a halo of tiny flowers. With its simple leaf formations, plantain is recognized as an ancient leaf, surviving through the ages, one of our ancestors. It is canny, surviving lawn mowers and grazing animals.

The overriding quality of plantain is soothing and calming, relaxing and restorative. Restorative to the mucous membrane, and soothing irritated tissue, it is perfect for cases of hay fever, allergic rhinitis, sinusitis or any inflammation in the membranes of the body. As a herb of Saturn, plantain has the ability to support both emotional and physical boundaries. This is particularly notable with regard to the mucosa within the body. Our mucosa represents a boundary, a place where external pathogens, food and gases come into contact with our internal environment. Through healing and supporting damaged or inflamed areas,

plantain restricts what enters via the mucosa. Before the invention of the telescope, Saturn was the boundary of space, the limit of what could be seen with the naked eye.

Plantain's membrane-toning and healing qualities are also helpful for the digestive system, soothing inflamed tissues and helping with conditions ranging from ulcers to leaky gut and irritable bowel syndrome.

When you chew up the leaves, a distinct earthy taste comes through, reminiscent of porcini mushrooms. This taste we ascribe to the plant constituent aucubin, a compound present in many of the herbs classified as nervines. The mushroom-like taste indicates the calming, cooling effect that plantain has on the nervous system.

Plantain leaves make an excellent antidote to insect bites or stings. Simply chew up a leaf and once it has been broken down a little by your saliva, rub it on the irritated area.

On an emotional level, we use plantain when people are highly flighty and in need of grounding. When people are lost in their thoughts and appear to be "in their heads", plantain offers a beautiful relaxing quality, slowing racing thoughts.

As you tear off plantain's leaves, you may notice the stretchy white string inside each vein. These elastic strands reflect plantain's wonderful ability to adapt to its environment, survive adverse conditions and heal. It can work wonders when you need to be flexible.

The immune-supporting effects of the polysaccharides present in plantain have also been researched and are invaluable for a wide variety of ailments, from hay fever to colds.

The lymphatic system is home to immune cells and is supported by good hydration, the kidneys and a strong immune system. Plantain supports the free flow of water in the system through its protective action on the mucous membranes and by improving elasticity, both physically and energetically, in the body. This gives us the ability to be more flexible. Plantain helps to ground and focus us, as well as aiding the flow of fluid.

COUNTERING HAY FEVER

Come spring, pharmacies triple their stocks of antihistamines. Hay fever is on the rise, it has been suggested because of nutrient-depleted diets and high levels of pollution. Rather than relying on pharmaceutical drugs, we recommend plantain – common, accessible and offering cooling anti-inflammatory properties. Our Earth Clarity Drops, for sufferers of hay fever or any over-reactive state, such as asthma or eczema, combine plantain and elderflower. Plantain contains and grounds airy thoughts by providing a soothing coating to the digestive tract and other mucous membranes. Growing near to the ground, it helps us to stay in touch with the Earth's energy. Elderflower, in contrast, acts on the head and throat, with a drying,

clearing action on a physical and emotional level. It is light, airy and expansive, useful for stuck, congested emotional states.

PLANTAIN RITUAL TO CREATE BOUNDARIES

Gather on a Saturday (Saturn's day) close to the full moon. Before harvesting, write down exactly where you need stronger boundaries in your life. Perhaps you are always saying yes. Or perhaps you seem to catch every cold that goes around. Craft an affirmation, such as "I am comfortable saying no." Or "I have strong protective boundaries letting positive beneficial energies flow in and out and keeping negative detrimental energies at bay."

Harvest 50–60 leaves, repeating your affirmation each time you pull up a stem. When you have your harvest, create an altar, place your writing in the centre and make a border of plantain leaves around the altar. You can enhance this ritual by rubbing a dab of plantain oil (see opposite) on your pulse points each morning, reciting your affirmation.

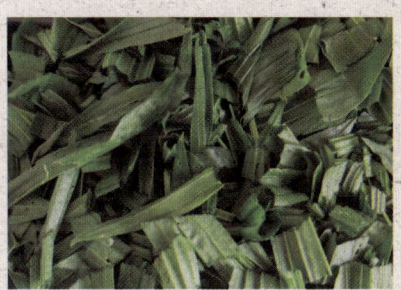

PLANTAIN OIL

This is a perfect base oil for ointments and creams or can be used as a simple oil, particularly if you have an insect bite or sting; just rub a little bit on the affected area a few times daily.

1. Harvest the leaves on a bright sunny day, after the dew has evaporated.
2. Dry them on newspaper overnight to remove the water, otherwise the oil will go rancid.
3. Fill a jar with the leaves and cover with almond oil.
4. Leave in the oil for one lunar cycle, then strain, bottle and label.
5. Store in a cool, dark space, where it will keep for a year or more.

PLANTAIN BALM

This plantain balm is soothing and healing for stings and bites.

*100ml (3½ fl oz/scant ½ cup)
plantain-infused oil (see left)
50g (1¾ oz) cocoa/shea butter
25g (1oz) beeswax
20 drops lavender essential oil*

1. Melt the oil, cocoa butter and beeswax in a bain-marie and stir well.
2. Stir in the lavender oil.
3. Pour into sterilized jars and leave to cool. Store in a cool, dark space, where it should keep for at least a year.

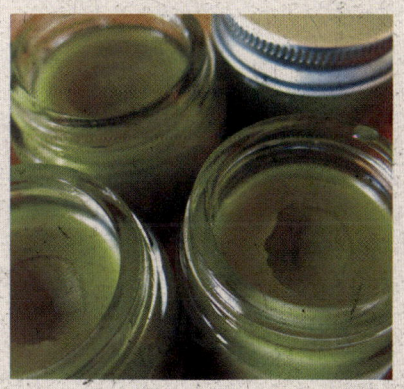

PLANT CHARACTER: PLANTAIN

I AM PLANTAIN

Gently hugging the Earth
My elastic tramlines
Signposted linear destination

Earth talking soothes the sting
Disbanding reactivity

Air flowing freely
Through cleared channels
My head haloed
Governess of boundaries

Plant Character

She has led an extremely long and interesting life with plenty of unwanted drama but always manages to remain calm. She has the ability to stretch in order to absorb potentially harmful overheating effects, cooling and calming herself and all those around her. Looking at her linear structure and stable disposition, you would never guess that she has survived and thrived through three ice ages! There is something that attracts people to her, and her ever-giving nature. Never flustered, she is flexible in any situation. After visiting Plain Jane Plantain, people feel soothed and calmed, bolstered by her kindness and care. They often offload all their worries onto her. But she can take it. She is grounded, open-hearted and loving.

CLEAVERS

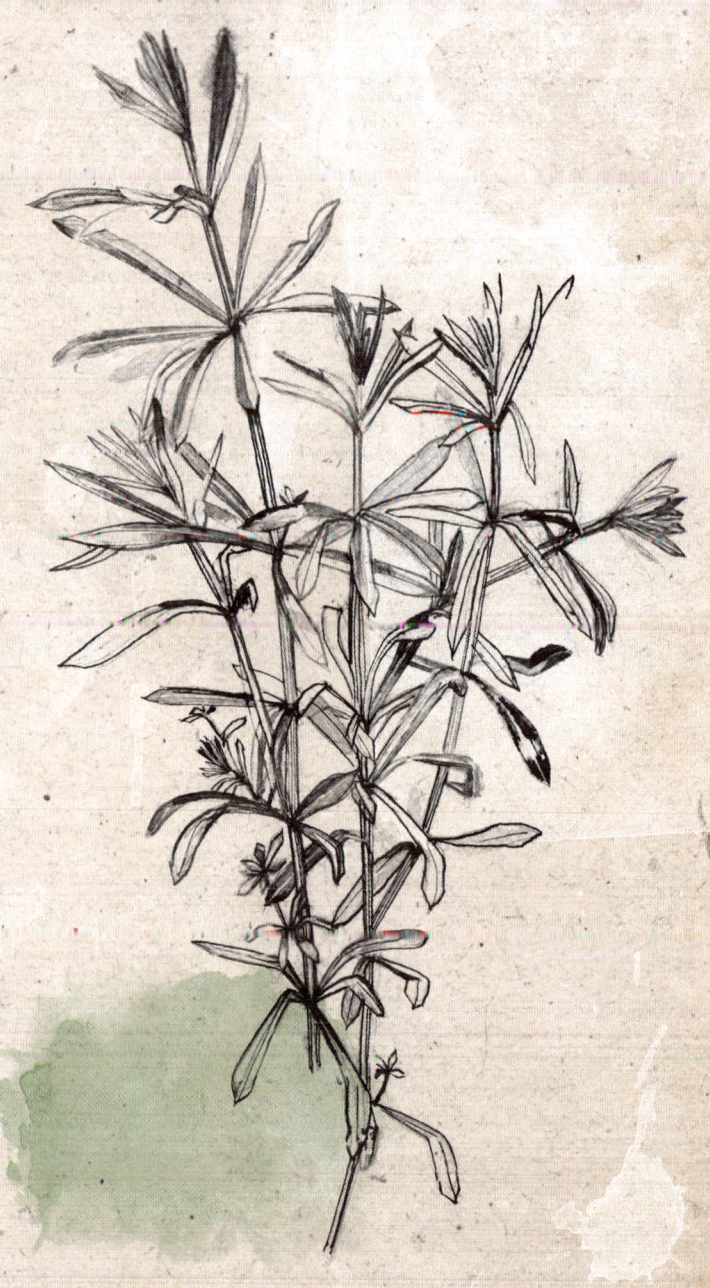

LATIN NAME:

Galium aparine

FAMILY:

Rubiaceae

ASTROLOGICAL SIGN:

Moon

SENSORY EXPERIENCE:

Spicy, crunchy, watery

From early spring, cleavers (also known as goose-grass or sticky willy) is poking through the earth. It is ready to begin its travels, climbing up by clinging on to fellow plants with fine crook hairs or trailing along the ground. Wonderfully copious, you can find cleavers growing in most hedgerows, forest clearings, field edges, gardens and parks. This vibrant green herb is vitally full of life, but almost as soon as it's picked it starts to wilt, losing its juicy water.

Because of its watery properties, cleavers may seem cooling at first, but when you taste the plant, a distinct hot pepperiness stays in the mouth and throat. Cooling to the body and watery in nature, cleavers also has the warmth to stimulate and move water within the body. Cleavers is part of the coffee (*rubiaceae*) family, and the ripe seeds of late summer and autumn have been roasted and used as a coffee substitute, as they contain caffeine and are naturally stimulating.

This herb looks a little like a bottlebrush; it's long and thin with whorls of leaves encircling the square stem. In fact, its effects on the lymphatic system are a bit like those of a bottlebrush, drawing and clearing out toxins, and giving the immune system a good scrubbing. This is why cleavers is referred to as a lymphatic. Its overriding action is helping to detoxify the lymph fluid and remove unwanted debris. It is very useful for swollen glands or tonsillitis. It is also helpful, where immunity is reduced, to help stimulate the flow and productivity of the lymph; it is therefore cooling to the body. It is used to bring down fevers – an "anti pyretic" – and to treat burns. This lunar herb has the ability

Choosing a Juicer

The wonderful thing about juicing herbs is that you can freeze the juice for future use, allowing you to obtain the herbs' healing properties all year round. It's therefore well worth investing in a juicer, but be aware that there are two types of machine available – centrifugal or masticating. A centrifugal juicer spins at high speeds, grinding fruits and vegetables to a pulp and forcing the juice away from the pulp. A masticating juicer is more efficient at squashing out the juice, working at lower speeds and with no spinning action. The high-speed action of a centrifugal juicer can produce too much heat, which can damage or possibly even kill the health-promoting enzymes in the juice.

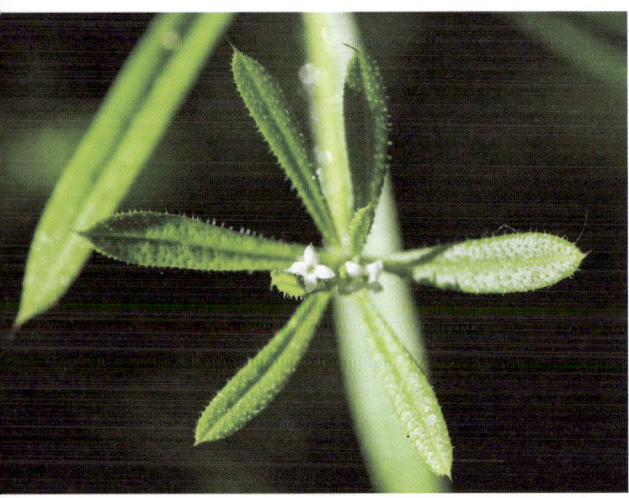

Tiny leaf hooks enable cleavers' climbing action.

CLEAVERS RITUAL TO CLEAR OUT WHAT NO LONGER SERVES YOU

Around the spring equinox, spend some time thinking about what no longer serves you, what you can leave behind, and then with this in your mind go and harvest a basket full of fresh cleaver shoots.

Create a matting from the plant material – cleavers shoots stick together brilliantly – as a ritual sieve to clear out what no longer serves you.

With any leftover plant material, brew a strong cleavers tea. While it is brewing pour 3 litres (5¼ pints/12½ cups) of spring water through the sieve, imagining that all old negative patterns of behaviour are washing away, cleansed.

Finally, strain the brewed tea through the sieve into a cup and drink in the cleansing energy of cleavers.

to balance waters in the body like the moon herself balancing the waters of the Earth. Cleavers can reduce any retention of fluids in the tissues.

We harvest lots of cleavers and juice them because the herb has a far better action fresh than dried. A juicer is a great way to get all the goodness out of your harvest. The fresh juice of plants is very much like the juice of our cells and therefore drinking juiced fresh greens can be especially rejuvenating. Fresh green juices contain live enzymes and bioactive vitamins and minerals, which are easily assimilated into the body. Cleavers is at its optimum for a relatively short period, in the spring before flowering.

HERB VINEGARS - CLEAVERS

Vinegar has many healing powers. It helps lower cholesterol, improve skin tone, moderate high blood pressure, prevent or counter osteoporosis and improve metabolic functioning. Herbal vinegars are a super-effective marriage, combining the healing and nutritional properties of vinegar with the aromatic and health-protective effects of mineral-rich green herbs. Spring greens are ideal for making into vinegars, as they are rich in minerals and these minerals are easily extracted by the vinegar.

Herbal vinegars can be used in a variety of ways. Add a tablespoon to water (sweeten with molasses if you like) for a daily drink, pour over beans or grains, use in salad dressings or to season stir-fries and soups. Regular use boosts the nutrient level of any diet with very little effort and they offer an easy way to keep calcium and other mineral levels at an optimum. Adding vinegar to your food helps build bones because it extracts minerals from the vegetables you eat. A spoonful of vinegar on your broccoli, kale or dandelion greens increases the calcium you get from eating them by one third.

1. To make cleavers vinegar, simply harvest some fresh vibrant cleavers as close to the full moon as possible. Choose a warm day, when the dew has evaporated.

2. Chop them up finely, place in a jar and cover with apple cider vinegar.

3. Leave to macerate for a couple of weeks then strain the herb out and bottle up your herb vinegar ready to use.

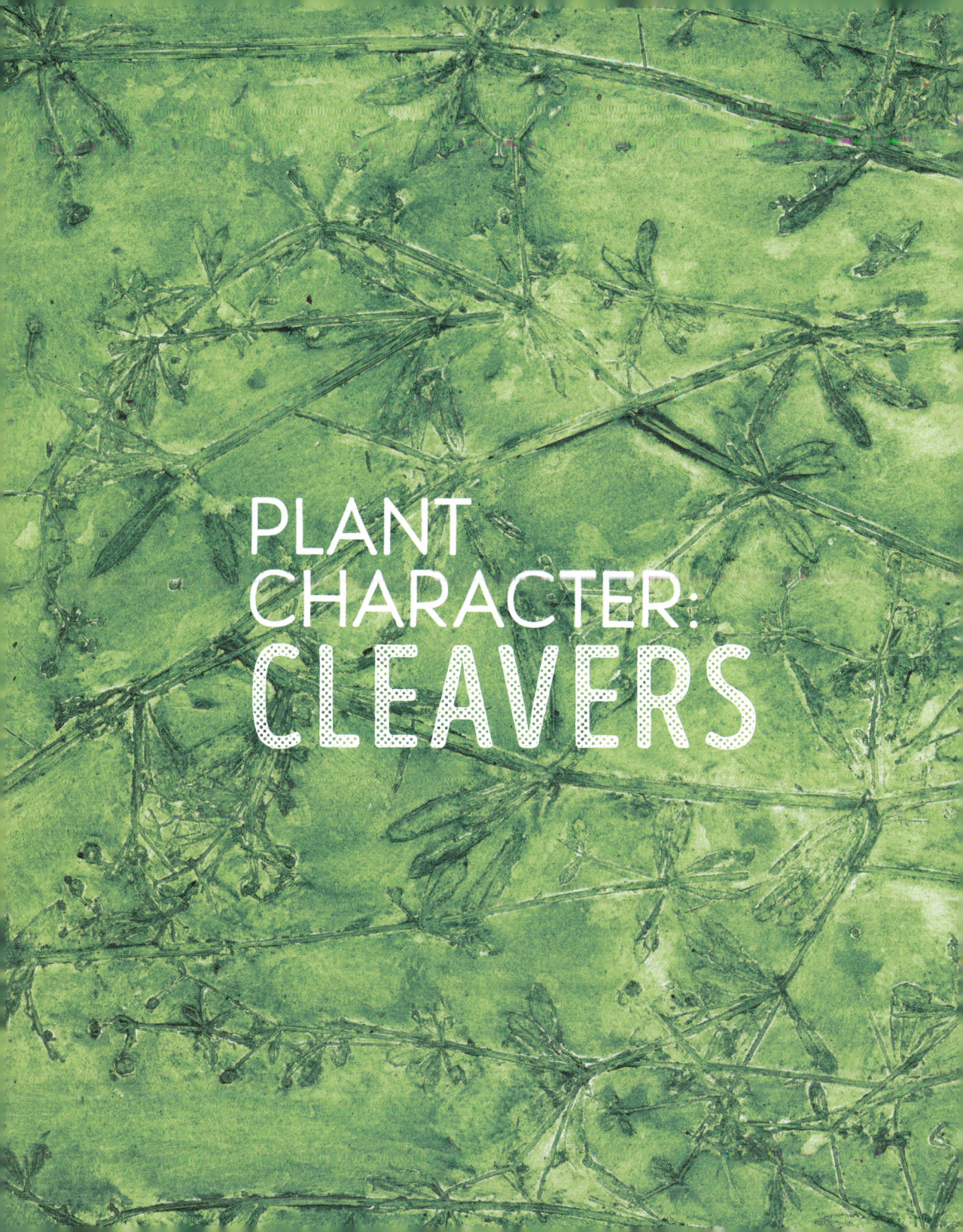

PLANT CHARACTER:
CLEAVERS

I AM CLEAVERS

I am lush Luna lucidity
Succulent flow
Creeping to and fro
Square-stemmed social climber
I am travelling through time
Hitching a ride
To hook you in
With my sticky, stimulant seed
A secret to reveal
Beneath my cool, cleansing water
Balancing
A coffee kick, spicy heat
I am moon medication
In vibrant green
My tiny button, a memory badge

Plant Character

Cleavers is a mover and a
shaker, rarely still, a traveller
in search of enlightenment,
making his way around
the place and leaving an
unforgettable impression. He
enjoys loud repetitive beats,
looks deceptively straggly,
weak and weedy, with his
sharp, grasping edges. He
has a spicy enlivening kick
that will have you up and
dancing with this "party
animal" all night long.
A very clingy type – cleavers
is almost impossible to
shake off!

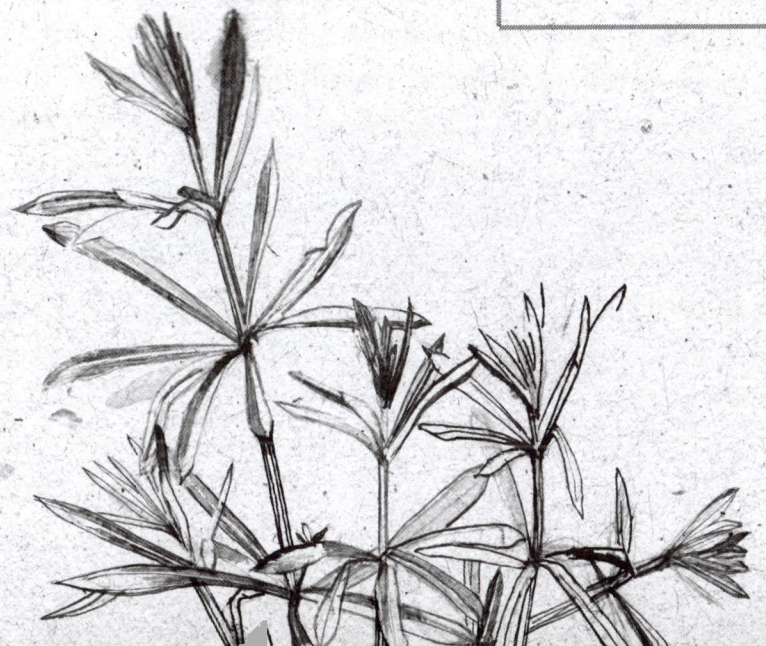

ROSEMARY

LATIN NAME:
Rosmarinus officinalis
FAMILY:
Lamiaceae
ASTROLOGICAL SIGN:
Sun
SENSORY EXPERIENCE:
aromatic, warming, pushy,
movement, direct focus, menthol,
eucalyptus-like, sage-like

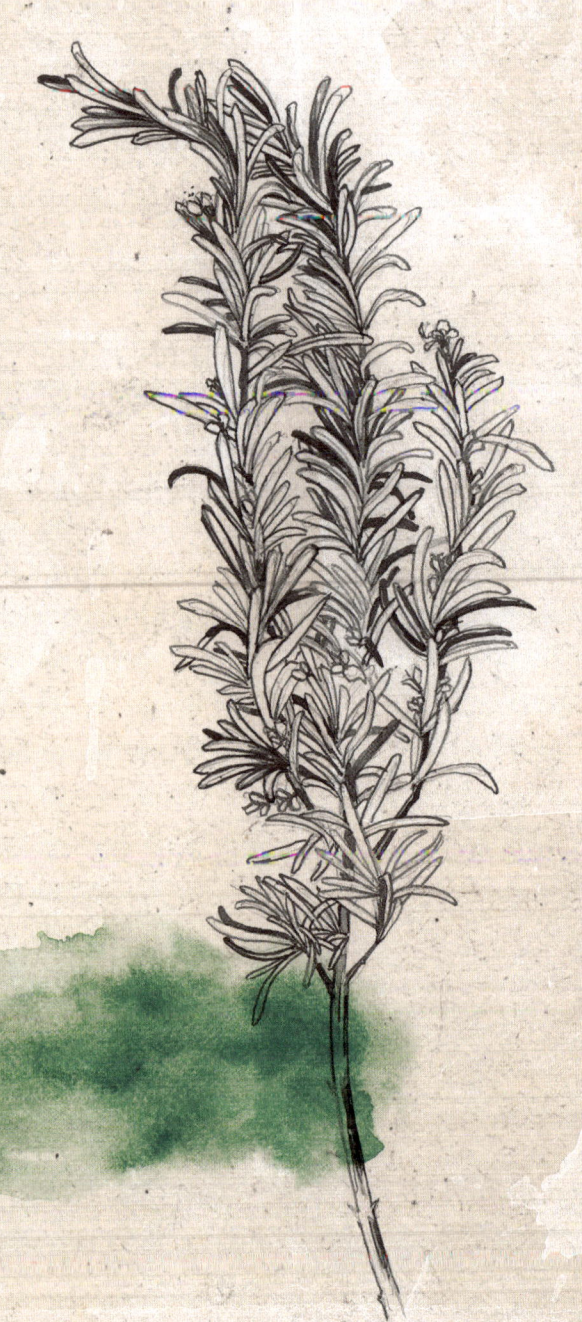

The word rosemary means "dew of the sea", from the Latin *ros*, "dew", and *marinus*, "sea". In southern Spain, there are cliffsides stretching for miles covered in aromatic rosemary. It hangs there with its purple-hued flowers, a reflection of the colours of the sea. If you fondle its needle-like leaves, you are greeted with uplifting aromas. Dew collected from any plant in the morning holds a memory of the herb and can make a powerful essence for medicine. Rosemary is a protective, warming, circulatory, brainpower-enhancing, aromatic, digestive plant. The memory-enhancing properties of rosemary, held in the sea dew on its morning leaves and flowers, can be potent medicine indeed.

Rosemary has a great variety of associated folk uses and mythology. Its essential oil is said to be one of the ingredients (along with clove, lemon, cinnamon and eucalyptus oils) of the Thieves' Oil developed by perfumers in 15th-century France to protect themselves as they looted the houses of victims of bubonic plague. It has been strongly connected to memory and remembrance since ancient times. The main historical medicinal uses of rosemary have been as a tonic to the brain and as a gently cleansing liver medicine.

A garden favourite, rosemary is always on hand to harvest, flavouring roast potatoes with its pungent aroma. It is not just for taste that we add rosemary to oily and fatty dishes though. It is a brilliant digestive herb, with bitter principles, beneficial to our whole digestive system by stimulating the production of bile and aiding the breakdown of fats. It also helps to reduce flatulence by targeting the muscles of the digestive tract.

A Natural Alternative to Coffee

Drinking coffee can lead to your physical body becoming dependent on caffeine to stimulate the release of adrenaline. Rosemary offers similar effects of mental alertness, without the addictive element! Try switching your coffee for a rosemary tea made by placing one small sprig of fresh rosemary in a mug of hot water – watch as it turns a bright green colour – sweetening with a little honey. However, as a herb of the sun, rosemary should be approached with caution for long-term use. We would never advise anyone to use one herb as much as many folk do tea and coffee. For a hot temperament or constitution, daily use of rosemary may be too heating.

ROSEMARY AND LEMON ZEST SEA SALT

A zesty seasoning for your cooking. We always opt for sea salt, as it is rich in iodine, essential for thyroid health.

85g (1 scant cup) coarse sea salt / 2 tbsp finely chopped / fresh rosemary zest of 1 unwaxed lemon, grated

1. Place the salt, rosemary and lemon zest in a blender and whizz up to a fine consistency. The mix will be slightly damp.
2. Spread onto a baking tray lined with baking parchment to stop any transfer of fats or flavours already on the tray.

3. Place in the oven on as low a heat as it will go with the door open for a couple of hours to dry out. Alternatively, leave it in an airing cupboard. If the mixture is lumpy after drying, blend again until fine.

As a herb of the sun with the energy to heat and circulate, rosemary is specifically indicated in depressive states accompanied by general debility and weak circulation. Known as the "tip-of-the-tongue herb", it has been used since ancient times to improve and strengthen memory. Students in ancient Greece and Rome wore rosemary garlands around their heads while studying, specifically for this quality. The plant brings freshly oxygenated blood to the peripheral arteries in the head.

Externally, rosemary has traditionally been used to ease muscular pain, sciatica and neuralgia. An infused oil of rosemary is a component of our own Ache-Ease Balm, as well as of many other liniments used to relieve rheumatism.

The wonderful herbalist and holistic veterinary medicine activist Juliette de Baïracli Levy always revered rosemary as one of her two favourite herbs. Her children have claimed in jest that she cured everything with rosemary. This is because of rosemary's incredibly wide-ranging applications, revitalizing all the systems of the body and protecting against pathogens.

During the spring months the evergreen bush rosemary will see a new growth of soft green stems and leaves. The leaves in particular are super active, full of new life and phytonutrients. The circulatory action of rosemary impacts on the lymph and will support other lymphatic herbs such as cleavers by working synergistically, strengthening the lymphatic action. We always include rosemary in spring cleanses and detoxes to support the emotions and mind, keeping people upbeat and determined to stick to the plan of health. Great strength is needed at these times of cleansing and rosemary really helps us to focus.

By growing this hardy perennial in a sunny space in the garden you will have a strong friend and nurse for any condition that needs warmth and invigoration. We use rosemary as a protection charm and often place it in bunches around the home.

ROSEMARY RITUAL FOR PROTECTION

Whenever you feel like a little extra support or protection, rosemary is the friend you need. We grow rosemary outside the front of our houses to make it super accessible for this simple and effective ritual. As you leave the house, simply pick a sprig to wear behind the ear, or in your hair or lapel, to encourage clear thoughts and bring you protection.

Try this when going into a new situation, if nervous about public speaking, or for support with social anxiety, when talking to a friend or loved one about an emotional issue, or taking an exam – or just for an extra boost in the morning.

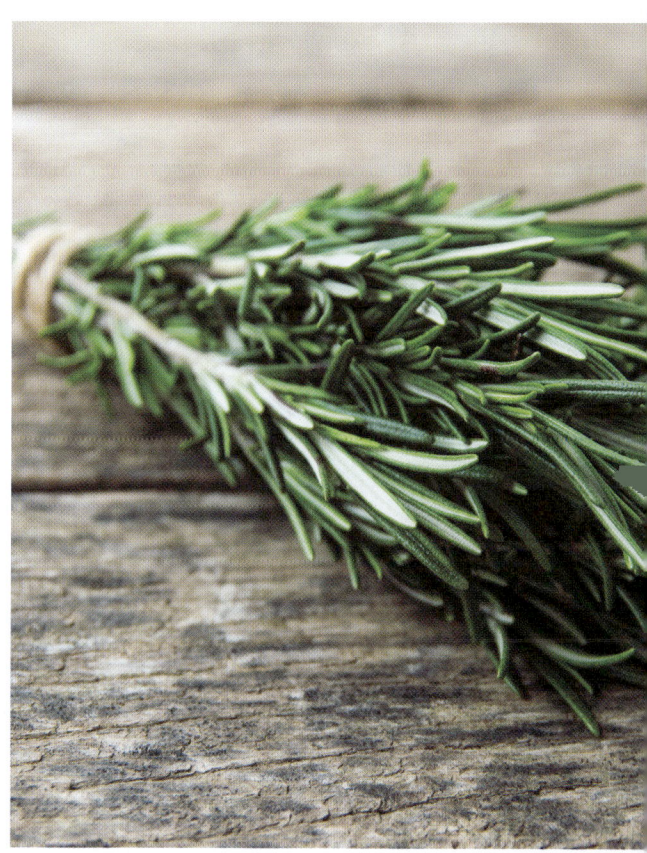

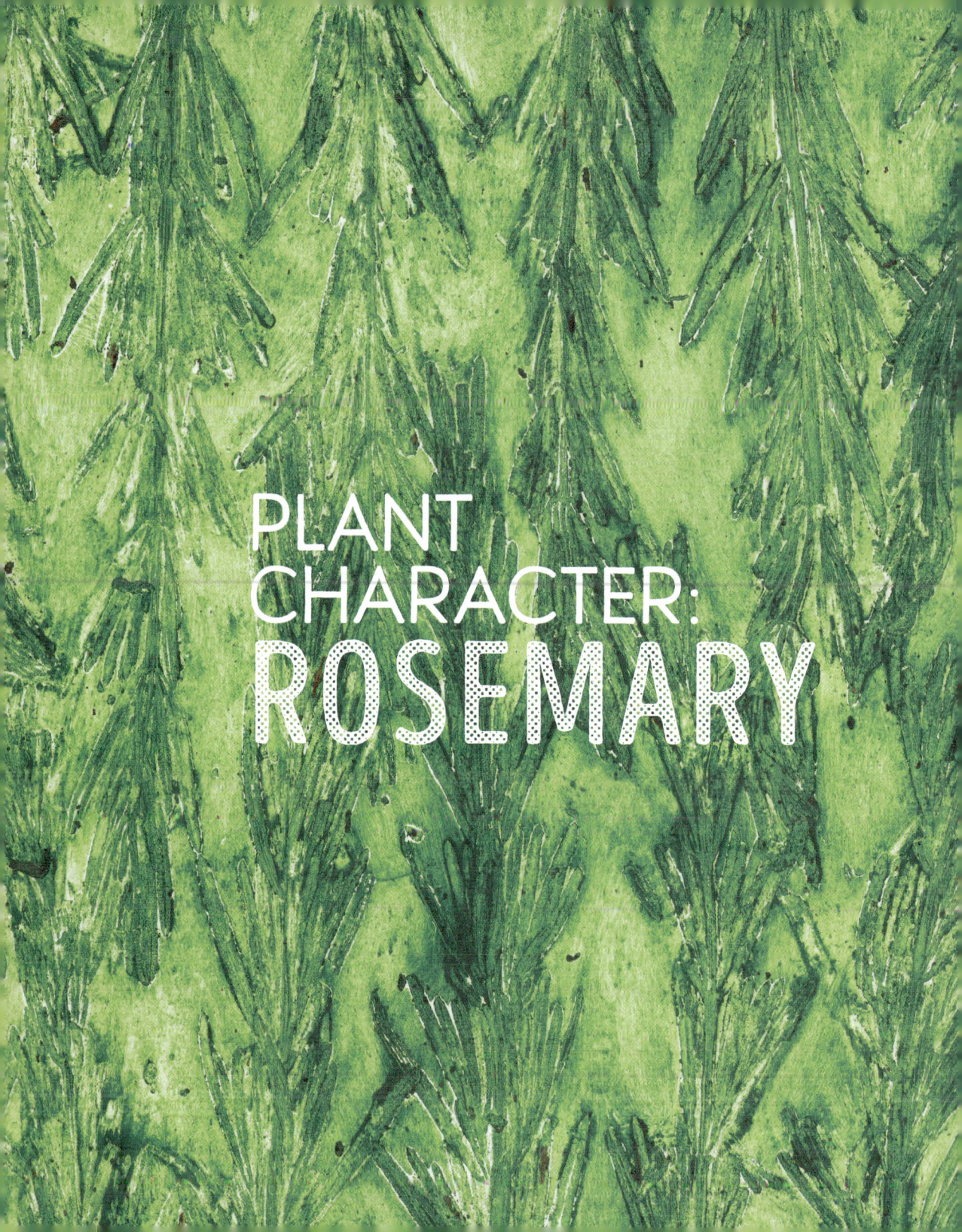

PLANT CHARACTER:
ROSEMARY

I AM ROSMARINUS

Evergreen rose of the sea
Purple-blooming femininity
Straight-lined sprigs of strength
Gifting crystal memory
Solar surge
Tactility offering stimulant scent
Aromatic circulatory

Holding amulet protection
Gypsy-lore luck
On waves of adventure
Merge with inside energy
Creating synergy
Courage on a cliff edge

I am rosemary

Plant Character

Rosemary is a gypsy fortune teller on the pier, her hair luxuriant and shining with health and her eyes deep inky pools reflecting your own soul back at you. Holidaymakers flock to her, year after year, for tales of their futures. She is a well-bringer of pure luck– it always seems to be sunny around rosemary. She has an incredibly sharp, active mind, remembering all the visitors she has ever met and their grandparents before them. She holds memories of every detail and protects these details lovingly. Bathed in a wondrous scent, she sells her homemade perfumes and facial water on her stall outside the booth. She loves music and dancing and rarely keeps still. She never married or had children; she pleases herself and is supremely free.

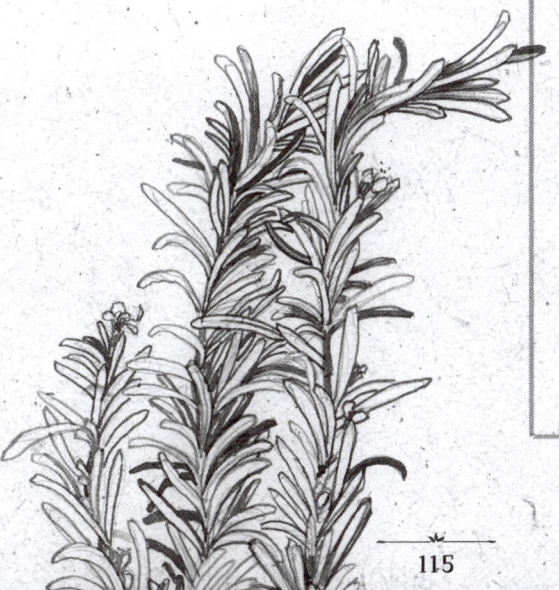

NUTRITION AND RITUAL WITH LEAVES

The leaves of spring hold the key to energetic health. In these lengthening days, the sun sheds its rays on a harvest of salad leaves. Leaves of tangy, citrusy sorrels, gently bitter dandelion leaves, nutty hawthorn leaves, fresh linden or beech leaves and a wealth of others are available at this time of year and provide excellent nutritious medicine.

SPROUTED SEED AND SPRING GREENS PESTO

Sprouted seed pesto with spring greens is healthy, delicious and versatile – and bursting with spring energy and sunshine goodness!

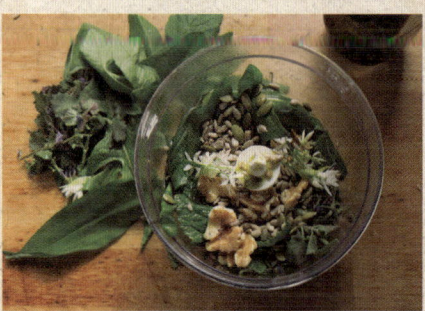

Get out and harvest some spring leaves, such as nettles, ramsons (wild garlic), dandelions, sorrel, plantain or beech leaves. Nettles are full of iron; ramsons are mineral rich and anti-infective; dandelions have potassium with cleansing and diuretic properties, and are also bitter, so support good digestion.

Put your spring greens in a blender or electric mixer with a good handful of rocket (arugula) leaves, a couple of cloves of garlic, and some alfalfa, cress or any sprouted seed of your choice. Pine nuts are a delicious addition to your pesto and give it a nutty flavour. Add enough olive oil or flax oil to achieve a consistency you are happy with, or use ground seeds and water instead. If you like, add black pepper to taste. Do experiment and feel free to combine whatever you like and feel you need in your pesto!

Whizz it all up again until smooth, then keep covered in the fridge where it will store for a couple of days.

By connecting with the rituals and leaves of spring, we can enhance our lives with this season's verdant energy. Harvesting the spring leaves connects us with this energy of new growth and new beginnings, and a renewed sense of purpose and activity. The water-enhancing effects of the leaves featured in this chapter offer us a variety of qualities – plantain with its earthy energy, cleavers with its cleansing wateriness and rosemary with its fiery, protective nature.

With the support of plantain oil you can create strong clear communication and boundaries that allow relationships to flourish. We can learn to listen to our internal compass, and clearly communicate how we feel. Using cleavers in juice and as a vinegar will support rituals designed to cleanse away old habits and invite in new, more nourishing pursuits. Rosemary sprigs can become a regular tool

that offers you additional support day to day in tackling some of the more challenging situations in life. We all need to feel supported and protected at times and rosemary can be an aromatic friend for life

Establishing clear boundaries and communication, washing away unhelpful habits, and connecting with the flow of the water element and the lymph and urinary systems, will set you in good stead for creating spring health and vitality.

Spring is a perfect time to focus on washing away all the heaviness, sluggishness and stasis of the winter and beginning to invite new growth and new ideas into your life, leading to the birth of new projects. The table below looks at some of the rituals we can perform at this time of the year. Consider: what do you need to clear from your life? What would you like to nurture or grow?

Spring Rituals

MARKERS	Spring equinox, bud and shoot
NATURE REFLECTIONS	Growth and new life, greens
FOCUS	Leaving the dark behind, welcoming new light and ideas, clearing out the old
MOON ASPECT	Waxing
RITES	Using running water to cleanse and wash away old habits to leave room for positive growth. Planting a particular seed with an intention of growth for a new project.

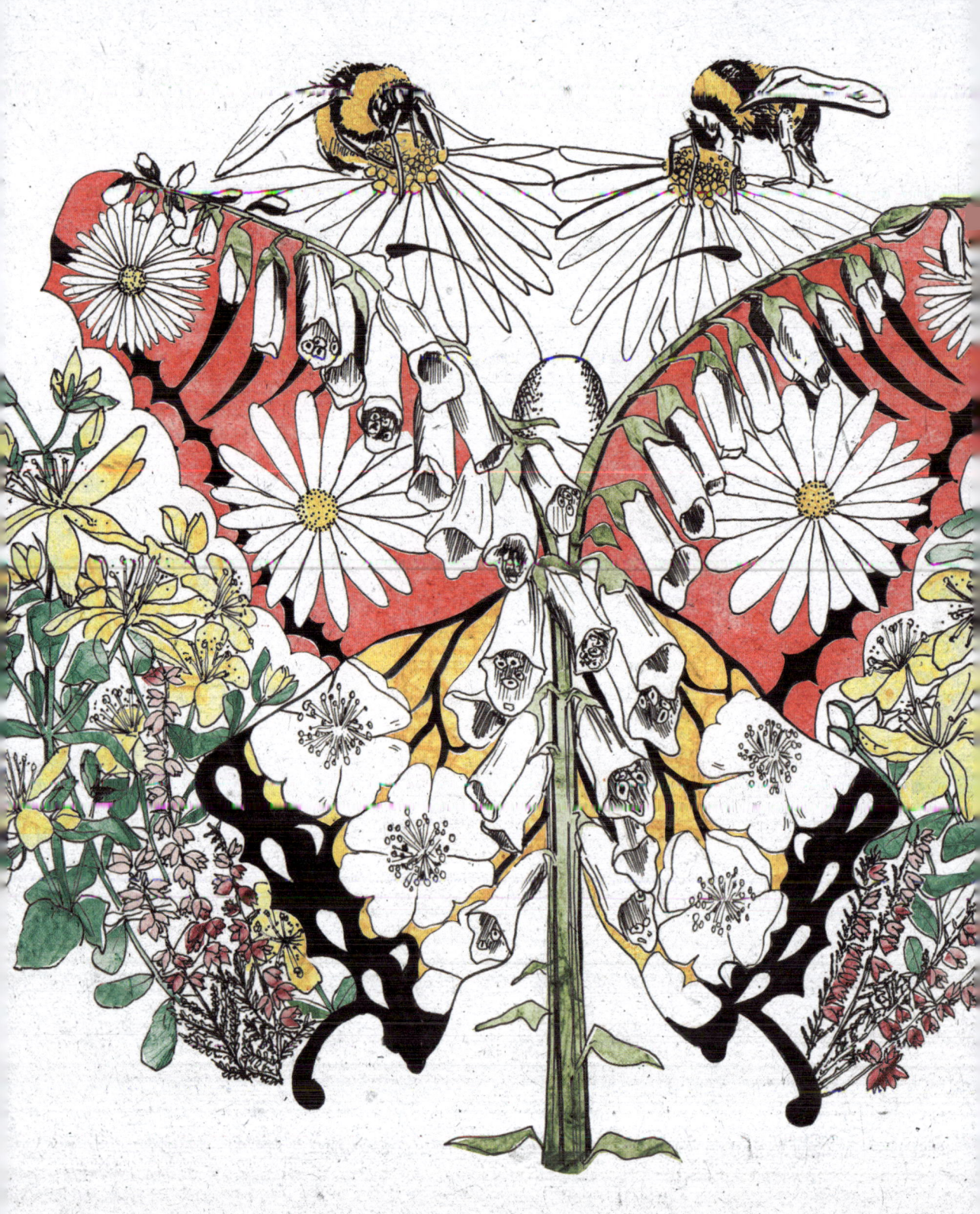

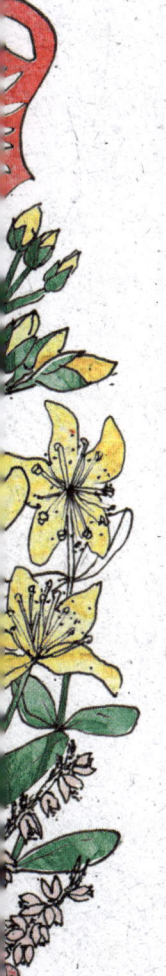

SUMMER FIRE FLOWERS

IGNITE OUR PASSIONS, ATTRACTING POSITIVE MOVEMENT AND GROWTH

As spring comes to a close, the seasonal cycle enters the lightest, warmest time of the year – the summer. It's a time of festivity, of long hazy days and balmy evenings, when a wonderful riot of scent and colour fills our senses. The theme for summer in Sensory Herbalism is passion, and the aspect of the body that this season closely relates to is the cardiovascular system (CVS). Our hearts beat with the exhilaration and celebration of this high-energy time.

SUMMER / FIRE

While spring is all about the renewal of life and growth in nature, summer is the time when plants turn to attraction and pollination. Flowers galore bloom to invite pollinating insects to work their magic. Herbs, especially those containing volatile oils, are often at their most powerful medicinally, bursting with the sun's energy.

Summer solstice (midsummer) is the celebration of light and the bountiful beauty the sun brings to life. Traditional celebrations include building bonfires over which people leap to bring fertility, purification, health and love into their lives. Midsummer is aligned with the energy of the full moon – it is a time of bright light and magnetism, of amplification of emotions and wild abandonment. Harvesting flowers around the full moon nearest to the summer solstice will create very powerful medicines.

FIRE

The element of fire brings action and movement, both creative and destructive. Fire represents warmth, attraction, nourishment and protection. People have been cooking on fires and gathering around them to share stories for millennia. Warding off danger and the darkness of the night, fire is central to the home, just as the sun is to our planet and our solar system. Fire's physical form can only manifest in the presence of earth (the wood) and air (oxygen). It has the power to heat metal, converting it from a solid to a liquid. It is the transformer, the magician, the alchemist. It purifies.

The Fire Element in Sensory Herbalism

ELEMENT IN BALANCE	ELEMENT IN DEFICIENCY	ELEMENT IN EXCESS	ASTROLOGY	EXAMPLE OF HERB
Passionate	Apathetic	Jealous	Aries, Leo, Sagittarius	Daisy

FIRE EXPRESSED ENERGETICALLY AND EMOTIONALLY

If fire is expressed in balance in a person, they are likely to be passionate and loving, vibrant and vital, possibly with many interests and a strong drive to achieve goals. The astrological signs associated with fire are Aries, Leo and Sagittarius. Anyone who has these signs prominent in their astrological chart is likely to express fire in balance when they are feeling healthy and vital.

Daisy has planetary associations with both the sun and with Venus. As a herb that restores joy and enthusiasm, daisy is indicated where there is a lack of fire. You can engage with daisy in many ways, from making syrup to creating daisy chains to just lying down in a patch of daisies.

FIRE EXPRESSED IN THE PHYSICAL

Sensory Herbalism links fire with the heart and circulatory system. In the body, fire is expressed as movement and the initiator of life, through the beating of the heart and the movement of our blood through the circulatory system. Our hearts beat more powerfully when we feel passionate – whether about a cause, an interest or a loved one. The excitement results in blood flowing more quickly and freely through the body.

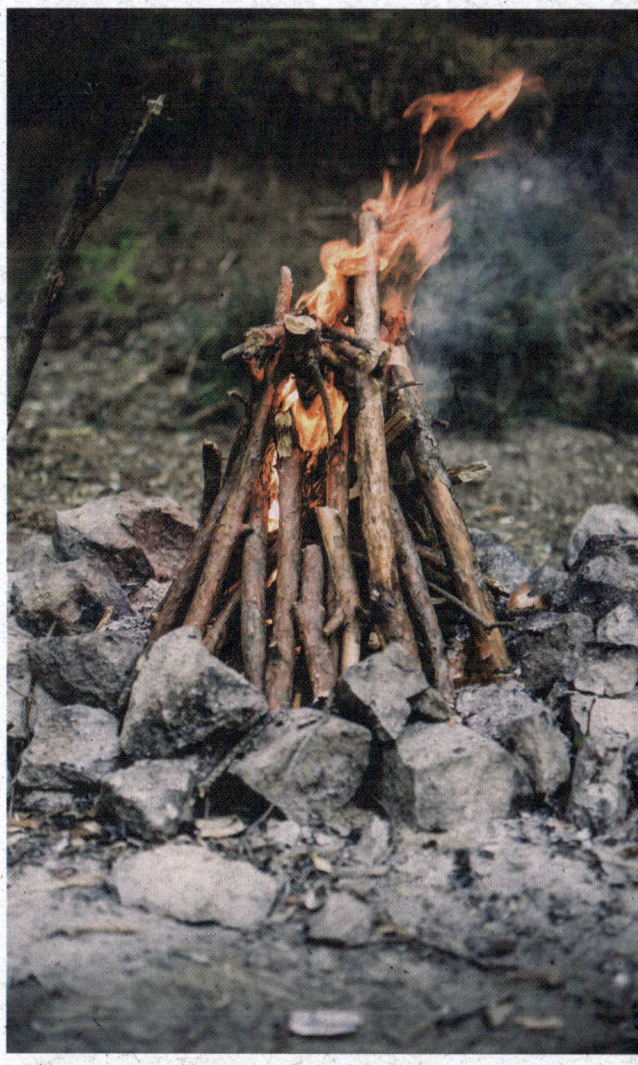

We are still drawn to gather around fire today, just as our ancestors were millennia ago.

CARDIOVASCULAR SYSTEM

The heart is one of the earliest functioning organs. In human embryos, it begins to beat at about 22–23 days, with blood flow beginning in the fourth week. In many ancient forms of medicine, such as Traditional Chinese Medicine, the heart is seen as governing the mind or spirit.

Between the 1970s and 1980s medical science discovered that the heart produces, and responds to, certain polypeptides (chains of amino acids involved in the endocrine system). It influences other organs that are involved in heart regulation, such as the kidneys. This changed the centuries-old idea that the heart was merely a pump and it is now also recognized as an organ that responds to hormones. This is interesting because we can sense emotions in our heart. We can feel heart palpitations, for example, when our heart responds to stress.

The rhythm of our heartbeat – baboom, baboom, baboom, baboom – is hypnotic. We spend months in our mother's womb surrounded by the sound of her heart. We are programmed to respond to rhythm and so when the rhythm of our life is disturbed, so is our heart.

Our heart emits electromagnetic energy. Electrical signals cause it to beat in rhythm and squeeze sequentially to send blood into our arterial system for transport around the body. Electromagnetic energy emanating from the heart is many times stronger than that emitted by the brain. It is measurable up to several metres away from the body and changes in frequency when it comes into contact with other people's energetic field. We are constantly merging electromagnetic energy fields with those around us. As this occurs, measurable differences in electromagnetic wavelength have been noted. This concept is reflected in the notion of the heart chakra. If we imagine that our heart waves, although ceasing to be mechanically measurable, emanate out into the world around us, we can connect with the idea of universal love.

Our energetic hearts can be said to have the ability to receive and process information from the world around us. When opening energetically in the giving and receiving of love, it is beneficial to reflect on how, and with whom, the energy is shared. Reflective exercises and meditation can maintain our energy in a safe and flowing way. If we choose to shut down our emotions as a way of protecting ourselves, the energy can become blocked. Remaining open to receive, but with awareness, can help to support deep, loving relationships.

Heart Conditions and Treatment Strategies for the Practising Herbalist

CAUSES	Stress (work, relationships, life), diet and nutritional deficiencies, congenital, environmental, drug induced, lack of courage
CONDITIONS	High/low blood pressure, valve defects, palpitations, varicose veins, poor circulation, cholesterol/vessel wall changes, heart attack, angina
THERAPEUTICS	Relax blood vessels for high blood pressure; stimulate circulation for low blood pressure; consider root causes and when you need to refer the patient to other medical professionals, such as doctor, physiotherapist, etc.
HERBAL ACTIONS CONSIDERED	Cardio-tonics, circulatory support with blood vessel relaxants, circulatory stimulants, nervine relaxants, adrenal support, nutritive herbs, diuretics
OTHER TOOLS	Nutrition, exercise, destress techniques (e.g. meditation, counselling)

When we are knocked emotionally, the heart is affected. The electromagnetic pulse alters and we feel "out of sorts" or crushed by emotion. The emotional response can have a knock-on effect on the functioning of other systems in the body, such as the digestive system, the kidneys and the nervous system. When a strong emotion occurs, receptors on the heart respond to the neurotransmitters produced in response. Palpitations may be felt, indicating a rise or fall in blood pressure. Prolonged stresses may lead to cold hands and feet, as well as varicose veins. Emotions may include feeling cross, angry or confused – or indeed emotionally numb. We have many varied defences for an emotionally damaged heart depending on our experiences and environment, as well as diet and coping tools.

COMMON SYMPTOMS OF CARDIOVASCULAR IMBALANCE

These include: palpitations, varicose veins, poor circulation, high/low blood pressure, cold hands and feet.

SUPPORTING THE CARDIOVASCULAR SYSTEM

HERBS

* **Hawthorn** berries have a normalizing effect on heart health with the ability to

balance blood pressure, bringing it back to its optimum. They have been shown to strengthen the force of the heart's muscular contraction while relaxing the blood vessels, avoiding extra pressure. A lack of courage may precede a weak heart, or vice versa. We use hawthorn, a herb that supports the blood vessels that feed the heart muscle, for giving courage. We often recommend carrying a few dried hawthorn berries in the pocket to play with like worry beads if a little courage is needed.

* **Rosemary** is a circulatory stimulant, clearing and motivating the mind and the brain. Bear in mind, however, that this is a pushy herb and should not be used if blood pressure is high.

* **Yarrow** is a blood-vessel dilatory herb encouraging the flow of blood and other herbs around the body. With the support of yarrow's dilating, opening energy, we can learn to act from an emotionally open place without feeling vulnerable.

* **Rosehips** are nourishing and restorative, rich in flavonoids that support the strength of the blood-vessel walls, and maintaining cardiovascular health as well as supporting the immune and nervous systems.

* Try Heart and Soul Tea to overcome anxiety and for uplifting heart support, blending lemon balm, hawthorn, lime blossoms and rose.

NUTRITION

* Incorporate garlic in your diet to maintain blood flow and avoid coagulation in the blood vessels. Garlic is associated with anti-platelet activity.

* Eat a rainbow of foods each day to ensure a variety of plant phytonutrients for anti-inflammatory and antioxidant activity.

LIFESTYLE

* Meditation and yoga for relaxation and maintaining a steady resting pulse

* Regular exercise

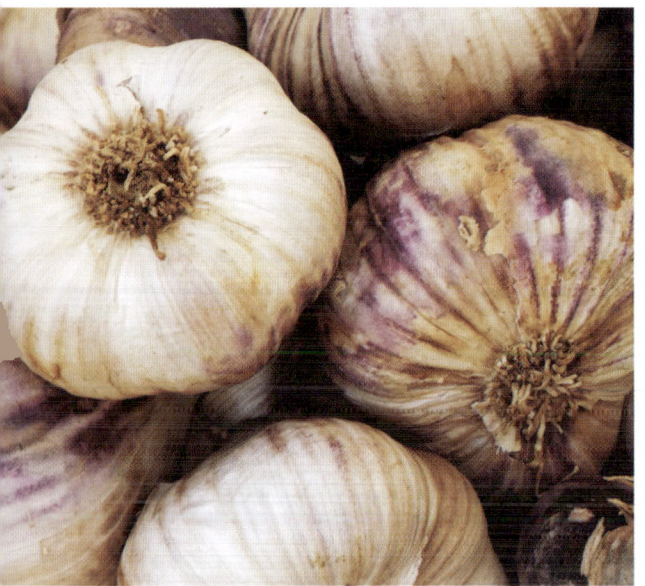

Garlic supports the cardiovascular system, promoting the free flow of blood around the body.

BLOOD

Blood flows throughout our bodies via our blood vessels. Made up of red and white blood cells and plasma, it carries oxygen to all our cells, collects carbon dioxide for excretion and transports nutrients. Good supply and circulation of blood is essential for health.

Interestingly, as shown in this illustration, the structure of haemoglobin in human blood and chlorophyll (liquid chlorophyll is a plant's "blood") is incredibly similar, an indication of how closely related we are to our plant ancestors. Chlorophyll contains oxygen, carbon, nitrogen, hydrogen and magnesium, while haemoglobin contains the same but with iron instead of magnesium.

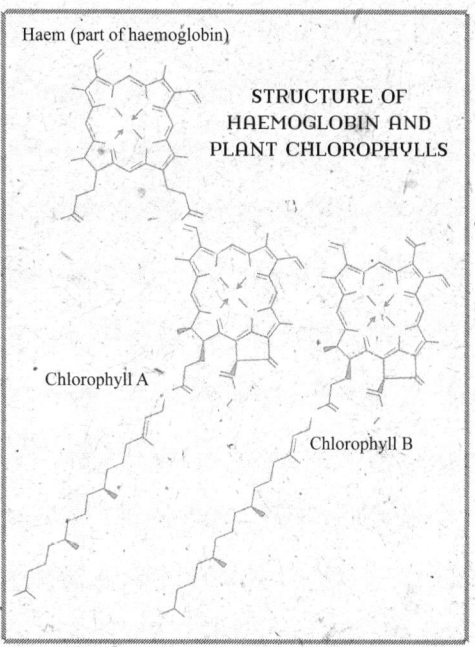

Haem (part of haemoglobin)

STRUCTURE OF
HAEMOGLOBIN AND
PLANT CHLOROPHYLLS

Chlorophyll A

Chlorophyll B

Blood Conditions and Treatment Strategies for the Practising Herbalist

CAUSES	Infection, physical obstruction, misshapen blood cells, increase or decrease in certain blood components
CONDITIONS	Anaemia (pernicious and iron deficient), haemophilia, septicaemia, blood-borne viruses (HIV, Hepatitis C), leukaemia
THERAPEUTICS	Aim to restore composition, consistency or flow
HERBAL ACTIONS CONSIDERED	Circulatory, antiviral, antimicrobial, lymphatic, styptic, nutritive, alterative
OTHER TOOLS	Nutrition

FLOWER

The energy of flowers is uplifting and exciting; their bright colours and diverse shapes provide visual stimulation. Many flowers, whether complex or simple, are designed specifically to attract insects and other pollinators. These carefully selected insects will complement the structure of the flowers and facilitate the movement of male sex cells in the pollen grains to the female stigma. Here the pollen grains germinate and release male sex cells, which eventually fuse with a female ovum. This then develops into an embryo enclosed within a seed.

It is an uplifting experience to walk through wild spaces blazing with colour –

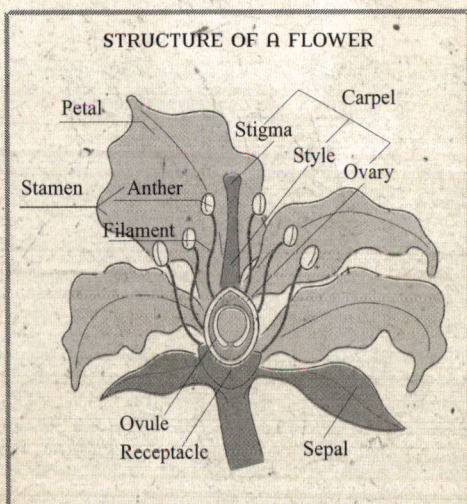

STRUCTURE OF A FLOWER

Petal
Carpel
Stigma
Style
Ovary
Stamen
Anther
Filament
Ovule
Receptacle
Sepal

purples, yellows, whites, blues, reds and oranges. Flowers used in herbal teas provide this joy with flashes of bright colour, so we try to balance herbal teas with a hint of colour to provide a healing feast for the eyes.

Take a moment to consider the feelings that different colours evoke in you.

* What is your favourite colour?
* Why are you attracted to this colour?
* What does it remind you of?

Your answers, which may change from day to day or week to week, may give you clues as to where you are at emotionally in your life at the moment.

Flowers have been brought into the home and used to decorate and bring joy to spaces for millennia. The idea that different flowers could offer us different energies is supported by the knowledge that the flower colours that our eyes recognize are in fact lights of varying wavelengths; each colour has its own individual wavelength and vibration.

Floriography – the language of flowers – was very popular in Victorian times. This coded communication allowed the expression of feelings that it was not socially acceptable to say aloud We still draw on some of these meanings today; think red roses on Valentine's Day and white lilies at funerals.

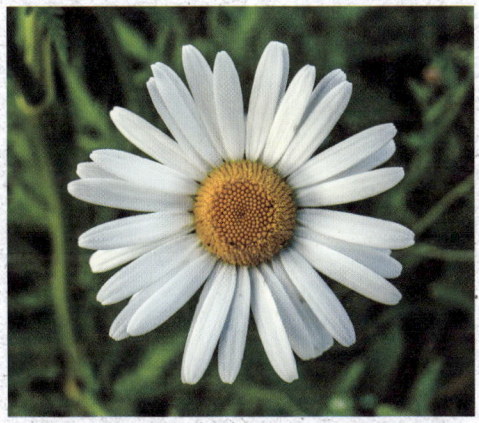

I AM FLOWER

I am flower

Delightful, delicate bloom
Attracting attention

I am the attraction,
Attract you
Trap you
I ignite your passions
Your fire

Come closer
Sniff my tantalizing scent
Dust your nose with my pollen
Beautiful, elegant, intricate
Tasty, tantalizing treat

I am perfect for you in every way
Come to me, creature, insect, human prey
Want me, take me

Sex, fire, passion, lust
Healing, warmth, love

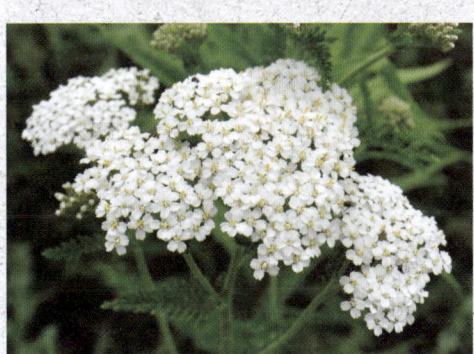

Flower shapes of daisy, heather and yarrow

THE HERBS
THREE SUMMER FLOWERS: DAISY, HEATHER, YARROW

DAISY

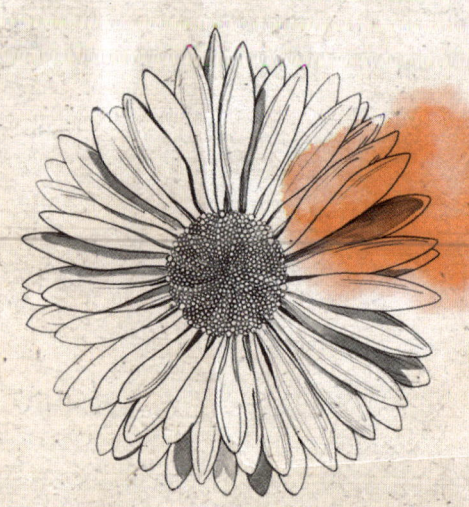

LATIN NAME:

Bellis perennis

FAMILY:

Asteraceae (Compositae)

ASTROLOGICAL SIGN:

Sun/Venus

SENSORY EXPERIENCE:

Metallic, soapy

Daisy was one of the first herbs that allowed us to respond truly to our intuition (see pages 11–13) and guided how we would work with plants in the future. It is representative of all beginnings, a little, wide-eyed, innocent baby, completely pure, loving and open with no sourness, bitterness or regret in its character. If it is downtrodden, it can bounce back. Have you tried standing on a daisy?

It leaps back, unscathed. You can mow a lawn and still see daisies popping up straight afterwards. It soothes emotional bruising and brings joy back into life.

The white-rimmed yellow pupils of this watchful eye flower, "the day's eye", stare up at the sky, tracking the sun. This action indicates the eye-strengthening and soothing properties possessed by this versatile plant when used as a wash for the eyes.

Daisy is in abundance throughout a good portion of the year, arriving in its multitudes in early spring, but it can be found hiding in much smaller numbers in any month. It's often found growing alongside its friends, plantain, dandelion and yarrow.

A strongly metallic flavour is evident after nibbling a flower head. A metallic flavour represents transformation (metal being an element that can be transformed from liquid to solid). With great kindness and gentleness daisy transforms bitterness into playfulness and joy as with ease it speaks to our hearts.

As you pick daisy, the sound and sensation of a light "pop, pop, pop" of the daisy heads is addictive. Despite knowing you have enough daisies for your tea, syrup or balm, you still feel compelled to pick more. This is a reminder of daisy's use on an emotional level for compulsions, of which you may be aware, but unable to stop. Daisy lightens the load and works to release compulsive behaviour patterns. It was once believed that putting a daisy chain around a child would protect them from being stolen by the fairies.

Also known as bruisewort, daisy is similar to arnica, known as a bruise-healer. It contains saponins, the compound responsible for making soap bubbles. When we fall or knock ourselves, inner tissues become damaged and blood leaks into the surrounding area, creating a bruise. Saponins break down the blood to help it to disperse. Thus, applied externally as an ointment or cream, daisy promotes the healing of bruises. The actions of the herb on the body are indicative of emotional and spiritual properties, too. Daisy helps us to bounce back from emotional bruising, strengthening resilience and character.

If you make a strong daisy decoction (simmering the flower heads in water for 10–15 minutes) you will notice that when you stir your tea or pour it from one cup to another, it quickly froths up like a head on beer. The saponins in the daisy make it a wonderful remedy for the lungs to help expectorate any stuck mucus. The saponins also have a reflex action via the digestive system. Key to this is the vagus nerve, which travels from the brain through the body and has a big role to play in linking up different physiological systems and coordinating their actions. The word "vagus" is derived from the Latin for "wanderer". The saponins in daisy irritate the gut lining and the message is relayed to the lungs via the vagus nerve to expectorate phlegm.

DAISY RITUAL USING FLOWER ESSENCE MADE AT FULL MOON

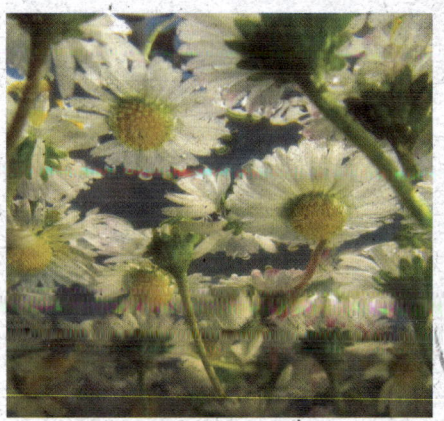

Daisy medicine reminds us to lighten up and go with the flow. Try making your own daisy flower essence to use in the daily ritual described below. Harvest your flowers on a bright day around full moon for best results. You will need a clear glass bowl, spring water, a glass dropper, bottles, a funnel, some labels for the bottles, and brandy as a preservative.

First, spend some time observing and connecting with the daisies. Then fill the bowl with water and place it outside in sunlight. Pick the daisy flower heads and place in the water until the surface is covered. Leave the bowl in the sunshine for a few hours.

Fill your sterile dosage bottles halfway with brandy. Remove the flowers and any debris from the water. Add this water to the bottles, filling them to the neck, sealing and labelling them. It's a good idea to include the date and also to note the phase of the moon and/or astrological sign under which the essence was prepared. You now have what is referred to as a mother tincture. Potentiate the essence by moving the bottle in a figure of eight, the infinity sign.

For a daisy flower essence for everyday use, fill a 30ml (1 fl oz) bottle with half brandy and half spring water, add two drops of the mother tincture and take drops throughout the day, or as needed.

Over a lunar cycle, take the daisy essence drops daily and consider how you would like to be more open-hearted and receptive to yourself and others and more connected to all of nature. Ask daisy to aid your journey to be able to see through child-like, innocent eyes. Request resilience and strength of character, and the power of bouncing back. Think about what you can do in return for daisy.

Daisy can be deployed if there is a need to connect people to a time that felt joyful and to remind them of their innate ability to be playful; daisy connects us with our inner child. Making daisy chains is one of the first experiences many people have of playing with plants. One participant at a workshop said, "Daisy will bring you the perfect childhood you never felt you had."

Daisy is useful for repeated patterns of behaviour, such as obsessive-compulsive disorder (OCD), depression, melancholia and paranoia. If people talk of feelings of defeat or oppression, daisy is indicated.

DAISY DELIGHT SYRUP

A delicious syrup to drizzle over food. You can use it for the treatment of coughs (take 1 teaspoon three times daily for up to five days) and to heal emotional bruising, taking several drops daily alongside an affirmation.

A harvest of fresh daisy heads
1 vanilla pod (optional)
450g (1lb/2¼ cups) brown sugar per
450ml (16 fl oz/scant 2 cups) water

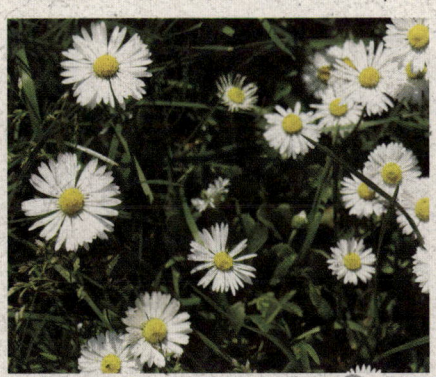

1. Harvest a small bowlful of daisy heads. Place the daisies in a pan and pour water over them until they're covered (you can also add a deseeded vanilla pod).

2. Bring the water nearly to the boil and keep just under boiling temperature until it turns a pale green-brown colour. Sieve the liquid into a measuring jug, watching as the soapy bubbles form on top of the tea.

3. Now add the sugar, placing the mix back in the pan and gently warming until all the sugar has dissolved. Keep over the heat for a further 5 minutes or so to make sure the sugar is fully incorporated.

4. Pour into sterilized bottles and label.

PLANT
CHARACTER:
DAISY

I AM DAISY

Watching attentively
The solar wheel
Clocks of light

Pure resilience
Release the past,
Bounce back

Dispelling bruise residue
Blood breakdown
Start anew
Youthful repartition
Chains of fertility
Curious naivety

The beguiling innocence
    of fairy's delight
I am daisy

Plant Character

Daisy is a little child, full of songs, giggles and boundless energy through the day. Playing and bouncing around, she never tires while the sun shines. As soon as the sun sets, however, she closes her eyes and rests all night. She is wide-eyed, naive and full of laughter and silly rhymes, and can make everyone smile. Her energy for recreation is infectious and she often has lots of friends around her playing countless creative games. If she falls and hurts herself she examines her injuries, takes stock, shakes herself off and carries on. Daisy always bounces back with resilience from any challenge or emotional set-back she encounters.

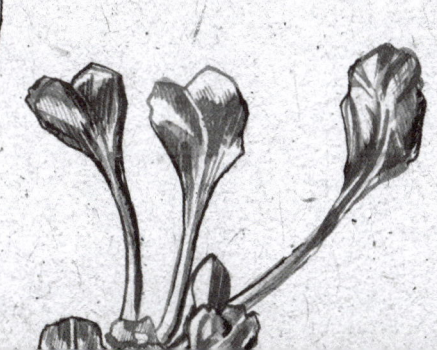

HEATHER

LATIN NAME:

Calluna vulgaris

FAMILY:

Ericaceae

ASTROLOGICAL SIGN:

Venus

SENSORY EXPERIENCE:

Astringent, sweet, nutty, mineral

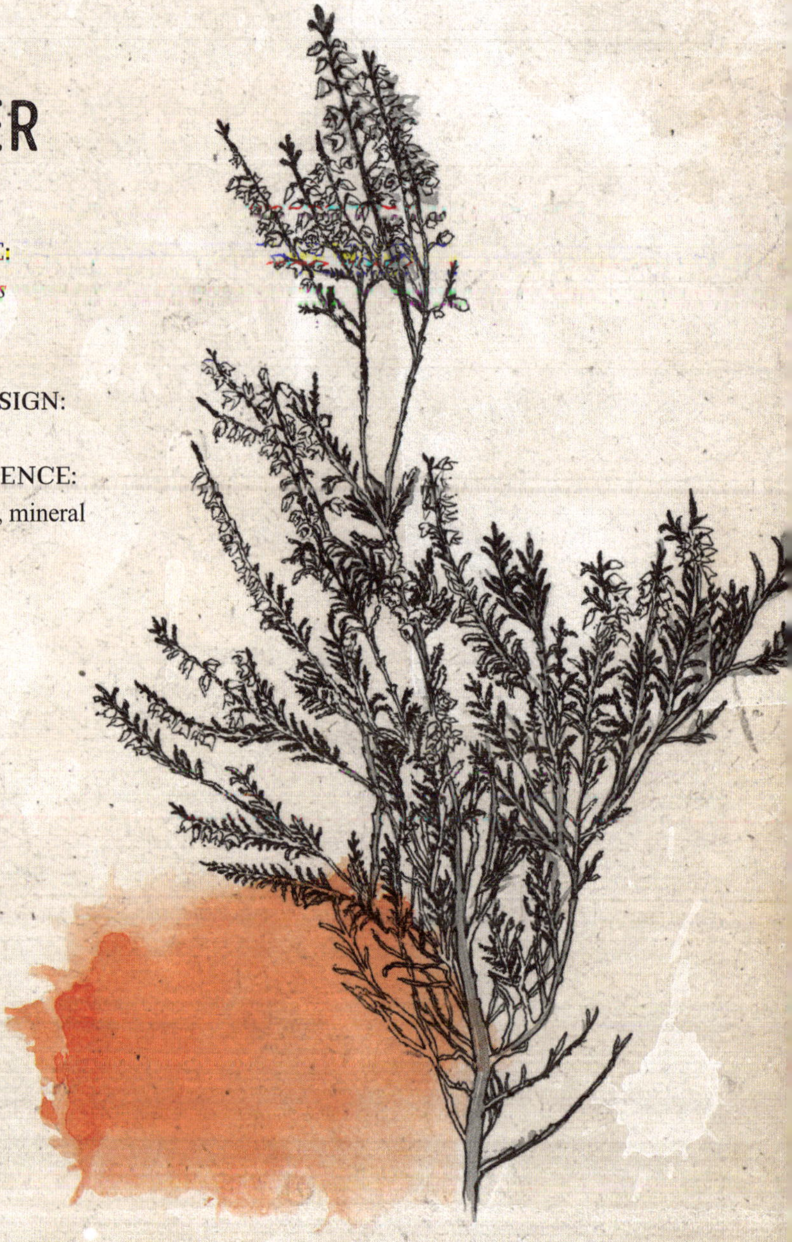

Heather (both the Calluna and Erica genera) has become unfashionable in modern herbal medicine. Perhaps its purple rinses are just too passé for some, but watch this space as it is becoming fashionably retro! Heather is connected to the later years of life, to wisdom and the crone phase. It is purple in colour, which in the chakra system is linked to intuitive knowledge, the third eye. This comes into its own especially once the reproductive years of a woman's life draw to an end and the fertility process ceases, allowing her to tap into innate states of being. Heather can be found growing in community with its kind. Up on moorlands and by sea cliffs, swathes of purple, violets and mauves dance in high winds, loving the acidic ericaceous soils. Heather is a gnarly, ancient, miniature tree, clinging onto the earth and unmoved by battering weather. It flowers in late summer, and harvesting the flowers is usually a quest, taking you out onto the hills to find this hardy medicine. Heather counsels perseverance. All its aerial parts are papery to the touch, therefore taking little time to dry and to process for making remedies.

Heather is anti-inflammatory, antimicrobial and diuretic, an excellent remedy for the urinary system and for aching joints. We use its flowers and leaves dried in our joint and urinary tea mixes, also as an infused oil in Ache-Ease Balm, as a tincture in kidney tonics and in our Clear Vision Drops.

Heather contains arbutin, a compound that is in part responsible for its antiseptic effect on the urinary system. This compound is also present in its more commonly used cousin bearberry, also in the plant family Ericaceae and famous among herbalists for being a urinary antiseptic. The anti-infective and diuretic action heather has on the kidneys indicates its use in encouraging harmony within relationships. Any herb connected to the kidneys, a paired organ, usually means it can be used where there is a difficulty with communication in relationships, especially partnerships. The kidneys – and kidney herbs – also have a connection with our ancestry, as the kidneys are the "house of ancestral chi" (see page 93). Heather can therefore shine a light on how our blood lines can affect us in this lifetime.

Heather offers us the gift of seeing clearly what is really happening in any given situation, being able to take a step back and witness in an objective way. It has the added quality of promoting positive communal living, which is indicated by the bees' love of heather. Bees have been long associated with communities and the social order that is reflected in a hive, which is viewed as one organism within which each bee has a clearly defined, specific role. Bees cannot function in isolation.

Heather is a strong survivor, exposed on the moors, yet thriving. It has a special type of mycorrhizal fungus that lives symbiotically with other plants of the same family (such as bilberry), making vital nutrients available. This mycorrhiza, *Ericoid endomycorrhiza*, is able to pass nitrogen and carbon into plants for nourishment, enabling the species to exist in harsh and sandy environments, where few nutrients are available. So heather teaches us how to survive.

Heather gives us the ability to intuit clearly and communicate unknown or unseen phenomena through its conversation with our hearts and its association, through its purple colour, with the third eye energy centre and psychic abilities. Our hearts are organs of perception and heather is a herb capable of amplifying our perceptive natures. We love this majestic purple oracle. We could all use its deep insights and perseverance from time to time.

Seeing this purple beauty about on the moors fills our hearts with joy and hope. Interestingly, the heart is at greater risk of disease if kidney function is compromised. We utilize heather, as a herb of the kidneys, for relationship challenges. It is no surprise that relationship issues are felt in the heart and can subsequently affect the urinary system. No one system is experienced in isolation. Chinese medicine draws links between the heart and kidneys in an energetic way and allopathic medicine has now noted the physiological links between heart disease and kidney disease.

Look for Your Local Herbs

From the late 15th century global trade routes have been explored in search of exotic spices, such as black pepper, cloves, ginger, cardamom and many others. Since this period, many of our useful and prolific local herbs have fallen out of fashion. This is the case with the heather flower, once so prevalent in apothecaries but now almost lost to the modern university-trained herbalist. Few herb shops stock heather as a loose herb, yet the heaths and moors are covered in its purple hues!

Today, everything we want is at our fingertips, and online shopping means goods from distant parts of the world are available with just one click. It is beneficial, however, to step outside sometimes and wonder at all that grows around us.

PISS-EASE TEA

This tea is incredibly supportive to the kidneys and tissues of the bladder and particularly useful when cystitis is an issue. We always incorporate heather for its plethora of useful actions: anti-infective, anti-inflammatory, mucous membrane restorative. Combine with other herbs such as horsetail, cornsilk, goldenrod and marshmallow leaf.

1. Harvest the herbs and dry them out in an airing cupboard or other warm area.
2. Lay them out on some paper and turn regularly until dry, which usually takes a few days, then store in an airtight jar.
3. For cystitis, steep 2 teaspoons of the herbs in boiling water for 10 minutes to make a large pot of tea. Drink three times daily until symptoms abate.

LUCKY HEATHER POSY

Creating a special heather posy to carry or give to friends is a lovely way to work with this auspicious plant. Collect the heather blooms on a dry day around the full moon. White heather is especially lucky so try to add some to your purples, to make use of the different types. These posies will attract peace, harmony, positive energies and protect against getting lost – so super helpful for travelling (we make posies to hang in the car!). And in addition, when your posy dries out, burning it is said to increase fertility …

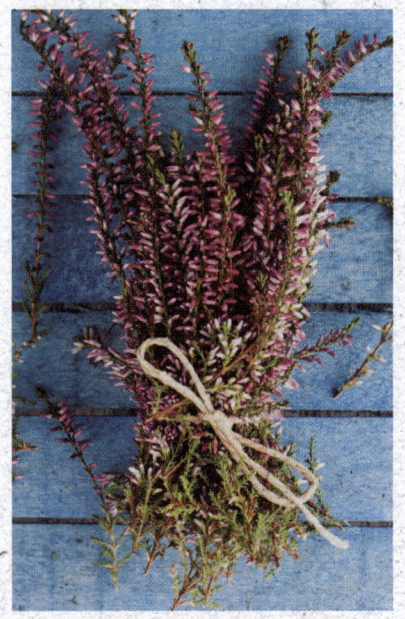

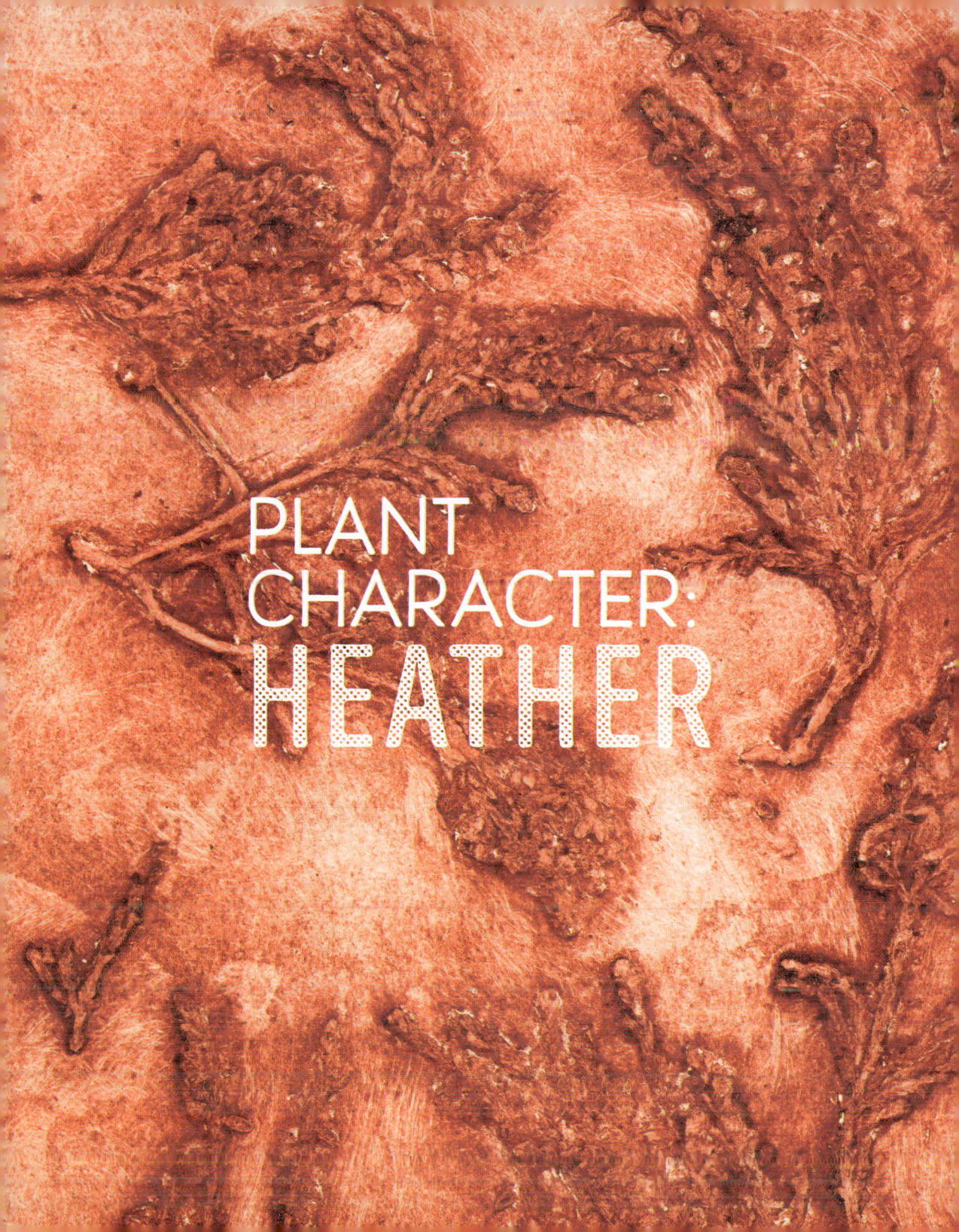

PLANT CHARACTER:
HEATHER

I AM HEATHER

Cushioning your fall
Bouncy bonsai worlds of purple
   and green
With Votes for Women co-create
Our own rules to make and break

Buzzing bees,
The lucky life, the plucky life
Honeyed laughter
Recapitulation
Divination down the lane
Paired in deep reflection
Neutralizing water pain
Joyous ways on darkest days

I am heather

Plant Character

Heather, with her purple
rinse, is a resilient old bird
full of gifts of humour and
a deep, dirty laugh that
bubbles up, often with witty
quips. She has a spring in
her step, this youthful crone.
She is a psychic, full of
prophetic insight. Her magic
is feminine and she can gift
babies. She holds memories
and healing in her waters.
Listen carefully to her joking
ways; there are pearls of
wisdom in there, wise words
to solve relationship woes.

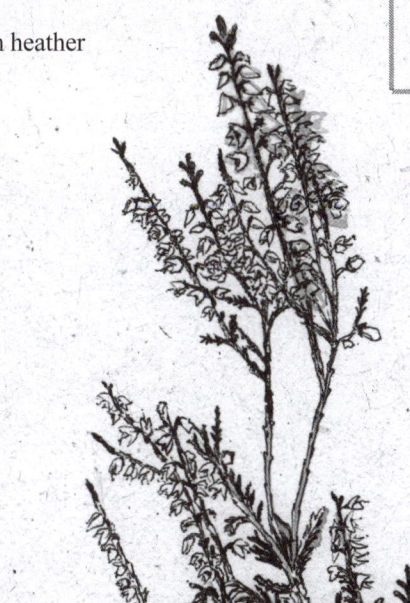

YARROW

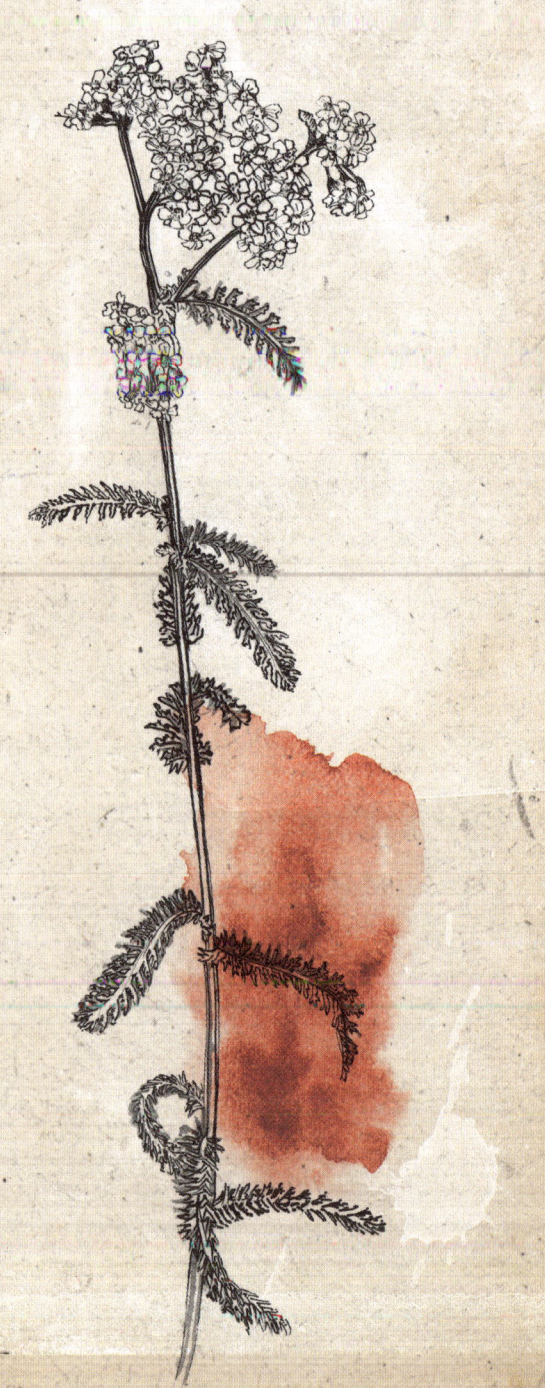

LATIN NAME:
Achillea millefolium
FAMILY:
Asteraceae (Compositae)
ASTROLOGICAL SIGN:
Mercury/Venus
SENSORY EXPERIENCE:
Bitter, pungent, aromatic, opening

Yarrow's leaves are made up of many tiny
strands feathering out from the erect stem
(hence the species name *millefolium*, which
means "thousand leaves"). It has protective,
dense umbrellas of flowers that are aromatic
and plentiful.

This herb contains a rich deep blue
essential oil, azulene – which is surprising
to see, given that the flowers are white, pink
or yellow! Azulene has been used since
the 15th century, isolated from German

chamomile, but wasn't discovered in yarrow until the 1800s.

Yarrow's Latin botanical name, *Achillea millefolium*, refers to Achilles, the warrior from Greek mythology. Achilles was dipped in a pool of magical protective water as a baby, which rendered him invincible except for the spot from which he was held – his heel. His heel was his weak spot (the original Achilles heel) and ultimately his downfall; he died from the wound made there by a single arrow during the Trojan War.

Achilles was known as a great healer and used yarrow on the battlefield to staunch and clean the wounds of his fellow soldiers. Yarrow holds the warrior spirit, it is a protector and has long been used to patch up areas of the aura that might be damaged and admitting unwanted energy. There is a flipside however. While having a great warrior on your side is beneficial, when pitched against him, it's essential to find his weaknesses. We use yarrow on an emotional level to help get to the root of our own Achilles heel.

Known as "nosebleed" due to its styptic property (it staunches the flow of blood), it can be chewed and applied up the nostrils to stem the bleeding. In contrast, it is also used to promote blood flow in the body, specifically to the womb and digestive areas, when taken internally as a tea or tincture. It relaxes and dilates blood vessels, thus aiding circulation. The white flowers taste bitter and aromatic; they support digestion, relieving congestion and promoting blood flow to the whole pelvic area. With its high number of essential oils, yarrow is a wonderful antiseptic for the whole system. It is a great addition to any cough, cold or flu tea.

ALTERNATIVES FOR THE CALPOL GENERATION

Yarrow flowers are one of the best remedies we've found for reducing fevers. We give teaspoons of a yarrow tea until a temperature is brought back to a comfortable place. Yarrow dilates the blood vessels, promoting blood flow and circulation, thereby encouraging heat to move to the surface of the body. This herb is a good alternative to the children's medicine Calpol®. It is essential that we are aware of alternatives to Calpol – and indeed why children might have a fever in the first place (see pages 142–3).

Calpol contains paracetamol and is used for all manner of childhood ailments including reducing fevers and teething pain and often just if children are feeling a little out of sorts. Over the past few years its sales have been among the fastest growing of all medicines and the brand has expanded its range to include ibuprofen products as well.

Because of our dependence on this sticky pink liquid, the phrase "Calpol Generation" has been coined. In excess of £60 million is spent in the UK on Calpol each year, a figure that is rising; 84 percent of children have been given this medicine by the time they are six months old.

Sales of Calpol are helping to boost the thriving paediatric pharmaceutical industry, which was worth £137 million in 2015 in the UK, and has been predicted to grow by more than £20 million by 2020. With these statistics in mind, we need to question whether Calpol is as beneficial for our children as we have been led to believe.

For example, research has linked the prevalence of asthma and eczema in adults and children with paracetamol sales in European countries. The study, published in the *European Journal of Public Health*, put forward the theory that paracetamol may reduce levels of the chemical glutathione in the lungs and blood, resulting in damage to the lung tissue.

Calpol doesn't contain paracetamol alone. It is a mixture of sweeteners, flavourings, preservatives and colourants, all making the product appealing and palatable to young children. There was a call to ban many of these substances after a study, funded by the Foods Standards Agency, showed links between hyperactivity and chemical additives. Calpol and other brands of children's paracetamol contain some of these substances, such as E122 and E218 (a synthetic food colouring and synthetic antibiotic respectively).

Being such a mixture of ingredients, it's not surprising that Calpol has the potential to cause allergic reactions, such as skin rashes and hay fever-like symptoms, as well as tiredness, unexpected bleeding or tendency toward bruising, headaches and nausea.

THE ROLE OF FEVER IN DEVELOPING RESILIENT IMMUNITY

Normal body temperature is 98.6°F (37.0°C) excluding individual variations or the fact that children tend to run slightly hotter than adults. Anything between 97.0°F and 99.4°F (36.1°C and 37.4°C) can be considered normal. Fever can be alarming for a parent to witness in a child, and it may feel natural to reach for the widely available and commonly recommended Calpol. The difficulty is that many parents and carers are not aware of the important role of fever in our natural immune process or that using paracetamol to treat fever may result in a child having a seemingly endless round of colds, as the body's natural fever response is not being allowed to kill the virus. A child's natural immunity can be reduced through repeated use of Calpol and it is imperative for the future health of our children that the role of fever is recognized as important, and the prolific use of medicines such as Calpol urgently addressed.

Fever is a symptom of a disease. It could potentially derive from an infection, bacterial or viral, or from pain such as teething. In infection, fever aids the immune system in disabling pathogens. It impairs viral or bacterial replication by heating the system and supporting the body's innate inflammatory responses.

Fever promotes sweating, fasting and sleep, three important measures for the healing of many transient illnesses. When a fever is artificially suppressed by using medicines like Calpol, the body's defence system cannot be fully activated. Repeated use of medicines of this kind risks leaving the immune system weakened and less able to respond effectively.

Fever serves another valuable role. Our children are not born with mature immune systems and fever is one way of activating and "educating" the immune system to respond when needed.

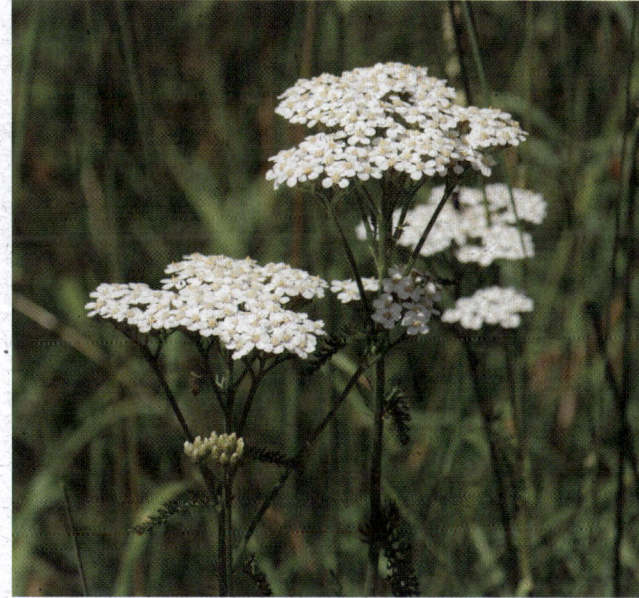

Diaphoretic yarrow offers us natural and safe fever reduction.

TREATING FEVER NATURALLY

Bear in mind that temperatures are usually worse at night and can spike for several nights in a row before the infection abates. Any time body temperature increases, salt and water are lost via sweating. Stores of energy and vitamins, especially the water-soluble ones, are burned up. During moderate fevers, we can compensate for these losses by drinking appropriate fluids, ingesting nutritious foods or taking vitamin supplements. Herbs can be used to lower prolonged or worryingly high fever, and cool flannels can help make the discomfort more bearable for a little one. Yarrow and other herbs that have diaphoretic qualities (the ability to induce a healing sweat and break a fever) such as elder, lime blossoms or sage, can be given in teas. Cooling sponge baths can also help to bring down a high temperature.

While most children can experience a fever over 39.0°C degrees without any adverse effects, if you are concerned about a child's condition for any reason, contact a health practitioner to seek advice and support.

YARROW RITUAL – SMOKE SHIELD OF PROTECTION

Yarrow has long been revered as a protective herb. The herbalist Christopher Hedley often spoke about its ability to help a person heal after "elfshot". Imagine a group of fairy folk opening fire on you with their bows and arrows. You would be covered in tiny little holes. These holes in our auric field let our energy flow freely out. This is sometimes why we feel completely exhausted. We can feel other people when they come close to us, even if we have our eyes shut. We sense their electromagnetic field; our auras intermingle. Yarrow has the properties of magic glue and can plug up and repair any holes in our auric field.

For this incense ritual you will need to harvest yarrow in full flower during a summer full moon. It is lovely to work with your personal intention for this work, so create some words as you are harvesting. This could be something like: "Yarrow, please gift me an invisible forcefield of protection."

Make yourself a strong brew of yarrow flower tea with some of your harvest and as you drink the tea, really think about the flavours and scents of the herb. Prepare the rest of the flowers for drying, laying them out on newspaper to dry or hang them in bunches somewhere with good airflow. When the plant is completely dry, take a pair of scissors and chop the flowers up finely and store in a glass jar.

You will need a charcoal disc on which to burn the yarrow flower "incense". Repeat your affirmation "Yarrow, please gift me an invisible forcefield of protection." As the yarrow burns, waft the smoke around your body and give thanks for the healing this herb has given you.

YARROW OXYMEL

This yarrow flower oxymel is a delicious healing mix. Vinegar extracts are brilliant for drawing out minerals and vitamins from a herb, and apple cider vinegar and honey themselves offer a wide range of benefits for a whole host of ailments, in addition to those of the yarrow flowers. Hippocrates spoke highly of oxymels, especially for children, and he suggested heating these mixtures gently before consumption during cold weather. Dose for a fevering child: a teaspoon in warm water, which can be repeated every hour.

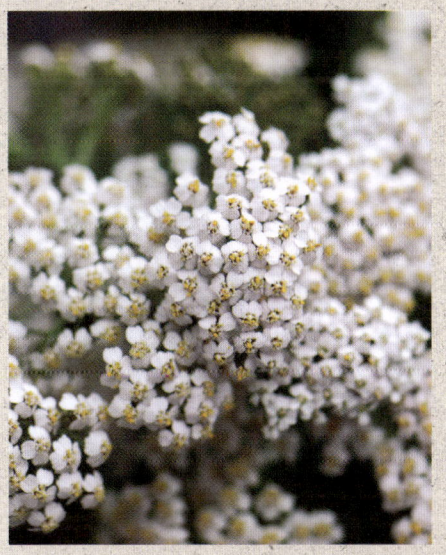

1. To make the yarrow vinegar, fill a jar with fresh yarrow flowering tops, harvested around the full moon, cover with apple cider vinegar and leave for two weeks maximum (or the herb will degrade). Strain the vinegar and discard the herb onto the compost heap.

2. To make the yarrow honey, fill a jar loosely with fresh yarrow flowering tops, also harvested around the full moon. Pour the honey over the herb, making sure it has settled and all the air bubbles have come to the top (adding more honey as needed) before sealing. Once or twice a day, turn the bottle on its head to "stir" the mixture. Strain after two weeks.

3. To make the oxymel, simply combine your yarrow vinegar with your yarrow honey at a ratio of one part vinegar to two parts honey.

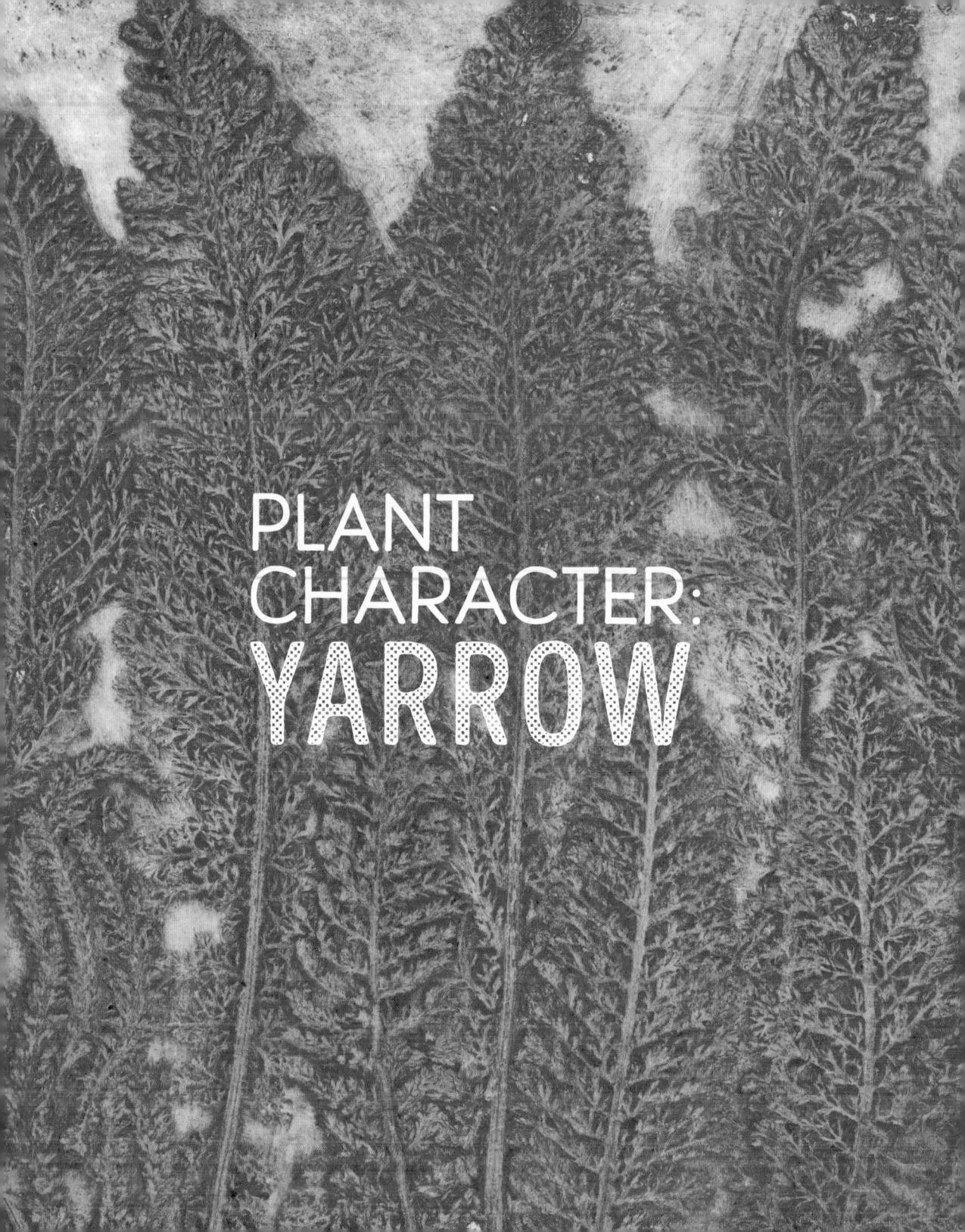

PLANT
CHARACTER:
YARROW

I AM YARROW

I am the greatest warrior
Sprouting from the cauldron
    of immortality
I open you up
Revealing the Achilles heel
Under umbrella shields
Tactile millefolium caterpillars
Ascending to
Blue-armoured light
I act on you

I am yarrow

Plant Character

Azul the warrior – painted blue like the Picts of old – is super tactile, often found purring like a pet cat with soft warm fur, which is difficult to resist stroking. Everyone wants to be near to caress Azul, and he loves it, humming in delight. Azul is protective and kind, always on hand with his umbrella to offer shelter, and warm you with his soothing hugs. He carries a first-aid kit on his person wherever he travels and loves to help heal cuts, scrapes and nosebleeds.

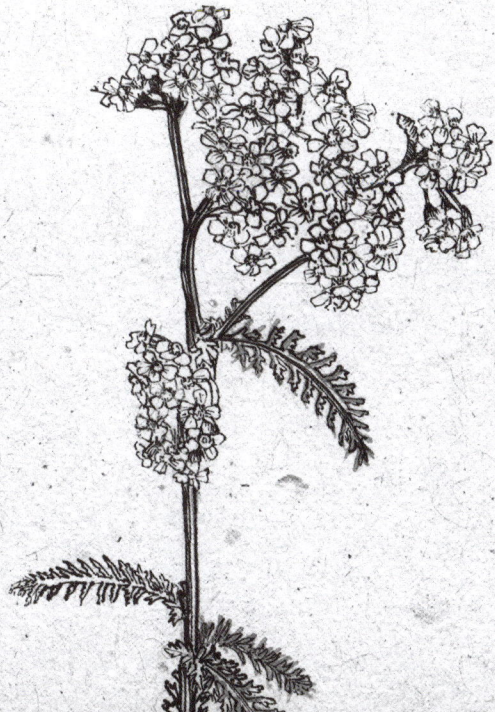

NUTRITION AND RITUAL WITH FLOWERS

The summer is an effervescent time, offering us so many edible healing flowers to enhance salads and cakes. They can also be dried and baked into bread, or frozen into ice cubes.

If we consume a full spectrum of colour and literally eat a rainbow, we are getting the broadest possible range of useful food compounds, as well as enjoying a delectable feast for the eyes. The first rule of pharmacy in Arabic medicine was to make the medicine beautiful. In this way, our eyes begin the healing process. Similarly, if we incorporate colours and flowers in what we eat, our foods become an art form, even more pleasurable to eat and, in turn, lift our souls. Here are some edible flowers we use (try the recipe below, with calendula and daisy petals):

* calendula
* dandelion
* rose petals
* violets
* rosemary
* nasturtium

* daisy
* jasmine
* honeysuckle
* lime flowers
* apple blossom
* wild garlic

RYE SOURDOUGH BREAD WITH PETALS

50g (2oz) sourdough starter / 500g (1lb 2oz/generous 4 cups) flour (rye and white spelt 1:1 mix) / 2 tsps sea salt / small handful of calendula petals / small handful of daisy flower petals / 1 tbsp fennel seeds

*1. **Day 1:** Mix 200ml (7 fl oz/scant 1 cup) water with the starter, stirring thoroughly. Then stir in 200g (7oz/generous 1½ cups) of the flour. Cover with a plate (to avoid it drying out) and leave overnight.*

*2. **Day 2:** Stir 200ml (7 fl oz/scant 1 cup) water and the salt, petals and seeds into yesterday's mix, then stir in the remaining flour. Adjust to make a sticky dough.*

3. Cover and rest for 30 minutes, then repeat. Leave, covered, for an hour to rise. Scoop into a greased bread pan and leave until risen (doubled in size). Sprinkle with flour.

4. Preheat the oven to 240°C/475°F/Gas Mark 9 and bake for 50 minutes, until dark brown.

Connecting with the rituals and the beautiful blooms of summer, we can enhance our lives with this season's full-fire energy. Harvesting the summer flowers connects us with the intense energy of attraction and helps to rekindle and ignite our passions. The fire-enhancing flowers featured here offer us a variety of qualities – daisy with its connection to childhood playfulness warming our souls, heather with its slow, burning patience and wise counsel, and yarrow with its fiery, protective gifts.

With the uplifting energy of the daisy syrup you will develop an ability to bounce back to health from any respiratory illness, as well as rebound emotionally from any stresses. Use the yarrow oxymel as a protective tonic in times of infection and as a tool to discover your own personal Achilles heel in order to become more self-aware and thus stronger in health. The heather posy can become a regular in your purse or car as support and an attractor of positivity.

Developing your passions and attracting plenty of positive energy are actions connected with the burning desires of summer's fire element, and the heart and the blood – and focusing on passion and positivity in this season is especially good for bringing health and vibrancy into your life.

Summer is a wonderfully energetic time to focus on what we want to attract into our lives. The table below looks at elements of rituals you might like to perform at this time. In summer we focus particularly on the idea of attraction. The fire vibes of summer also make this season perfect for burning away negative patterns of behaviour. Highlight one unhelpful type of behaviour that you exhibit. Then consider: what is it you would like to attract into your life? What would you like more of?

Summer Rituals	
MARKERS	Summer solstice, blossom
NATURE REFLECTIONS	Full energy and attraction, pollination, light Bright yellows, oranges, reds
FOCUS	Celebration and passion
MOON ASPECT	Full
RITES	Burning negative habits in the flames of the fire. Celebration and gratitude for all the gifts of nature. Attraction spells. Dancing/movement to create rising energy.

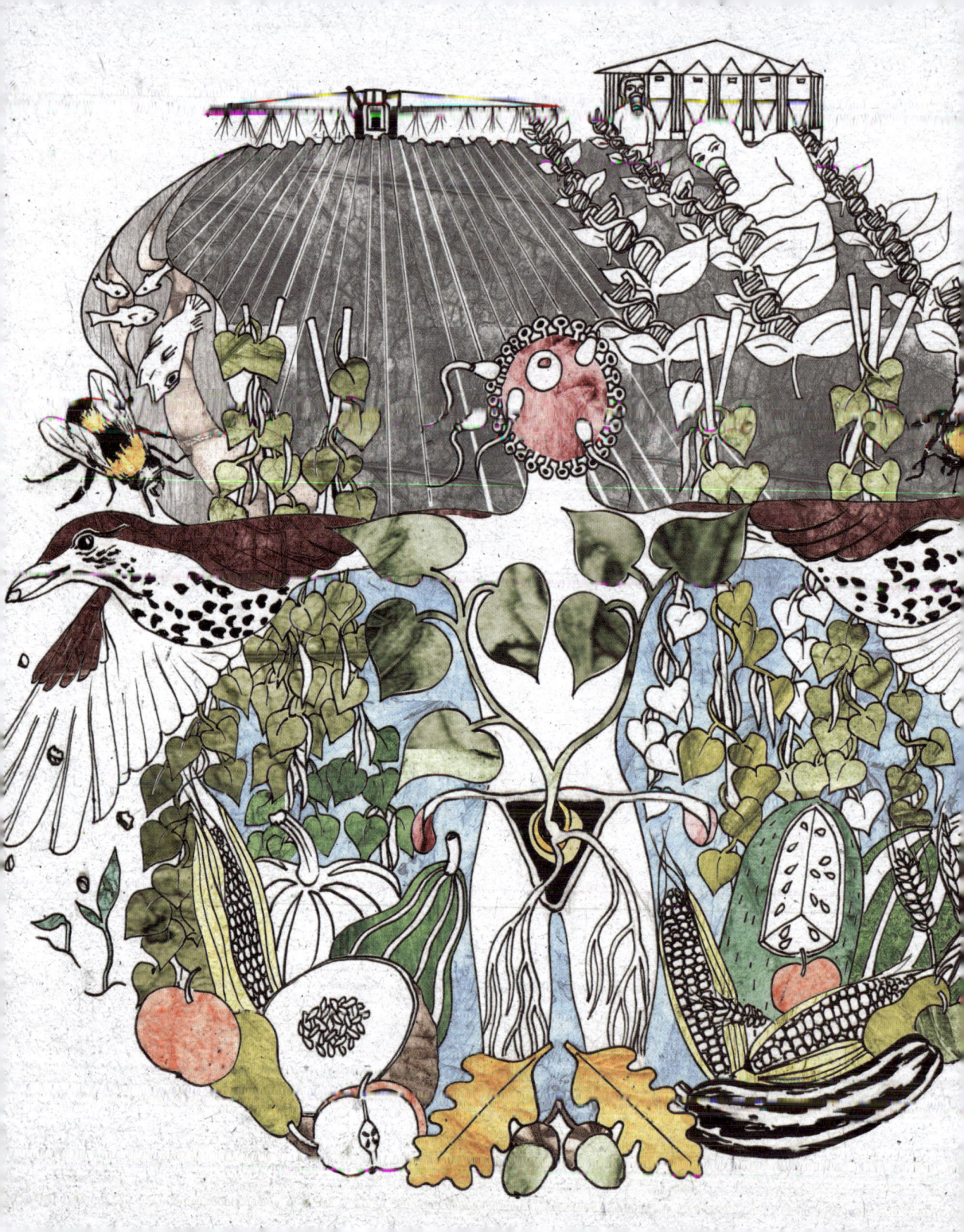

AUTUMN
AIR
SEED

BLOW IN THE SEEDS TO INSPIRE, FILLED WITH THE POTENTIAL ENERGIES OF GENERATIONS TO COME

After summer's fertile passion culminates in an abundant fruit harvest, autumn arrives. Fertilized plants produce seeds and berries aplenty and the hedgerows are now full of the potential of future generations.

The theme for autumn in Sensory Herbalism is the breath of life, which connects the respiratory and nervous systems with the element of air.

AUTUMN / SEED

At the autumnal turning point, the equinox, the lengths of the day and night are exactly equal. The days will become shorter than the nights from this point on as the energy from the sun continues to wane. The beauty of the summer plants has begun to decay, growth has slowed, and already many plants will have gone to seed. Apples weigh down the boughs in the orchards, hips redden on the rose bushes. The bees must work hard now, searching for late blossoms to provide nectar and pollen to stock up their honey supplies for winter.

The plant cells bow gracefully to the laws of the universe. As autumn progresses and the trees head toward their winter slumber after a busy time of reproduction, the leaves fall and a carpet of reds, yellows, purples and browns covers the ground. A human cellular process has been named after this phenomenon that occurs so magically in trees: apoptosis, from the Greek word meaning "to fall off". This is programmed cell death and illustrates the intelligence of nature moving around the ever-turning wheel of life and death.

Apoptosis is a rather mechanical term for a necessary and beautiful aspect of nature, present in living things, which allows for renewal and regrowth. Billions of cells in the human body are given up every day in this way to allow for regeneration. If our life force is flowing freely and strongly, apoptosis functions efficiently. When it happens within our body, this exquisite process connects us with life cycles occurring in nature, and is essential for the healthy functioning of the human organism.

AIR

Invisible to the eye, autumn's element, air, can be felt in the wind, through movement and sound. Associated with the planet Mercury, air is able to travel quickly, carrying and communicating information, smells and sounds. We therefore associate air with inspiration, new ideas and concepts, wit and the power of communication. The wind of autumn carries seeds full of potential, waiting to grow into new life.

AIR EXPRESSED ENERGETICALLY AND EMOTIONALLY

If air is in balance in a person, that person is likely to be breathing well, be a clear communicator, full of ideas and able to hold lots of information in the mind at once.

The air element may be expressed in balance in any of the astrological signs that come under the domain of air. However, if

The Air Element in Sensory Herbalism

ELEMENT IN BALANCE	ELEMENT IN DEFICIENCY	ELEMENT IN EXCESS	ASTROLOGY	EXAMPLE OF HERB
Communicative, inspired	Unimaginative	Ungrounded, flighty	Gemini, Libra, Aquarius	Fennel

there is a lack of air, it can present as lack of inspiration, as someone feeling unimaginative or flat. Fennel is a perfect example of an air herb with a useful seed (the autumn plant part). This plant will bring inspiration, creativity and flair, and can also instil a sense of balance and emotional harmony. Drinking a delicious fennel tea accompanied by an affirmation of feeling inspired, such as "I am open to new ideas and inspirations," or simply chewing a few fennel seeds with conscious awareness, can help lift spirits.

AIR EXPRESSED IN THE PHYSICAL

Sensory Herbalism links the nervous system and the respiratory system with the element of air. The quick wit, changeability and intangibility of air is expressed beautifully here. The nervous system perfectly represents the element of air through its ethereal quickness and its ability to inform our communications. Often if we are nervous or depleted we literally look like we contain air, as we shake or tremble.

Vital life force (known as chi in Traditional Chinese Medicine and as prana in Ayurveda) fills the lungs and breathes new life into our being. The breath represents the vital life force. We inhale on entry to the world and release a final exhalation at death.

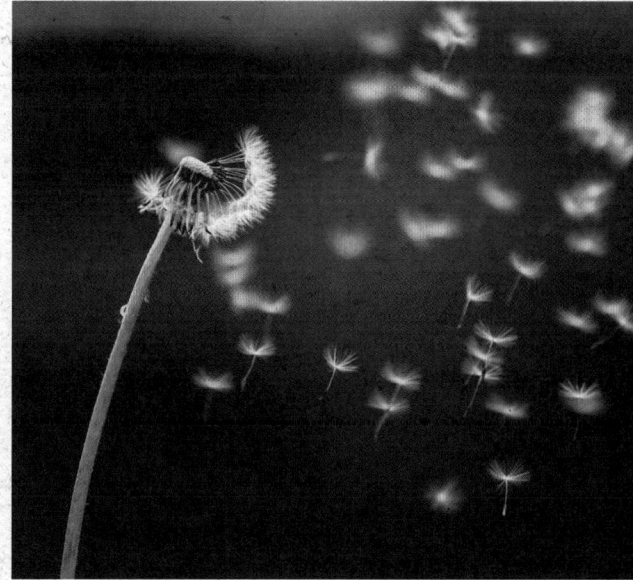

Wind-blown seeds spread the potential of new life.

NERVOUS SYSTEM

Our nervous system, governed by the element air, is influenced by our life of experiences so far. Emotions affect the nerves and the state of the nerves affects our emotions. Our nervous system can keep us cool, calm and collected in stressful situations, or it can throw us into anxiety. The brain, heart and intestines are all centres of nervous activity, closely linked to our external environment. These are the areas where feelings and tensions are often experienced. The heart and intestinal tissue all stem from the same origin as our brain tissue; we can feel with our hearts and our gut. We hear this in phrases such as "gut instinct" or "heartache".

The brain is the major processing organ of the electrical impulses that run along neural pathways from the peripheral nervous system (PNS) through the central nervous system (CNS) and back, to all organs and the extremities of our bodies. This can be likened to telephone wires carrying messages through our bodies, travelling through a central hub – the CNS. Hearts and wombs also have the potential to receive messages via neurotransmitters, minute carriers of information throughout the nervous system. The messages carried by our nerve cells are then perceived by the brain as feelings, emotions or actions that need to be taken. Psychoneuroimmunology (PNI), a branch of modern medicine, considers that specific neurotransmitters and hormones affect, or can be related to, our emotional and spiritual health. It looks at the idea of "mind over matter" in a medical context. Stress and negative states of mind are often the "root cause" of many illnesses. When the nervous system is overtaxed, messages can get confused. When people are continually stressed without periods of rest (physically and emotionally), there is a knock-on effect on physical and emotional health.

One of the first places that stress or anxiety affects us on a physical level is the digestive system. Prolonged nervousness and anxiety felt in the stomach can lead to accelerated peristalsis (movement of the

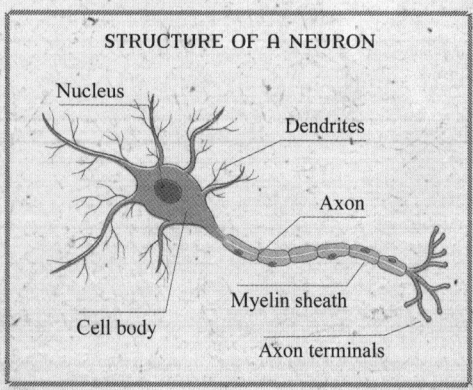

STRUCTURE OF A NEURON

Nucleus

Dendrites

Axon

Myelin sheath

Cell body

Axon terminals

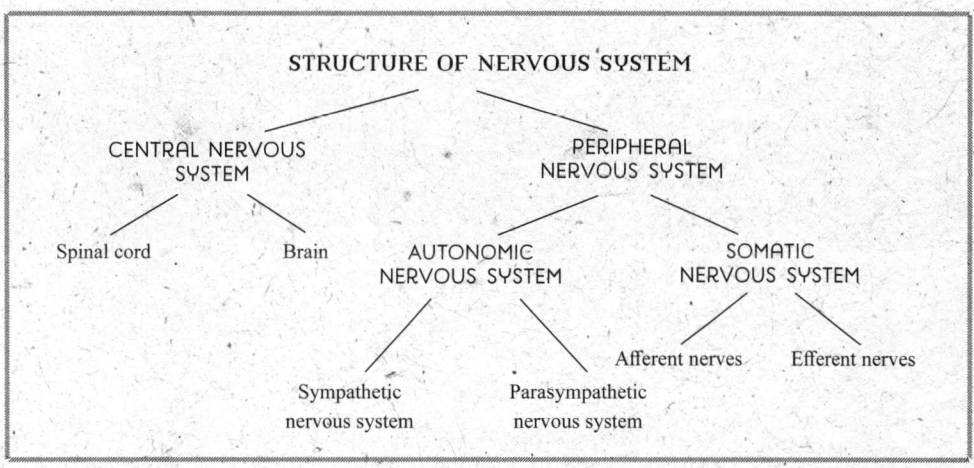

STRUCTURE OF NERVOUS SYSTEM

CENTRAL NERVOUS SYSTEM

PERIPHERAL NERVOUS SYSTEM

Spinal cord   Brain

AUTONOMIC NERVOUS SYSTEM

SOMATIC NERVOUS SYSTEM

Afferent nerves   Efferent nerves

Sympathetic nervous system

Parasympathetic nervous system

intestines) through hyper-stimulation of the nerve pathways. This can cause nutrients to be lost because food is travelling through the gut so quickly that absorption is inefficient. This means that people who are not coping with their stress may be lacking nutritionally even if they are eating a relatively healthy diet. Stress can also be the cause of stagnation and constipation. Prolonged release of stress hormones such as cortisol acts to draw blood to the vital organs needed for the fight-or-flight response, such as the heart. As a result, the digestion slows down as the production of digestive juices decreases. This could be seen as representing the holding on to emotions.

This link with digestion flows both ways. If the diet is not nutritious then the nervous system does not benefit. Wholesome food can really help to ground and support the

nerves, while stimulants can fray and damage nerve tissues by preventing absorption of B vitamins, vital for nerve function.

Considering that our health is so linked with our state of mind and our state of mind can be affected in many different ways, the spiritual, emotional and physical root causes of the presentation of experiences within the body must be considered. If one of these aspects is thrown off balance or challenged in a way that cannot be managed, disease sets in.

The first manifestation of a condition will often relate to a shock or trauma or a period of prolonged stress. It is the skill of the Sensory Herbalist to identify this and ascertain on which level this occurred and at what point it became a physical issue. Treatment will focus on restoring, nurturing, past injuries and healing.

ADRENAL GLANDS

The adrenal glands sit on top of the kidneys and are representative of strength and resilience. They help us to cope with the inevitable stresses of everyday life, from day-to-day temperature changes to major emotional upsets. In response to the nervous system, the adrenal cortex produces several hormones to manage metabolism and various body characteristics. The most important are aldosterone (a mineralocorticoid), cortisol (a glucocorticoid), androgens (of which testosterone is one) and oestrogen (sex hormone produced from androgens).

* Aldosterone helps the kidneys regulate the amount of salt in the blood and therefore also in the tissues of the body.
* Cortisol helps the body manage and use carbohydrates, protein and fat, causes changes in metabolism and is important in how the body manages stress. It suppresses the immune system. Cortisol also helps to maintain our circadian rhythm, giving a welcome boost at the start of the day.
* Testosterone is an androgen (male sex hormone). Androgens are the precursor to oestrogen (female sex hormone). They create the physical changes at puberty and possibly help regulate other organs.

All adrenocortical hormones are steroid compounds derived from cholesterol. This means that a certain level of cholesterol is needed by the body to produce these hormones. The hormones produced by the adrenal medulla are called catecholamines. They manage the body's response to stress. The two most important catecholamines are:

* Adrenaline, released during times of short-term stress (such as a sudden shock or fear), increases heart rate, blood pressure and blood sugar level.
* Noradrenaline, like adrenaline, constricts blood vessels. It also increases heart rate, blood pressure and blood sugar levels.

When the adrenal glands are subjected to continuous strain, the system becomes sluggish and we strive to maintain the demands of daily life.

ADAPTOGENS

Adaptogenic herbs are used to improve the health and function of the adrenal glands. The word "adaptogen" was first used in 1947 by the Soviet scientist Nikolai Lazarev, who was researching ways to enhance the productivity, performance and health of soldiers, athletes and workers without the negative side effects that come from the use of synthetic stimulants such as cocaine and amphetamines.

An adaptogen has come to mean a substance that boosts the body's ability to resist multiple stressors and therefore exerts a normalizing influence on physiology. The adaptogen is a relatively new way of referring to a type of remedy commonly found in traditional forms of medicine. For example, chi and kidney yang tonics are used in Traditional Chinese Medicine to restore balance and health. Ayurveda has *rasayanas*. The idea of using tonic remedies to restore balance and health in a person is an ancient one.

All plants are conscious, intelligently responding to their environment. If a relationship with a plant is created, it is possible that it will be able to uniquely "adapt" its function to a system's specific needs. This implies that all herbs have the potential to be in some way adaptogenic. Herbs are constantly adapting to their environment, as are we. Every time we step from a warm building to the cool chill of the air outside or experience heightened emotions, we need to adapt to some degree.

So far research has focused on Chinese or Indian adaptogenic herbs. Rosemary – a Mediterranean plant that has been naturalized in many parts of the world – can also be considered as an adaptogen. A wonderful, balancing herb, it strengthens the nerves, promotes immunity, and has protective and uplifting qualities. However, there is no reference to rosemary as an adaptogen in any literature, simply because the research is yet to be done.

COMMON SYMPTOMS OF AN IMBALANCE OF THE NERVOUS SYSTEM

These include: anxiety, depression and low mood, fatigue, blood sugar issues, poor concentration, sleep disturbance, cold sores and shingles, tingling extremities, reliance on alcohol and stimulants.

SUPPORTING THE NERVOUS SYSTEM

In any condition presenting in the nervous system (e.g. anxiety, depression or viruses that live in the nerves of the skin such as cold sores or shingles), supporting the nerves physiologically with herbs and diet is essential.

HERBS
* **Fennel** balances emotions, lifts glum spirits and calms nervous excitability. It also seems to be adaptogenic in nature, supporting the body to be more adaptable to life's strains.
* **Rose** encourages nurture and relaxation.
* **Valerian** helps to calm frayed nerves and can encourage relaxation and deeper sleep.
* Try a Tension Tamer Tea blend of fennel, plantain, mugwort and rose to relax and soothe nerves.

NUTRITION
* Increasing the intake of omega oils (essential fatty acids) is beneficial,

Conditions of the Nervous System and Treatment Strategies for the Practising Herbalist

CAUSES	Shock, prolonged pressure or stress, lack of sleep (incl. insomnia), vitamin and mineral deficiency (especially B vitamins), essential fatty acid deficiency, malabsorption of nutrients, excessive refined sugar intake, negative outlook, viruses, hyperstimulation (e.g from screens and caffeine)
CONDITIONS	Herpes virus (cold sores, shingles, chicken pox, warts), anxiety, panic attacks, depression, low mood, adrenal insufficiency, multiple sclerosis, chronic fatigue, myalgic encephalomyelitis (ME)
THERAPEUTICS	Nourishing the nerves, relaxing the tissues, lifestyle changes, addressing emotional factors, looking at digestive involvement
HERBAL ACTIONS CONSIDERED	Adaptogens, relaxing nervines (e.g. chamomile), nourishing nervines (e.g. oats), stimulating nervines (e.g. rosemary), digestives (including carminatives and bitters)
OTHER TOOLS	Meditation and breathing exercises, counselling, life coaching, exercise, connection to nature and time spent outside, massage, diet

specifically to the myelin sheath (the nerve coating that ensures smooth transit of nerve impulses). Omega-3 fatty acids are found in oily fish, such as mackerel and sardines, as well as in nuts and seeds.
* Vitamin B12 is important for nervous system function as it is needed to form the myelin sheath. B12 is found in animal foods: meat, fish, shellfish, eggs, dairy.
* Reduce intake of refined sugar and caffeine to help balance blood sugar.

* Choose high-quality, fresh whole foods to provide a wide range of nutrients.

LIFESTYLE
Reduce stress! Find what works for you:
* Spending time in nature
* Massage
* Meditation and yoga
* Regular exercise
* Good-quality sleep
* Self-care — time spent creating daily happiness for yourself.

RESPIRATORY SYSTEM

LUNGS

After birth, a baby takes his or her first breath, beginning their relationship with the external environment. This marks independence from the supporting environment of the womb.

Our breath both sustains us and represents our life force. The autonomic nervous system, as the name implies, monitors via the central nervous system the functioning of the body and regulates this accordingly. It connects both our conscious awareness and the subconscious workings of the body.

We breathe subconsciously, the autonomic nervous system (ANS) regulating how quickly we need to breathe in order to provide enough oxygen to our cells. We also have the ability to consciously guide the breath, altering the depth and speed to relax, to energize and to initiate altered states. The lungs ensure that there is enough oxygen in our blood but also provide a route of elimination of unwanted products from the blood such as carbon dioxide (CO_2).

Observing how a person breathes is a very useful diagnostic tool:

∗ Do they take short, shallow breaths?
∗ Do they take long, deep breaths?
∗ Is there any difficulty in breathing?
∗ Are there deformities in the chest area?
∗ Do they hunch their shoulders (which may be restricting their breathing)?

If someone is embracing life and feeling happy and relaxed they are much more likely to be taking deep, full breaths, with their shoulders moving gently back, creating lots of space for an open, receptive heart space. In contrast, someone feeling low, melancholic or nervous may hunch their shoulders to protect their heart or take shallow breaths and have difficulty breathing.

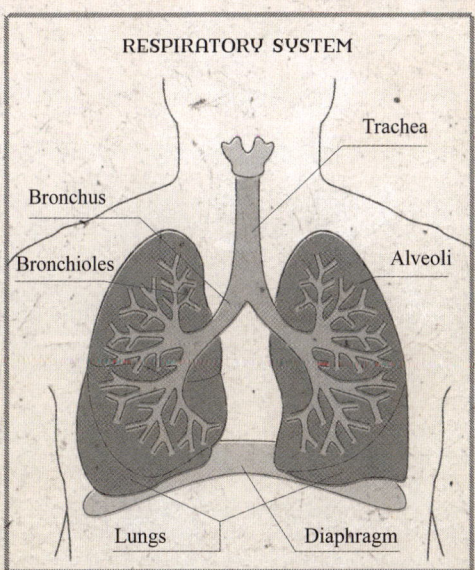

RESPIRATORY SYSTEM

Trachea

Bronchus

Bronchioles

Alveoli

Lungs

Diaphragm

Conditions of the Respiratory System and Treatment Strategies for the Practising Herbalist

CAUSES	Food intolerances, allergens, physical damage (from smoking, inhalation of pollutants, pesticides and other chemicals), stress, lack of exercises
CONDITIONS	Asthma, chronic pulmonary obstructive disorder, bronchitis (acute), cough, chest infection, tumours, certain heart conditions, pneumothorax, cystic fibrosis
THERAPEUTICS	Steam inhalations with essential oils and herb teas, breath work, exercise, stretches and yoga that will create more space around the chest area, massage, diet
HERBAL ACTIONS CONSIDERED	Expectorant (soothing/irritant), anti-inflammatory, demulcent, mucous membrane restorative, lung tonic, circulatory, antispasmodic, antitussive, digestive support (if food intolerances): bitters, hepatics
OTHER TOOLS	Removing allergens or food intolerances, identifying causes, rest, relaxation of system, restoration of lung tissue, removal of stuck mucus with herbs and inhalations, support with stopping smoking

Keeping the lungs clear, the membranes healthy and protected and ensuring there is enough relaxation in the lungs for deep, full breaths is important in any treatment plan.

COMMON SYMPTOMS OF RESPIRATORY IMBALANCE

These include: shortness of breath, pain on inhalation, fatigue, asthma, bronchitis (acute), cough, chest infection.

SUPPORTING THE RESPIRATORY SYSTEM

HERBS

* **Thyme** is a wonderful antimicrobial that is perfect for respiratory infections as it has an expectorant action to aid expulsion of mucous from the lungs.
* **Daisy** with its saponins is a gentle lung herb, useful with children and the elderly.
* **Elecampane** is anti-infective and strengthening, useful in respiratory issues.

* **Horseradish** is clearing and supports breathing, especially for sinus infection.

NUTRITION

* Consider cutting out mucus-forming foods such as dairy products, refined carbohydrates and sugars.
* Eat nutrient-rich fruit and vegetables to aid the immune and lymphatic systems.

LIFESTYLE

* Exercise
* Steam inhalations with essential oils and herb teas
* Pranayama (yogic breathing exercises)
* Stretches and yoga that will create more space around the chest area
* Massage

The 4-7-8 Breathing Exercise

This relaxing breath exercise, a natural tranquilizer for the nervous system, was developed by Dr Andrew Weil. When your exhalation is even a few counts longer than your inhalation, the vagus nerve (running from the neck down through the diaphragm) sends a signal to your brain to turn up your parasympathetic nervous system (PNS) and turn down your sympathetic nervous system (SNS). The SNS commands your fight-or-flight response. The PNS, on the other hand, controls your rest-and-digest response. When it is dominant, your breathing slows, your heart rate drops and your body is put into a state of calm and restoration.

1. Sitting up straight, exhale completely through your mouth, making a whoosh sound.

2. Close your mouth and inhale quietly through your nose to a mental count of four.

3. Hold your breath for a count of seven.

4. Exhale completely through your mouth, making a whoosh sound to a count of eight. This completes a one-breath cycle.

5. Now inhale again and repeat the cycle three more times, a total of four times.

Always inhale quietly through your nose and exhale audibly through your mouth. The tip of your tongue stays in position the whole time. If you have trouble holding your breath, speed the exercise up but keep to the ratio of 4:7:8 for the three phases. With practice you can slow it all down and get used to inhaling and exhaling more and more deeply. Do it at least twice a day. You cannot do it too frequently but do not do more than four breaths at one time for the first month of practice. Later, if you wish, you can extend it to eight breaths. If you feel a little lightheaded when you first breathe this way, take a break and it will pass.

SEED

While the leaves are slowly falling off the trees, seeds and fruit are beginning to form, products of all that passionate summer activity. The hips, haws, nuts, berries and fruit now hold the genetic potential of the future generations. Before the period of stillness and death of the winter months, there is time to "get the house in order" and gather in and store the harvest. We can still benefit from autumn's nourishing gifts in the cold times to come, by preserving them as chutneys and as dried fruits, berries and seeds. And in six months' time, after the rest period, the spring will return, and we will be rewarded once again with new growth and budding life.

SEED POLITICS AND FOOD SOVEREIGNTY

Today, the sources of our food are, on the whole, controlled by agricultural companies. In the 1950s and 1960s it was felt there was a need to engineer seeds that would ensure higher yields from crops, to be able to feed the Earth's rapidly growing population. Unfortunately, higher yields became synonymous with the use of pesticides, fertilizers, genetically modified crops and terminator genes (a terminator gene is a specific genetic sequence inserted into a seed's DNA that renders the seed and the crop it produces sterile, meaning that the farmer must repurchase seed for the next season).

The history of F1 hybrid seeds and GM crops has been seen as one of great leaps forward, however there have been disastrous unintended consequences.

Although advances in agriculture have indeed been useful in increasing crop yields, they have also caused much suffering for farmers, many whom have lost everything across continents due to greedy profit-seeking agricultural giants.

Seeds are life. They are also a powerful tool that in recent years have been abused by big agro-farming companies seeking to take control of food growing all over the world. This has had devastating effects on some of the world's most vulnerable people.

Seed saving for the following year's crops has taken place since the dawn of agriculture. It is one of the ways that we have survived as static and self-sufficient communities. Farmers have always carried out some degree of selection and, as a result, until recent times there were always many strains of cultivars, with genetic differences, allowing crops to survive hostile climates or particular diseases.

In the 1960s, F1 hybrid seeds were sold to farmers in developing countries as a reliable way to grow uniform crops with high yields.

The new F1 hybrid seeds did indeed give amazing yields but had to be bought from the seed companies every year as only they had the means to produce them. Traditional methods of seed saving appeared have become redundant, as saved seeds would not produce such predictable large yields. What is more, the new seed required increased fertilizer inputs to give the higher yields, and the fertilizers were also supplied by the same seed companies. This dependence on purchasing from agro-business meant many farmers went bankrupt and even committed suicide.

More recently, these companies have also introduced genetically modified organisms (GMOs). Genetic modification means splicing the genetic code of plants with other plants or even unrelated organisms such as fungi or fish. This creates "super seeds" that can withstand various pathogens or insects, or use less water to produce crops in less time than through conventional methods. Although this is a desirable aim, these seeds can then be patented, which means that the company that holds the patent then owns that particular seed and all plants that produce it.

In the USA and Canada many farmers have suffered because of these patents. Organic growers are not allow to use GM seeds, but cross contamination has been found to have taken place between GM and conventional crops both in the field

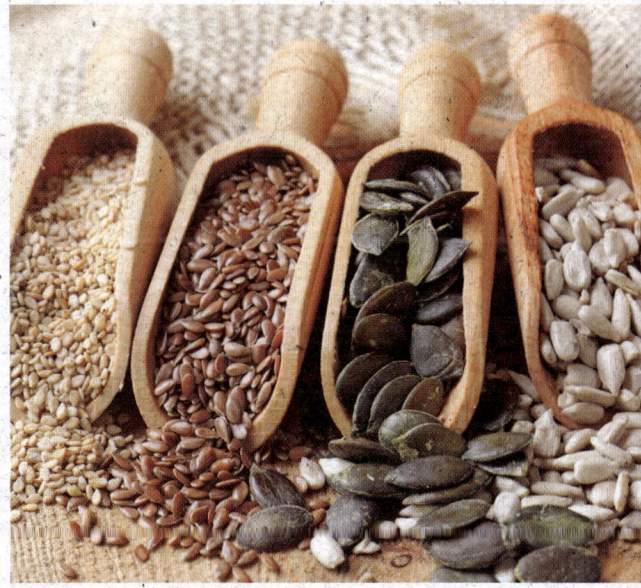

Seeds hold the key to life.

and when seed is transported, rendering the conventional crop worthless.

Small farms that back on to the large industrial farming areas where GM seeds are planted are at risk of cross-pollination and even subsequent suing if the small farm's crops start to resemble the GM neighbour's. Small farms have been swallowed up by the large agro-farming companies and people's dreams and livelihoods shattered.

The GM technology is only a couple of decades old and it is not yet clear how the cross-pollination of GM seeds will affect heritage seed strains, organic farming and the ecology of the countryside. What is certain is that there is no going back once GM crops are unleashed. Another concern is that GM crops may cross with closely-related wild species causing genetic contamination, altering their genetic make-up for ever and creating problems such as "superweeds".

At the time of writing there are no commercial GM crops being grown in the UK, but there are areas of test crops near Leeds and in Norfolk and other parts of the country. The future of the UK's farming and our native plants hangs in the balance. The ban on GM crops here and in Europe has been consumer-led thus far. It's important to keep up visible resistance to the infiltration of GM crops. The technology is only a couple of decades old and it is not yet clear how the cross-pollination of GM seeds will affect heritage seed strains, organic farming and the ecology of the countryside.

Now is the time to find positive ways of using the power of seeds to strengthen our communities. We must be robust enough to push forward belief in food sovereignty in creative, non-violent ways.

WHAT CAN WE DO?

* We can keep growing food and medicine, and keep sharing seeds in our communities. If we hold the seeds of the future in our hands, we keep the power. The act of exchange and sharing strengthens us and bonds us together.

* We can also harvest and use the seeds that our herbs produce. These will produce plants that are particularly good at growing in our local climate.

* Whatever you do, keep believing in our future and know that taking the time to care for the land we live on promotes personal, social and community health.

* Find positive actions to take, no matter how small, to keep feeling strong in the face of adversity.

SEED BALLS

Seeds encased in compost and clay are great for guerilla gardening. This term, coined in the 1970s in New York, refers to cultivating or rewilding derelict land, for political, practical and aesthetic reasons. Undercover techniques of the guerilla gardening movement include the seed ball phenomenon. Try packing a range of seeds in balls of clay and compost, and throw them onto abandoned land. The balls will crumble with rainfall and grow into useful or pleasing herbs and flowers, transforming the space.

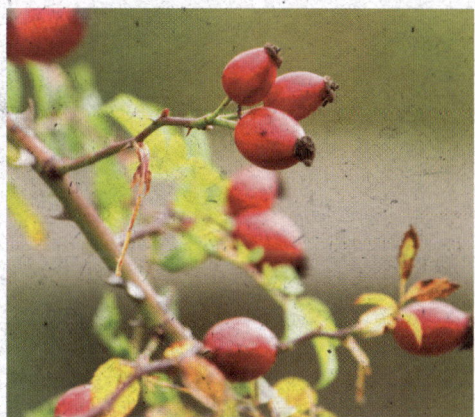

I AM SEED

Here in this moment all around me dies,
I stop,
Slow,
In my heart is the potential,
All-consuming passion for regeneration.

Contained but bursting.
Give me water,
Fire and earth,
I will transform.

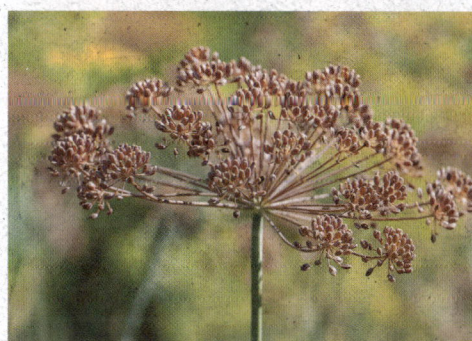

Come down from your lofty heights
Withered ways
Nourish me
As I in turn hold the promise of nourishment.

The axis between the worlds,
Fulcrum
Holding court with no one but me, myself
and I.

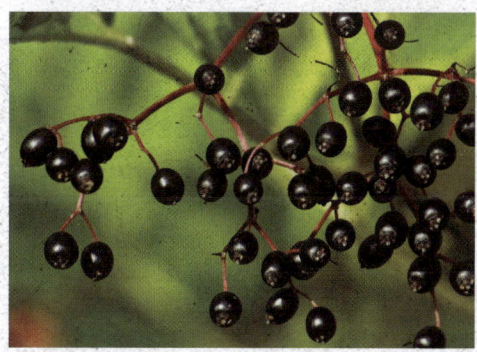

I balance all the energetic matter from the
sands of time
With the foresight,
The promise,
The potential,
The future.
Perfect preparation

Seed shapes of rosehip, fennel and elder

THE HERBS
THREE AUTUMN SEEDS: ROSEHIP, FENNEL, ELDER

ROSEHIP

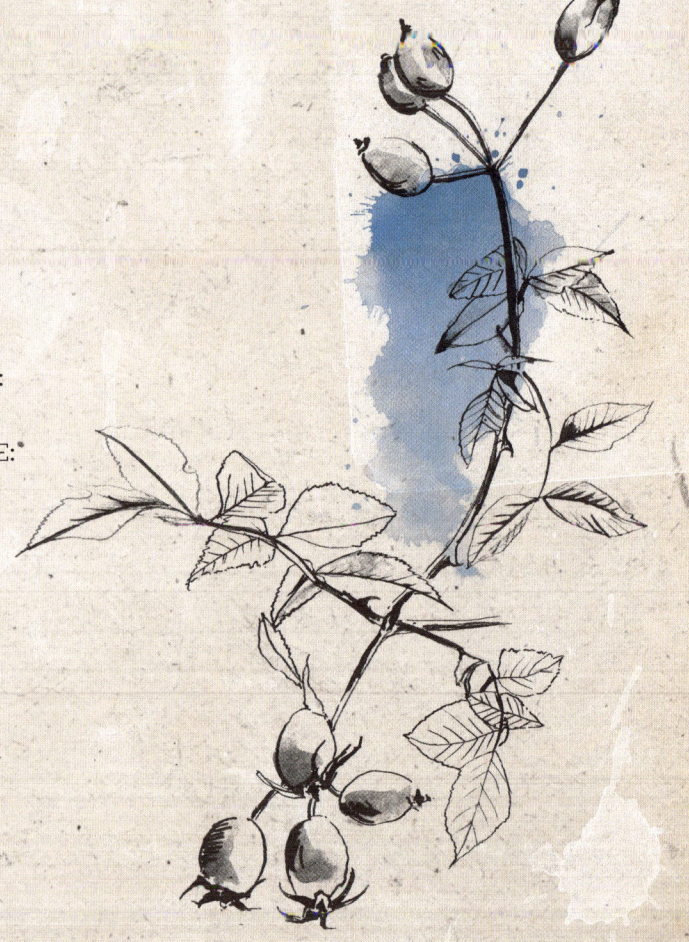

LATIN NAME:

Rosa canina (dog rose)

FAMILY:

Rosaceae

ASTROLOGICAL SIGN:

Venus

SENSORY EXPERIENCE:

Sweet, fleshy,
appley-citrus, tangy

Beautiful, delicious, nutritious rosehip! The varied red hues catch your eye in autumn as the hips bob their heads throughout the hedgerows, contrasting with the dark green serrated leaves. Nestled in their thorny briar, the blood-red hips are reminiscent of the fairy tale of Sleeping Beauty. They counsel the importance of protection, the good fairy godmother's magic of patience and rest, followed by the awakening.

These sensual, fruity hips represent the whole of the female reproductive system. Their womb-shaped nourishing shells are filled with thousands of seeds holding the potential of generations to come. We use them as a tonic for the female reproductive system and to nourish women with heavy periods. The gentle nervine quality in the hips encourages nurture and relaxation.

We use rosehip syrup (see page 169) in combination with rose and peppermint tinctures as a support through times of loss and grief. Ruled by Venus, rosehips help us express emotions. In times of shock, disconnecting from our emotions is an easy coping mechanism, but this has repercussions; we often see the onset of health issues shortly after a major difficult incident in life. Rosehip creates a nurturing space deep within us, enabling us to heal.

Rosehip shows us how important it is to protect ourselves, as she does with her thorns; how important it is to link arms with our communities, as she does with hawthorn, sloe and bramble in the hedgerow, creating a strong boundary. In this time of ecocide committed on our wild spaces, we can support each other, ever pushing forward, and always resisting any oppressor! We can respond to our grief in a positive, activist way, finding creative solutions to come together in opposition.

Emotionally, we use rosehips to restore the ability to nurture, whether in the home, at work or as a political activist. There is a particularly maternal quality offered by this constant giver. We see rosehip as a grandmother midwife, quietly supportive and clicking her knitting needles while she waits, but when the moment comes to bring that baby forth, she'll be there to encourage you, to give you nourishment and support.

Take care while harvesting rosehip, as the barbed thorns can be vicious, snagging the skin. When this happens we take it as a message to move on to another bush. When harvesting rosehip you can feel the mischief of children playing tricks with itching powder; the fine hairs between the seeds and fruiting flesh are an irritant to the skin!

The hips have a high vitamin C content, which supports the immune system through the autumn and cold winter months. We've seen rosehip syrup trigger memories from the time after the war, when there was little fruit from abroad, especially oranges. The government encouraged people to gather rosehips from the hedgerows to be made into syrup. Children were then given a teaspoon every day to prevent diseases such as scurvy.

The vibrant red colour of rosehips attracts the birds. After eating, the seeds are excreted, a process that increases the rose's potential for survival.

Rosehips are renowned for treating arthritic complaints, especially in the knees. They also heal the gut. They contain tannins (a polyphenol present in all the Rosaceae family), which bind to proteins and tonify tissues in the intestinal tract, improving absorption of nutrients. An unbalanced digestive system is linked to joint problems. Clinical research has highlighted rosehip's gifts as a medicine for osteoarthritis and rheumatoid arthritis. It has recently been discovered that the galactolipid compound is present in rosehips, and is in part responsible for their anti-inflammatory actions. Galactolipids are fatty acids and this research indicates how important good plant-based fats are in our diets (other oil-rich seeds are flax, nettle, hemp, pumpkin and sunflower).

Rosehips nourish and support us during the transition from autumn to winter, providing the vitamin and mineral boost needed at this time of year and also offering some of the nervine quality of rose buds and petals. Rose also offers us patience to deal with the pressures of the winter season.

ROSEHIP RITUAL FOR PATIENCE

Rosehips have much to teach about patience, and harvesting and preparing them can be a ritual in itself. Choose a time around one of the autumnal full moons and write the word "patience" on the container you take to collect the harvest.

As you harvest the hips, take the time to breathe, to sink into your physical body and to become aware of every detail of the felt experience of picking the rosehips. Fill your container with these red beauties, all the while being in the moment.

To dry your harvest of rosehips for tea, take a sharp knife and cut each shell in half. Lay them on newspaper and dry in an airing cupboard or warm place for a week. When they are dry, lovingly scrape out the seeds – a lesson in patience and care. Save these seeds for cultivation. You will be left with perfect fairy boats of patience. To make your tea, simply pour boiling water over your rosehip shells and steep for 15 minutes.

ROSEHIP SYRUP

A delicious syrup to add to pancakes, fruit salads or porridge. It can also be taken as a medicine to soothe frayed nerves or nourish the immune system. Simply take 1 teaspoon of the syrup three times daily.

Rosehips
Spring water
Apple juice concentrate

1. Cover the washed rosehips with spring water in a large pan and bring to the boil. Simmer for 10–20 minutes.
2. Mash with a fork or potato masher, adding a little more water if necessary. Pass the mash through a food mill, discarding the seedy pulp onto the compost.
3. Then pour through a jelly bag or muslin square, keeping the liquid and discarding the pulp.
4. Add the apple concentrate to the rosehip liquid at a ratio of two parts apple to one part rosehip liquid, and boil rapidly for 5–10 minutes.
5. Pour into hot sterile bottles and seal immediately.

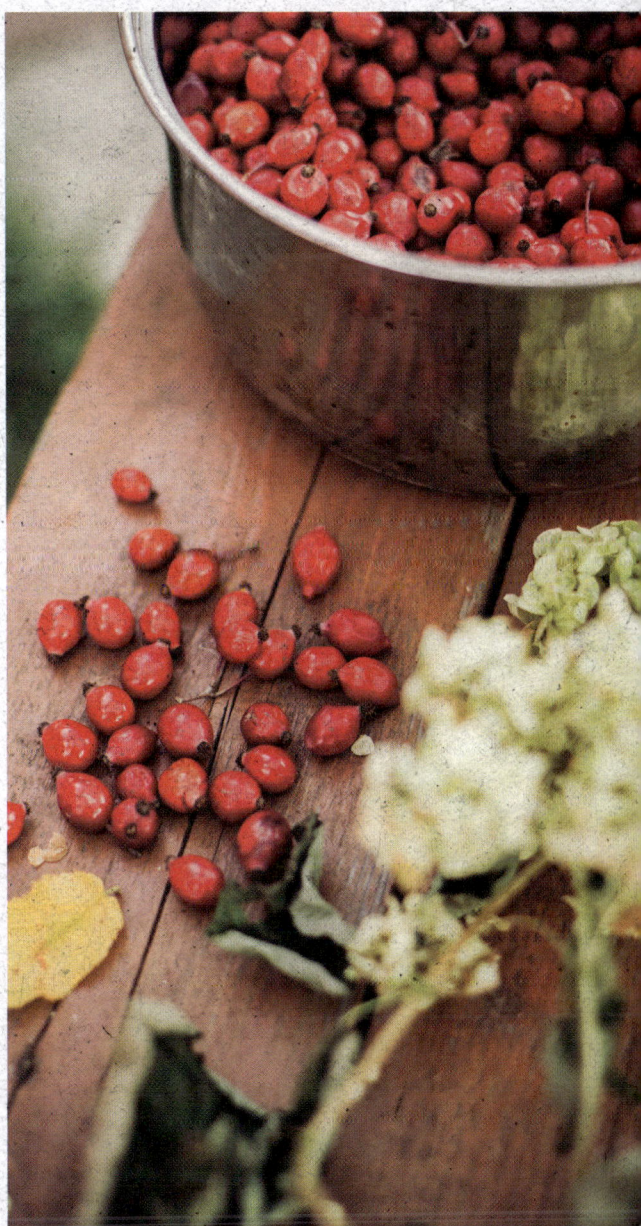

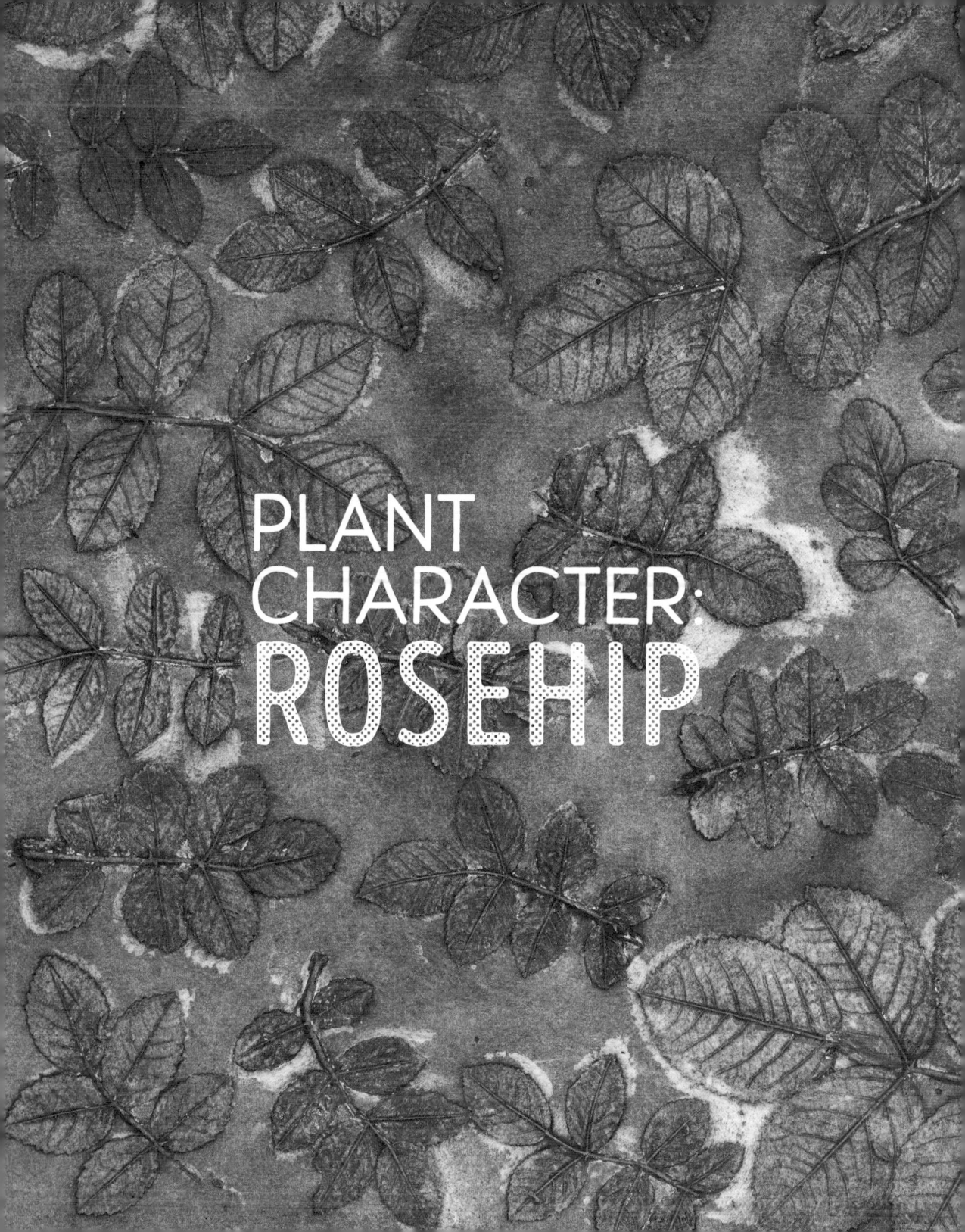

PLANT CHARACTER: ROSEHIP

I AM ROSA HEARTSPETAL

All aspects of time.
Midwife,
Death wife and all that go betwixt.

Great-great-grandmother, nurturer.
Delicately fragranced,
Smooth-skinned,
Protective,
Taking no nonsense.

Intolerant of impatience.
Bearer of deep, fertile secrecy,
Sanctuary,
Holder of chaotic grief.
Seed-filled nourishment,
Pure, loving abundance.

Attract you to hypnotic imprisonment,
Sharp lessons await.

Open your eyes and smell the roses.

Plant Character

Rosa Heartspetal is a grandmother and a midwife. She is incredibly wise, and both gentle and caring, but she takes no nonsense. She encompasses all aspects of the feminine through her own life cycle from bud and flower to hip and seed. She holds many a secret deep in her protective arms. She grows abundantly in all our hedgerows, often intertwined with her equally protective and prickly cousin hawthorn (also from the Rosaceae family). She offers a lovely warm hug to anyone who needs drawing into her soft bosom. She listens patiently to all your woes but does not tolerate self-indulgence or self-pity and soon becomes sharp with anyone who starts to wallow!

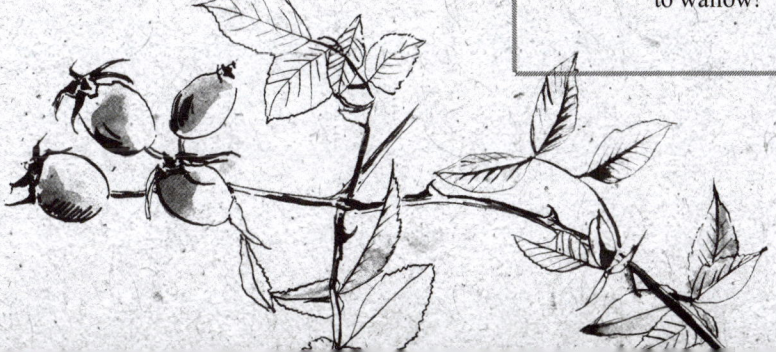

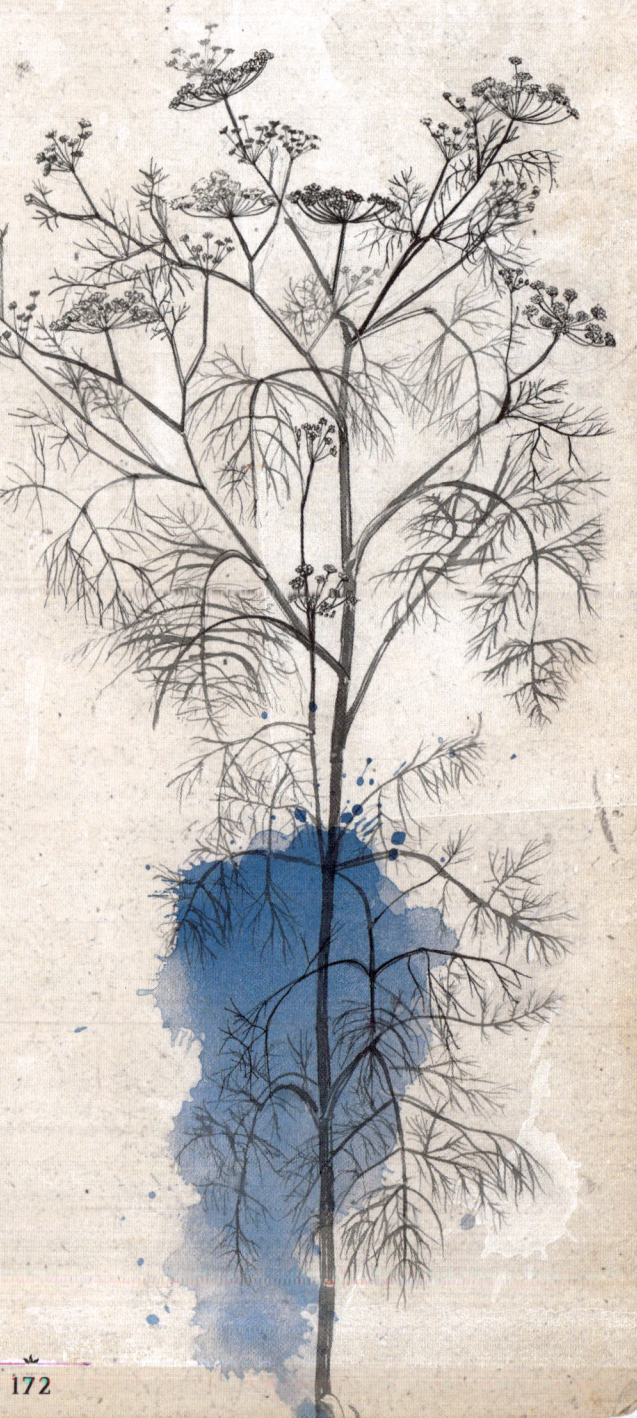

FENNEL

LATIN NAME:
Foeniculum vulgare
FAMILY:
Apiaceae
ASTROLOGICAL SIGN:
Mercury
SENSORY EXPERIENCE:
Sweet, aromatic, anise, tingly,
clearing, high energy

Tall, majestic, airy fennel is fresh, aromatic,
digestive, opening and expansive for the
head, a great boost to clear thinking. The
sweet, feathery leaves are an excellent
addition to salads, while the stripy seeds,
which promote digestion, are a delicious
complement to so many culinary dishes.

Home to many spiders and creepy-
crawlies, fennel enjoys well-drained soil,
plenty of sun and can easily grow to over
2m (7ft) tall. Fennel is a marvellous plant to

cultivate, with its remarkable structure that extends from a bulbous base to the delicate umbrella-shaped seed heads. When the tiny yellow flowers fade at the end of summer, tasty, aromatic, stripy seeds take their place, alongside the many spiders who seem to love creating their webs in the seed heads.

Fennel contains wonderful volatile/essential oils, which give this herb its signature sweet aroma. These are especially supportive and protective to the liver. Fennel is often applied to treat mild spasmodic gastrointestinal complaints such as flatulence, colic, indigestion, bloating or heartburn. Stripy seeds (caraway and aniseed are other examples) generally soothe digestion.

We use fennel as a nervine to balance emotions and lift glum spirits. Hildegard von Bingen, a nun and herbal writer of the 12th century, recorded that fennel was a herb for strengthening the eyes, brain, hearing and heart, and that eating it would make one happy. She is famously quoted as saying, "Fennel forces the spirits into the correct balance of joy." You will not usually find fennel mentioned as a nervine herb in modern herbals, but in our experience it is excellent at encouraging a lifting of the spirits, and also at calming nervous excitability. In general, fennel is wonderfully supportive as we move through the autumn months, a time when anxiety can set in as we see the light dwindling and know that the cold times are not far ahead.

In ancient Greece, Olympic athletes used the seeds to enhance their performance. In fact, the Greeks called fennel "marathon" for its association with strength, longevity and courage. Perhaps the adaptogenic quality of fennel seeds needs to be explored.

Fennel is a well-known galactagogue, promoting the flow of breast milk, and we have used it as a tea for many breastfeeding women. It can also soothe colic – if drunk as

Fennel as a Mood Lifter

Interestingly, you will rarely see fennel in herbal texts as a nervine; however, its mood enhancing properties are undeniable when this plant is consumed as food, herbal tea or as drops of a tincture. If you are feeling out of sorts, why not try consuming more fennel? It's a natural mood elevator and can really help to uplift and inspire positive change. The sweet, zingy taste of the seeds, so opening to the physical body, also nourishes the emotions.

a tea by the mother, it will be passed through the breast milk to the baby. It is possible that the effect of certain herbs is boosted by being passed via breast milk.

Fennel's power of physically restoring vision was known to the poet Henry Wadsworth Longfellow, who wrote:

Above the lower plants it towers,
The fennel with its yellow flowers,
And in an earlier age than ours,
Was gifted with the wondrous powers,
Lost vision to restore.

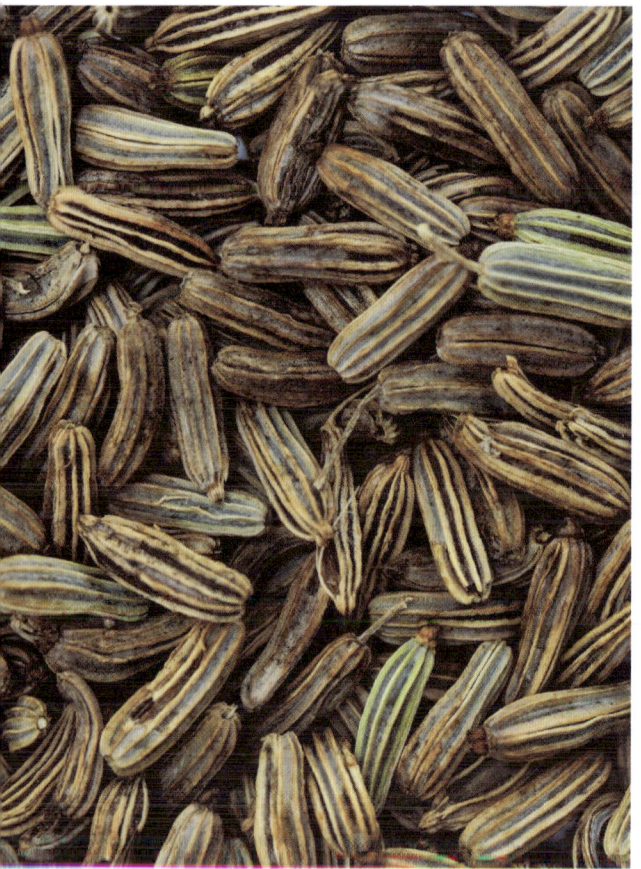

FENNEL RITUAL: SAVING SEEDS OF INSPIRATION

Collecting seeds in order to cultivate future generations of a plant is a very ancient human practice. Fennel is an especially inspiring plant to work with because of the sweet uplifting flavour of the stripy seeds.

Hold a few fennel seeds in your mouth and let yourself be inspired by the tastes. Then collect some seeds in a paper envelope. Add the date, the name of the plant and information about moon phase/astrological sign.

Now store the seeds for the spring season, when you can germinate and propagate new fennel plants as gifts of inspiration for friends and family.

ROAST VEGETABLES WITH FENNEL SEEDS

SERVES 4

Fennel seeds with their sweet anise flavour work super well in savoury dishes.
Why not try roasting them with some delicious organic vegetables?

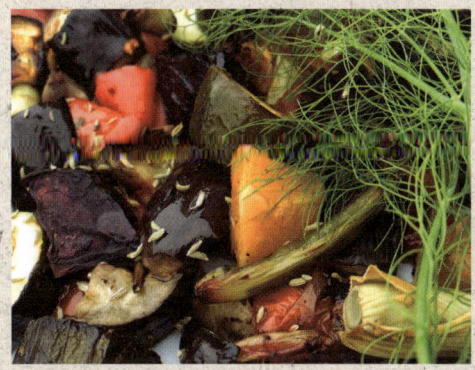

1 courgette (zucchini)
1 aubergine (eggplant)
3 tomatoes
1 large beetroot (beet)
1 large onion
1 garlic bulb
1 tbsp fennel seeds
olive oil
2 tbsp freshly squeezed lemon juice
salt and pepper

*1. Preheat oven to 200°C/400°F/Gas Mark 6. Chop up the vegetables into large chunks
and place in a large ovenproof dish.*
2. Break up the garlic bulb into whole cloves (no need to peel them) and add to the veg.
3. Crush the fennel seeds using a mortar and pestle and scatter over the veg.
4. Season and drizzle over some olive oil and the lemon juice.
5. Roast in the oven for 40 minutes or until soft.

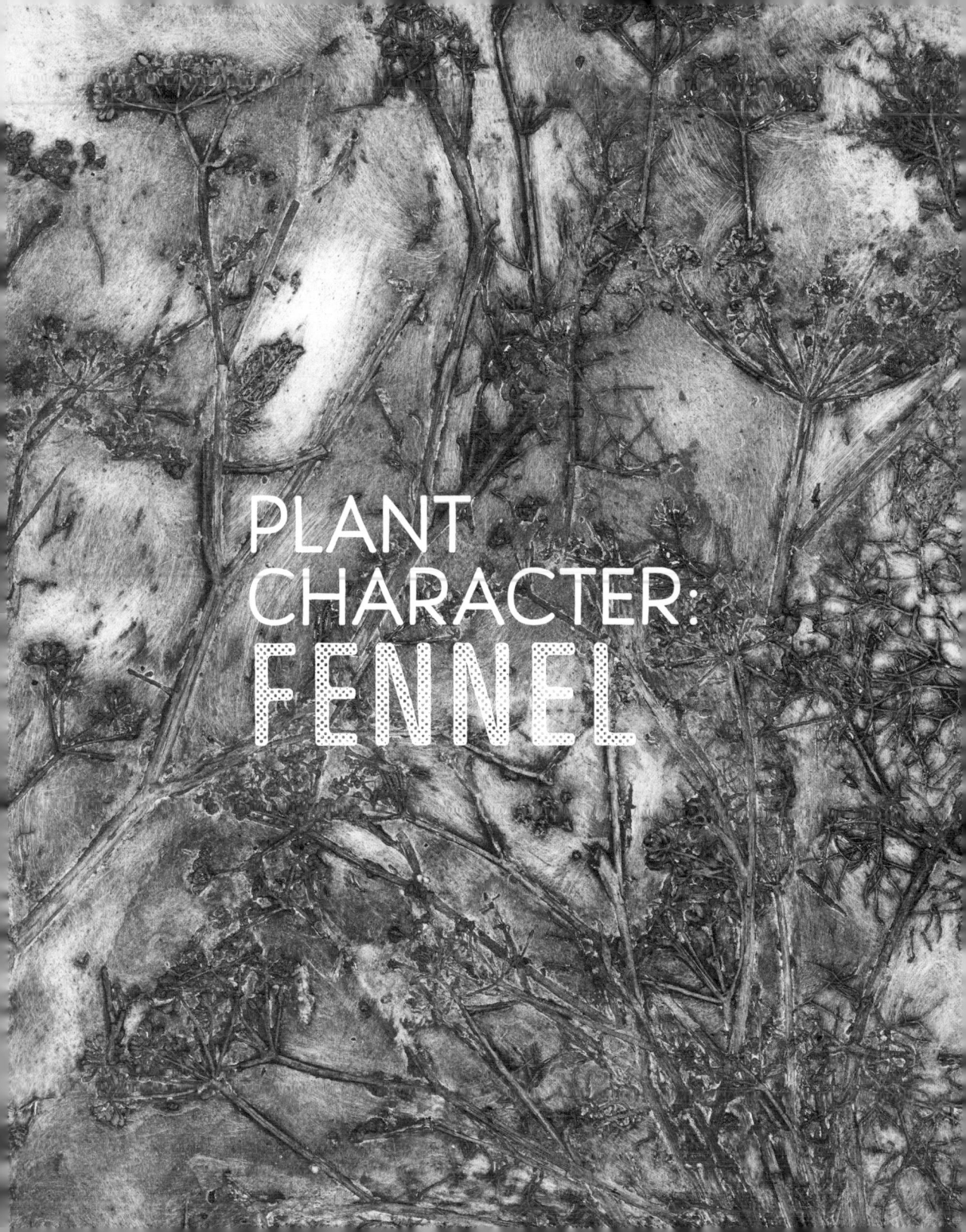

PLANT
CHARACTER:
FENNEL

I AM FENNEL

Uplifting
Mercurial
Flights of fancy
Wizardess of androgeny
Herding melancholy away
Balancing joy
Opening inspirational circuitry
Arachnoid astral homes
Webbing interconnectivity
Shooting stars of stripy seeds

I am fennel

Plant Character

Fennel is pure Mercurial inspiration, a free spirit, outrageously witty and droll. The life and soul of any party, he has his finger on the pulse of current affairs and the arts; he can wax lyrical on almost any subject. Thin and tall, incredibly camp and always immaculately dressed in some wonderful patterned fabric, his sweet nature and fine fashion lifts us up when we feel down. He can be relied upon as someone who can always point out the positives in a situation to help you release anxieties or tensions.

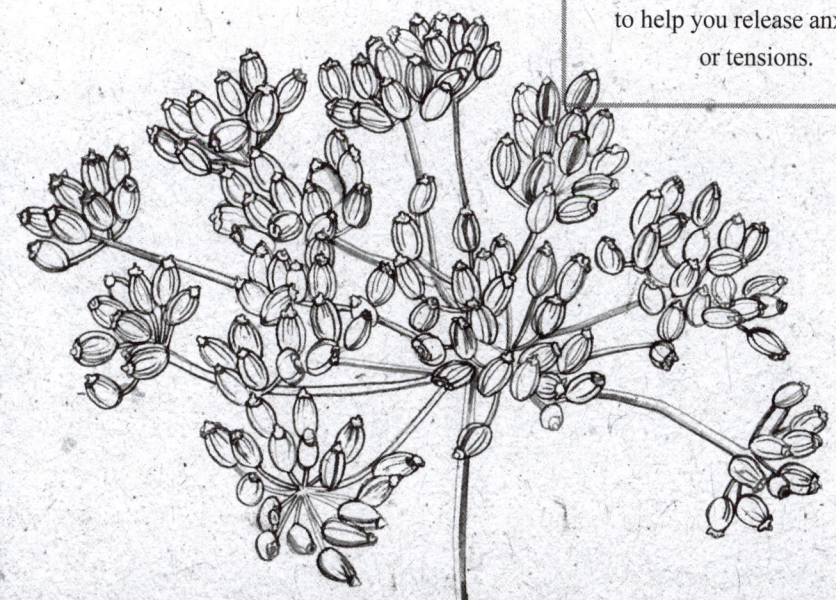

ELDER

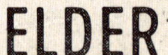

LATIN NAME:
Sambucus nigra
FAMILY:
Adoxaceae (Moschatel)
COMMON NAME:
elderberry, elderflower
ASTROLOGICAL SIGN:
Venus
SENSORY EXPERIENCE:
Pungent, warming, opening, flushing,
rising heat

Elder is widespread, found on railway
embankments and roadsides, in hedgerows
and parkland. This perennial tree is bushy and
relatively short, growing to a maximum of
15m (49ft) over a lifespan of around 60 years.
The bark is quite pitted, and the branches
and stems are hollow, making excellent

musical pipes and bellows for lighting fires. When rubbed, the dark green pinnate leaves emit a very strong fetid scent which is insecticidal, so they make an effective natural anti-insect preparation. The scent and insecticidal qualities of the leaves fade as the blossoms develop and bloom in late spring and the early summer months. These creamy beauties decorate the waysides with showy flowering umbels that are actually tiny petals in huge clusters. As the tree is hermaphrodite, the flowers contain both male and female reproductive parts; once pollinated, they are replaced by the red berries that darken to become completely black in the autumn. It is autumn's berries that are our main focus here.

There is so much to say about elder that Mrs Grieve (a prolific grower, writer and herbalist of the early 20th century) devotes 11 entire pages in her superb herbal to the many traditional uses of the elder tree. She tells us, for example, that the berries were boiled in wine to make a black hair dye, and that elderflower water used to be "a household word for clearing the complexion of freckles and sunburn, and keeping it in a good condition". We often follow her wonderful advice with cold elderflower tea, which was considered good for inflammation of the eyes.

Mrs Grieve also writes about the wealth of folklore and romance associated with this magical tree, such as its link to the symbolism of sorrow and death. It was also said that the fairies would take a baby sleeping under an elder tree and swap it for a changeling. The scent of elder certainly can be soporific and it can feel like you are being taken to another world as you lie beneath the tree.

Known as "the medicine chest of the people", elder is one of our most prolific and useful plants. For us to be healthy, it is essential for fluids and energy to move freely through our system, but times of ill health can lead to physical, emotional and spiritual stagnation. Elder opens the body's channels of elimination, cleansing the system and promoting flow. The diaphoretic action (from the berries and flowers) relaxes the blood vessels and promotes circulation, thus raising body temperature and causing sweating, which is useful in fevers. The diuretic action (from the berries) will increase urination, helping to detoxify through the kidneys.

Elder also has what we refer to as "heroic" medicinal actions. The laxative action (from the pips in raw berries) will clear the bowels. The emmenagogic action (berries) promotes blood flow to the pelvic region and can bring on delayed menstrual bleeds. The emetic action (from the leaves and bark) will trigger the vomit reflex and is useful in treating food poisoning (although this "heroic" method is now not commonly used in Western Herbal Medicine). These laxative, emmenagogic and emetic actions are best left to the experienced herbalist.

Elder's dark berries are full of vitamin C and antiviral compounds, and perfect for use in the autumn and winter months to protect against the onset of colds and flu. Much recent medical research has focused on the astonishing antiviral and immune-stimulating effects of elderberry, which has been shown to prevent replication of the human influenza (flu) virus and to stimulate the immune response, thus shortening the duration of illness as well as protecting against viral infection. This immune-stimulating effect seems to be linked to the regulating effect the berries have on cytokines, the chemicals released into the bloodstream when we become ill. It is cytokines that make us feel tired and achy, and force us to rest. Cytokines are a part of the immune system that is attacked by the human immunodeficiency virus, so elder is now being investigated for its potential in the treatment of HIV. The berries have also been shown to have the ability to prevent viruses from binding to a host cell and from replicating.

Vaccination against flu is now available, but only covers a few strains of the virus at a time. With more strains appearing year on year, it is important to consider what we can do as a preventative, alongside vaccination. Every year, tons of elderberries go to waste on the trees, which could instead be made into a virus-busting, immunity-boosting (and delicious!) syrup (see opposite).

BERRY ART

Pound a few elderberries in a mortar and pestle and use the resultant ink to express yourself creatively. If you have spent time with the plant and noticed how it grows, you may find this observation shapes what comes out on to the page to depict the energy of elder. Perhaps you have a sense of elder's personality or an image of a character that embodies her spirit; draw that in the ink or use the ink to colour her costume. As your fingers become dyed purple, you will really connect to elder's wonderful creative energy.

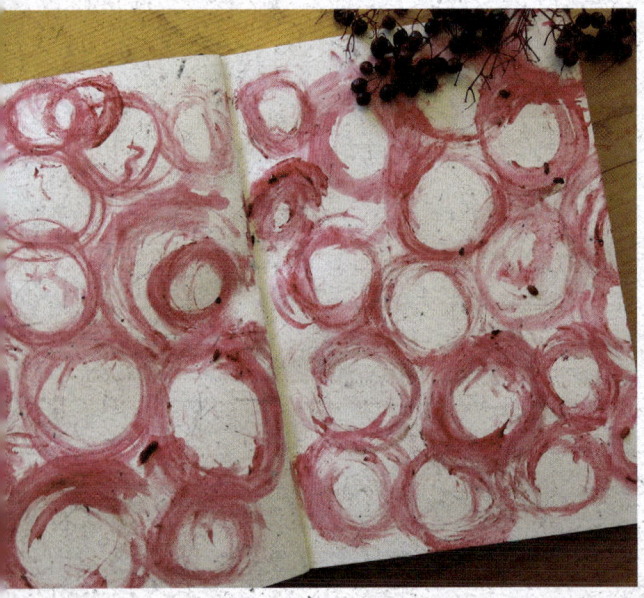

Elderberries make a wonderful ink for berry art!

ELDERBERRY SYRUP AKA VENUS ROB

Elderberries are dark black and ready for harvesting in late summer and early autumn. (Under-ripe berries will float to the top when you cover them with water; discard them as they can cause nausea.)

We like to harvest and work with the elderberries on Fridays (the day of elder's planetary ruler, Venus). Take a generous dollop in a cup of hot water with a big squeeze of lemon juice daily, to keep all viruses at bay. Up the dose to 3–5 cups daily if you are suffering with a cold!

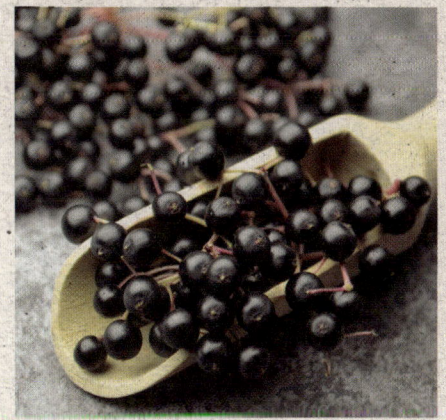

500g (1lb 2 oz) elderberries, forked off their stems / 1 cinnamon stick, 1–2 cloves or a 2.5cm (1in) piece of fresh root ginger, peeled and chopped / fairtrade sugar (500g/1lb 2oz/2½ cups to 500ml/18 fl oz/generous 2 cups of liquid)

1. Place the elderberries in a pan, along with the cinnamon stick, cloves or ginger – or any other warming spice. Cover with water and warm through gently until just simmering, then simmer for 20 minutes or so.

2. Mash up the berries, then strain through a piece of muslin in a sieve.

3. Rinse out the pan. Measure the amount of strained elderberry liquid as you return it to the pan and add the sugar.

4. Warm the mixture through until gently simmering, stirring all the time to stop it sticking to the pan.

5. When it looks nice and syrupy, pour into a sterilized bottle with a stopper. Store in a fridge for maximum life expectancy. Discard if you see mould forming on the surface of your syrup or it lets off gas when you open the bottle. A well-preserved syrup in a sterile bottle can last years and still be medicinally active.

PLANT CHARACTER: ELDER

I AM ELDER

My name is Samantha Bucosa Black,
Your elder, know me, the Crone,
The crack of breaking twigs underfoot
in the darkness,
That makes you run from your
own breath.
Be one with your fear.
I am death-filled terror,
Soporific nightmares, sweet
piped music.
Through death – rebirth.
The death scent lingers in my
laced flowers,
Again and again and again this
cycle goes on and on,
For those of you that choose to
drink my blood
Opening,
Pure medicinal movement is gifted
Provision of nourishment for
your soul
Should you dare to seek my
knowledge
Powers of regeneration,
Solitary ritual
Acceptance of your darkest fears.
The Earth Witches' twisted path
has called to you.
Each step carries great responsibility.

If you accept this weighted challenge,
prepare to face your deepest fears.
Root, grow, flourish, fruit.
Know me.

Plant Character

Samantha Bucosa Black is
an ancient, brimming over
with knowledge, but also
incredibly practical. She can
turn her hand to anything
from whittling whistles to
playing mystical music.
Lighting fires is one of her
passions and she brings the
gift of heat. She holds the
key to a great medicinal
armoury and can rebalance
any system, with a cure for
every ailment. She is fertile,
resilient and comfortable
with her underworld energy.

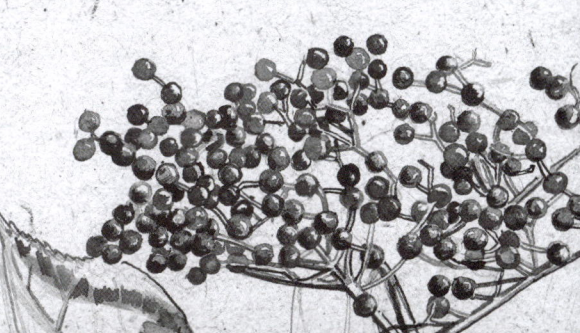

NUTRITION AND RITUAL WITH SEEDS

When the fruits and berries, hips and haws are ripening on the trees and bushes and the seeds are maturing on the plants, it is a perfect time to be incorporating seeds in your diet. Seeds such as pumpkin, caraway, nettle, borage and many more are full of the energy that will create new growth in the spring and an excellent boost at this time of year. Jams, chutneys and syrups are a way of preserving the riches of this season to store over the winter months, but we can also start to enjoy our rich pickings. Many seeds are full of omega oils, which are essential for cell health and replenishment, and are also packed full of phytonutrients that nourish our nervous system.

SEEDY FLAPJACKS

3 dessert apples, cored and sliced / 300ml (10 fl oz/1¼ cups) pressed apple juice 2.5cm (1 inch) piece fresh root ginger, peeled and grated / 1 tablespoon ground cinnamon / 250g (9oz/2½ cups) whole rolled oats / 25g (1oz) sunflower seeds / 175g (6oz/generous 1 cup) raisins / 100ml (3½ fl oz/scant ½ cup) rosehip syrup (see page 169)

1. Heat the oven to 180°C/350°F/Gas Mark 4. Place the apples (with skin left on – a good source of pectin) in a pan with the apple juice. Bring to the boil, reduce heat and simmer, uncovered, for 25–30 minutes, stirring occasionally, until the liquid is absorbed.

2. Pureé the apple mix in a food processor or with a hand-held mixer.

3. Line the base of a 22cm (8½in) cake pan with baking parchment (or use a square casserole dish, which won't need lining or greasing). Stir the ginger, cinnamon, oats, sunflower seeds and raisins into the apple pureé, mix well, then tip it into the cake pan and spread out.

4. Bake for 30–35 minutes until firm and golden brown.

5. Cool slightly, cut into wedges and leave to cool completely in the pan. Drizzle with rosehip syrup before serving.

By connecting with the rituals and seeds of autumn, we enhance our lives with the season's abundant energy. Harvesting seeds connects us with the energy of wealth, a sense of lavishness and helps us to celebrate autumn's gifts with gratitude. The air-enhancing seeds and fruits featured here offer us a variety of qualities – rose with her Venus-like, nourishing femininity, fennel full of inspirational Mercurial air and elder with this herb's deep insights.

Rosehip shells will help you to work with patience and perseverance in life. Using the fennel seeds in cookery and medicine will fill you with a lightness and quick-witted humour – the ability to laugh where once you may not have seen the lighter side! The elder syrup has stories held in the inky dark depths, which if you give yourself the time to explore them, will heal you from winter viruses and bestow the wisdom of the elders on you.

Breathing deeply, planning and preparing for the future, getting organized and communicating clearly, connecting to the air element, and balancing the respiratory and nervous systems, will set you in good stead for creating autumn health and abundance.

Autumn is a time to focus on preparation, from preserving the fruits, berries and other harvests that we reap during this plentiful season to gathering our selves for the darker months to come and getting our lives in order. The table below looks at some autumn rituals. Ask yourself, what is it you would like to bring into your life? What would you like more of? Who or what inspires you?

Autumn Rituals	
MARKERS	Autumn equinox, seed, fruit
NATURE REFLECTIONS	Harvest time as nature begins to die down, fruits are ripe. Planning ahead ensures stores for the winter months. Perfect balance. Muted reds, browns, yellows.
FOCUS	Inspiration, preparation and organization for the dark months (making chutneys, dried fruits, etc.)
MOON ASPECT	Waning
RITES	Seed saving. Preparing dried fruits, jams or syrups with intentions of protection over the dark months. Celebration of abundance. Spells of preparation and planning.

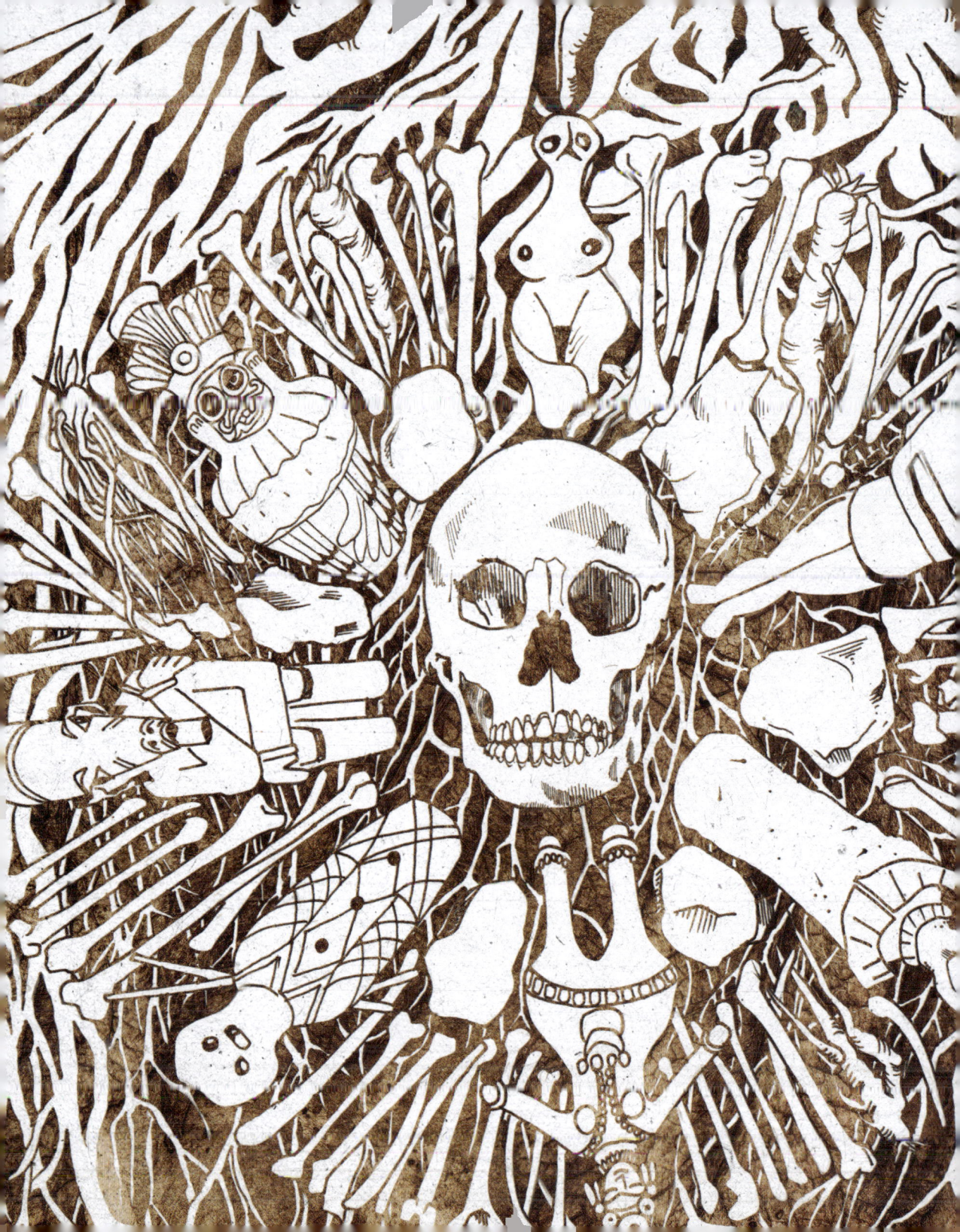

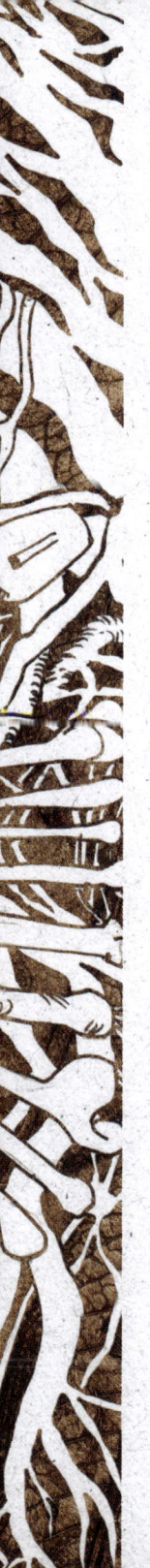

WINTER EARTH ROOT

NOURISH OUR ROOTS, CONNECTING AND HONOURING OUR ANCESTORS

This is the dark, cold season of contemplation, introspection and rooting down into our depths, when nature slows down and we retreat indoors. Sensory Herbalism connects winter to the element of earth, the plant part root, the musculoskeletal and digestive systems and the overall themes of nutrition, soil and ancestry. In this season we explore our "bare bones", the essential foundations of our health – the bones and skin that give us our form and mobility, and our digestive system that nourishes us.

WINTER / EARTH

Winter is the season of stillness and surrender. The deciduous trees are bare, berries have been picked off and nuts stored away. Nature's energy is deep underground. It is a time of retreat, rest and introspection, and often also of hardship, darkness and facing our fears. Winter is the season of the Crone, of the dark moon and of death.

There is a much higher incidence of death in the winter months. Death is part of nature's cycle, yet is often feared and misunderstood in Western society, removed from the home into hospices or hospitals. Traditional death rites used to involve the whole community paying respects and mourning. Open caskets are rare nowadays, so few people ever see a dead friend or relative, and dressing the dead is now attended to by an undertaker, not the family. Death is a sanitized event, something to avoid. We do not face the true horror and beauty of death.

The medical trend in hospitals from the 1950s has been to preserve life at all costs. In many cases, this creates intolerable suffering and dependence when death would be the natural solution. This trend is currently changing with the option "do not resuscitate". However, in many parts of the world choosing your own time to go is not legal, and nutrition fluids are often given intravenously if you stop eating and drinking. The growing "death café" movement is giving people a space where they can discuss attitudes to death and dying. Winter teaches us that death is a natural part of life and not something to be feared.

EARTH

Planet Earth is our mother, provider of life. Every creation myth has a mother and a father figure. The mother is often the Earth and the father the sky or the sun. The element of earth is the foundation, the darkness before the light, the energy of consolidating ideas, nurturing dreams and planning for the future.

To the naked eye, the earth is solid and unmoving, but the activity happening beneath our feet is astounding. Rain pounds on the earth's surface, filters down through the mud, and roots drink up the sustaining life force. The underground movement is relentless, rootlets searching for nourishment, stretching out and feeling their way in the dank darkness. Mycelia of fungi carry information and nourishment in a vast network of radical connection. Further below is the continuous movement of the tectonic plates.

Earth is physical, tangible and grounding. We are firm believers that we have been given this reality with which to work, and that

The Earth Element in Sensory Herbalism

ELEMENT IN BALANCE	ELEMENT IN DEFICIENCY	ELEMENT IN EXCESS	ASTROLOGY	EXAMPLE OF HERB
Pragmatic, practical, ordered	Lacking in will	Stubborn	Taurus, Virgo, Capricorn	Dandelion root

we have been given our senses to enhance this work. Nature is reliable – if not always predictable. Even in cities we see her bursting forth from any crack in the concrete.

EARTH EXPRESSED ENERGETICALLY AND EMOTIONALLY

If earth is in balance in a person they are likely to be steady, practical and capable of tenacity and order. They are able to build and create, to be solid, dependable friends and to keep a calm disposition.

The astrological signs that are associated with earth can be seen in the table above. Where someone has these signs predominant in their chart they may find the earth element expressed strongly in themselves. However, if earth goes out of balance, especially when a deficiency of the earth element can be seen, we reach for dandelion root. It will gently improve the production and flow of bile from the liver, literally giving more gall or will. It can be taken as a coffee substitute by roasting

and then grinding (see page 205); you can also boil the roasted root for ten minutes.

EARTH EXPRESSED IN THE PHYSICAL

* The body's earth associations are the musculoskeletal system, the digestive system and the skin. Our bones and the skin hold us up and keep us together. They are our foundations.
* The digestive system is where we process our food, releasing the nutrients that nourish our body, from which all else can be built.
* The earth element, like the planet Saturn, connects with our boundaries, our skin and mucous membranes and also with our bone structure. The digestive system is also where we sense and feel emotions first. If we keep our digestive system in good working order, thoughts concepts and ideas are easier to process. Our expression in the world becomes more clear and grounded; we literally become "earthed".

MUSCULOSKELETAL SYSTEM

Bones create our structure. They hold us up and give us our posture. They are solid but ever changing, constantly being renewed by the bone cells osteoclasts and osteoblasts. It is so important to care for our bones and all the tissues and ligaments that connect them together. Our bones will be here long after we have gone, offering clues to our life on Earth.

We may think of bones as hard and lifeless, because normally we only see them out of the context of a living body, but they are actually growing tissue. Three major components make them flexible and strong:

* collagen, a protein that gives bones a flexible framework
* calcium phosphate mineral complexes that make bones hard and strong
* living bone cells, which build, remove and replace weakened sections of bone.

Try this experiment. Put any bone into mineral-leaching cider vinegar and leave it for three days. When you take it out it will be rubbery – and the vinegar will be calcium rich. Vinegar is considered a mild acid, but it is strong enough to dissolve away the calcium in the bone. Once the calcium is dissolved, all that is left is the soft bone tissue.

This also makes vinegar an excellent medium in which to extract all the minerals in the plants for medicine (see page 107 for a recipe for cleavers vinegar).

COMMON SYMPTOMS OF MUSCULOSKELETAL IMBALANCE

These include: stiffness or pain in joints (including in morning), injury, swelling or heat in the joints, sore or tired muscles, shooting or stabbing pains down legs or in lower back, headaches.

SUPPORTING THE MUSCULOSKELETAL SYSTEM

HERBS

* **Heather** supports the kidneys, helps to clear the debris that can get lodged in joints and is a fabulous remedy against gout and other joint-inflammation diseases.
* **Rosemary's** warming circulatory effects are wonderful for joint health. It is also a staple as an essential oil in muscular rubs.
* **Comfrey** or knitbone is a primary herb for treating breaks or sprains. It is also a connective-tissue repairer so useful for tendons and ligaments. We use it in an ointment with heather and rosemary; these herbs potentiate each other perfectly.

Musculoskeletal Conditions and Treatment Strategies for the Practising Herbalist

CAUSES	Lack of exercise, hormone imbalances (e.g. reduced oestrogen in menopause), mineral deficiency, trauma
CONDITIONS	Osteoporosis, osteoarthritis and rheumatoid arthritis, physical damage (breaks and fractures), leukaemia, cancer
THERAPEUTICS	Remineralize the joints, improve blood flow to the area, remove debris and waste from the inflammatory process by supporting the kidneys, ensure digestion is functioning efficiently, address pain and stress levels
HERBAL ACTIONS CONSIDERED	Bone regeneration, remineralizers, connective-tissue restoratives, lymphatics, diuretics, anti-inflammatories, rubefacients (externally), circulatories, digestive support: bitters, hepatics
OTHER TOOLS	Exercise (especially yoga and walking), massage, diet

* Try Joint Juice Tea, blending chamomile, heather, marshmallow, lavender and nettle.

NUTRITION
* Eat more fruit and vegetables.
* Calcium-rich leafy green vegetables can help strengthen bones. They also contain vitamin K, which is essential for the movement of calcium around the body.

LIFESTYLE
* Regular walking strengthens the bones, stimulating bone-building osteoblasts. Habitual weight-bearing exercise, such as walking, signals that we need our bones to be strong, prompting the body to deposit fortifying minerals in the bones, especially in the hips, spine and legs.
* Vitamin D is essential for the absorption of calcium, so get out into the sun to top up your levels. Another benefit of walking!
* Reduce smoking and alcohol consumption.

If we consider that emotional patterns can influence physical wellbeing, you may want to ask some of the following questions if you (or someone else) experiences joint or muscular pain or inflammation:
* Who or what supports you and how?
* Do you ask for help when you need it? If not, why not?
* Do you feel able to move forward in your work, emotional challenges and projects?

SKIN

The nerve endings in our skin help us to see the world. Try closing your eyes and rubbing your thumbs gently across your fingertips, enjoying the sense of touch as the nerve endings are stimulated. The skin contains us and is our boundary with the world. It is the first thing that people see of us and a map to what lies beneath, both emotionally (as with blushing) and physically. When our organs are overloaded, the lymphatic system will excrete toxins via the skin, leading to skin conditions such as pustules and acne.

COMMON SYMPTOMS OF SKIN IMBALANCE

These include: itchy skin, rashes, spots or pustules, weeping skin, wounds that heal slowly or get infected easily.

SUPPORTING THE SKIN

HERBS

* **Dandelion** root encourages the production and flow of bile, aiding digestion and liver function, helping the body process toxins more efficiently. Dandelion root also aids the regulation of blood sugar, which in simple terms makes the blood less sweet and therefore less prone to infections that opportunistically reside on the skin and may enter the blood (as in septicaemia).

* **Horseradish** root promotes circulation and has a bitter action on the liver. Encouraging circulation supports the whole system in moving waste products to the liver or kidneys, ready for excretion.
* **Daisy** is an excellent lymphatic, clearing debris and inflammation from the site of infection. It also contains saponins, which help to break down areas of pooled blood (often seen as bruising). For bruising, use externally directly over the affected area.
* **Calendula** is more commonly used than daisy as a lymphatic and external skin healer; it is in the same family as daisy and similar in action, but with more antifungal resins and less saponin.
* **Lavender** is a wonderful anti-inflammatory and antimicrobial. Add a few flowers to a herbal brew to promote healing and calm.
* **St John's wort,** with its blood-red oil, is an excellent supportive herb for the blood. It also has specific action for any virus-related skin complaints, such as cold sores.

NUTRITION

* Juice regularly, focusing on green leafy veg with only a little fruit, for healthy skin.
* Celery and cucumber support the kidneys with their diuretic action, which has the knock-on effect of taking pressure off the

Skin Conditions and Treatment Strategies for the Practising Herbalist

CAUSES	Hormonal imbalances, poor diet, food intolerances, vitamin and mineral deficiency, stress, physical damage (UV radiation, cuts, bruising, contact with irritants), other sensitivities (e.g. dust mites), overheating of skin, compromised immunity, infection (bacterial, fungal, viral)
CONDITIONS	Eczema, psoriasis, infection, fungal (e.g. thrush, ringworm), bacterial (e.g. impetigo), viral (e.g. herpes, cold sores, shingles, warts, molluscum)
THERAPEUTICS	Consider digestion, address stress levels, observe what/who they're coming into contact with, look at family predisposition and emotional situation, support eliminatory organs (kidneys, lungs, liver)
HERBAL ACTIONS CONSIDERED	Lymphatics, digestive herbs (e.g. hepatics, bitters), alteratives, depuratives, circulatory herbs, diuretics, mucous membrane restoratives
OTHER TOOLS	Body brushing, stress management, creams, diet, salt scrubs, Epsom salts baths, saunas

skin as a dump for unwanted toxins.
* Fat-soluble antioxidants, especially carotenoids such as the beta-carotene in orange and red foods, maintain the skin.
* Eat a varied diet low in refined sugars.

LIFESTYLE
* Exercise to promote the flow of lymph
* Saunas and body brushing (see page 91), to promote circulation and lymph flow
* Increased water intake to support the elimination of waste

Ask someone you know whether you can touch their skin to gain an understanding of what is happening beneath the surface. For example, flushed skin in a relaxed person could indicate heat in the system, while pustules on the surface could mean the liver, kidneys and lymph need additional support.
* How does the skin feel to the touch?
* Is it soft or rough, clammy or dry?
* What colour is the skin: pale or flushed, grey, pink, brown, white, yellow?

DIGESTIVE SYSTEM

The gastrointestinal tract is a pipeline that runs from the mouth to the anus. It's lined with delicate mucous membranes that form an essential boundary between the outside environment and our internal environment. This pipeline is full of millions of bacteria, and we also host other single-celled organisms known as archaea, as well as fungi, viruses and other microbes. Research is currently looking at gut bacteria and examining how different bacteria support and inform the brain and nervous systems (the gut is often referred to as "the second brain"). Other major functions of our millions of microbes include informing the immune system, providing the correct nutrients for our cells, and preventing colonization by harmful bacteria and viruses.

The gut microbiome has been linked to a whole host of illnesses and diseases, such as autism, obesity, anxiety and diabetes, to mention just a few. It is also implicated in how medicines are absorbed and integrated into each individual's system, affecting how we respond to drugs.

Nutrients and water are absorbed through the membranes of our digestive systems at various points. The digestive pipeline of the human body starts at the mouth, where we use the senses of smell and taste to determine what we want to eat. Once we have taken in food, digestion begins in the mouth through chewing and the action of enzymes in our saliva. The pipeline then continues down the oesophagus to the processing area of the stomach, and into the small intestine, supported by the pancreas, liver and gall bladder, and then into the large intestine and, finally, out of the anus.

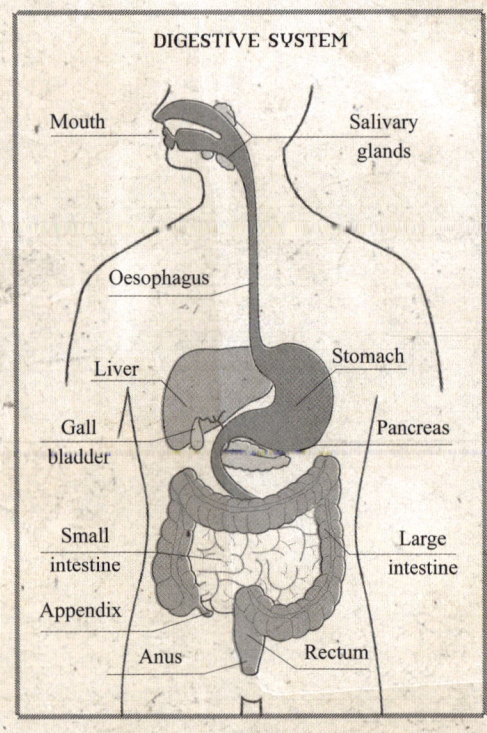

DIGESTIVE SYSTEM

Mouth

Salivary glands

Oesophagus

Liver

Stomach

Gall bladder

Pancreas

Small intestine

Large intestine

Appendix

Anus

Rectum

HOW IS YOUR DIGESTION?

We can see how efficiently we are digesting our food by studying our stools. Their structure, smell, volume and colour, and whether they float or sink can provide us with important information about the state of our digestive systems.

* Do you experience bloating, pain and flatulence?
* Are your stools easy to pass?
* What is the consistency of your stools?

If your stools are like small pellets and are hard to pass, it could be indicative of dehydration, a food-related or nervous system-related irritable bowel syndrome or intestinal worms; if they're loose and you find yourself going to the toilet more than three times a day, it may indicate a stress-related condition, again presenting as IBS-like symptoms, or an imbalance of gut flora as seen in candida overgrowth.

The digestive system, as the root or grounding element, bears the strain when anxiety and stresses take precedent in our day-to-day mental processes. If your digestive system is out of sync, it may be time to assess what stresses are in your life and how you could support yourself to deal with them in a nurturing way. Often people with cloudy minds or foggy brains, or those who find it hard to gather their thoughts, have poor digestion. This is a favourite subject of herbalists, who will talk quite openly about bowel movements at any gathering, much to other guests' amusement or disgust!

How can we hope to digest information and the lessons of the world around us if we cannot digest our nutrients efficiently? The digestive system is one of the most important systems to look at as the potential cause of many conditions. As the earth or foundation of the whole body, it needs good-quality fuel to function efficiently. More often than

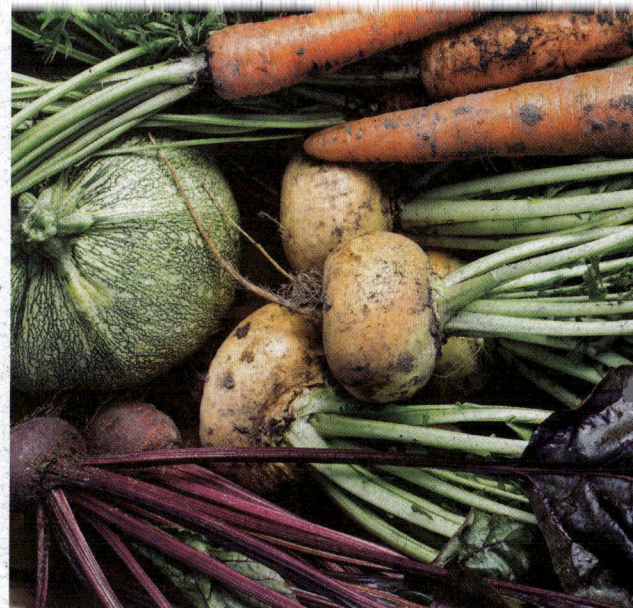

Locally grown food is optimum for digestive health.

not a treatment plan will start with digestive herbs and the introduction of a nourishing wholesome diet that is appropriate to the individual. In Western diets, foods and substances such as dairy, wheat, caffeine and sugar may need to be eliminated for digestive health. Supporting digestion with herbs can help a person make profoundly positive changes.

LIVER

The liver has hundreds of functions, including vitamin storage, the conversion, processing and metabolism of chemicals for excretion, the production of bile and the production of proteins important for blood clotting. If the liver is not functioning optimally, it can have a knock-on effect throughout the body.

This powerhouse uses a lot of energy to process toxins, hormones and nutrients. Where energy is used, heat is produced. When our livers are under strain they will be producing more heat, which can often be detected in a red face, or in a fiery temper. It makes sense, then, that those who drink more alcohol or eat more rich foods than is usual can have a florid complexion and be more irritable.

In Traditional Chinese Medicine, the liver is responsible for planning and creativity, as well as instantaneous solutions or sudden insights. It is therefore known as "the General in Charge of Strategy". The liver is associated with the positive psycho-emotional characteristics of kindness, compassion and generosity. Its negative attributes are anger, irritability, frustration, resentment, jealousy, rage and depression. It is often also described as the "seat of anger".

Low bile production (through lack of bitter foods in the diet, or through stress, poor diet or many other factors) can lead to sluggish digestion and therefore weakened digestive function. There may be gas, bloating, explosive or too-solid bowel movements, diarrhoea or constipation. All are indicators that digestion is suffering, and it is important to consider the liver in these cases.

Emotional factors are also inextricably linked to digestion; anxiety and long-term stress often cause irritable-bowel-type symptoms such as constipation or diarrhoea. It is therefore important to restore the production and flow of bile and all the digestive juices, together with a dietary plan. You may need to cool the liver, or warm the digestion, and this plan will determine which herbs you use.

HERBAL BITTERS

When the taste receptors in the mouth recognize the presence of bitters, we begin to secrete saliva, and an enzyme called amylase in our saliva begins the chemical process of digestion by breaking starch down into sugars.

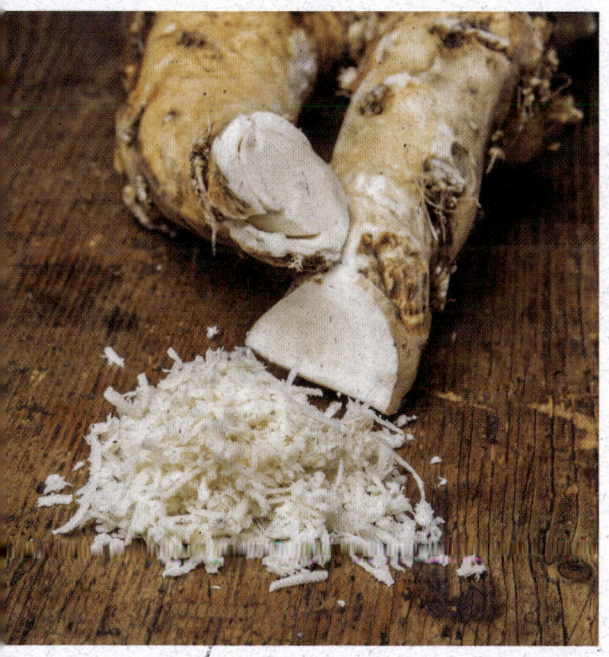

The bitter action of horseradish supports digestion

In the stomach, bitter herbs stimulate the secretion of the hormone gastrin, which regulates the secretion of gastric acid. Bitters also increase production of the enzyme pepsin, which helps break down protein, and intrinsic factor, which is essential for absorption of vitamin B12.

Bitters act on the pancreas, the liver and gall bladder. They can help to normalize blood sugar levels and promote the release of pancreatic enzymes and bile, which aid in digestion of fats and oils.

A healthy flow of bile helps rid the liver of waste, prevents the formation of gallstones and emulsifies lipids, breaking fats down into smaller molecules for processing by the small intestine. Bitters also optimize peristalsis and lubricate the intestine, restore the appetite and improve chronic indigestion.

Bitter herbs can be classified into the following five main types:

* astringent bitters (e.g. agrimony, avens)
* simple bitters (e.g. dandelion, burdock, centaury)
* aromatic bitters (e.g. rosemary, valerian, angelica, mugwort, wormwood)
* laxative bitters (e.g. aloe vera)
* spicy bitters (e.g. ginger, horseradish).

COMMON SYMPTOMS OF DIGESTIVE IMBALANCE

These include: abdominal pain and bloating, constipation/loose stools, fatigue, blood sugar issues such as getting shakes after not eating for a while. Skin rashes and spots may also be linked to digestive function.

SUPPORTING THE DIGESTIVE SYSTEM

* **Fennel** seeds are calming to the gut and help to dispel trapped or excess wind. They also have that balancing effect on mood, which is extremely helpful when digestive issues are linked with stress and the nervous system.

Digestive Conditions and Treatment Strategies for the Practising Herbalist

CAUSES	Physical stagnation (long periods sitting), lack of digestive enzymes, stress, diet, intolerances, rushing while eating
CONDITIONS	Irritable bowel syndrome, inflammatory bowel disorder (Crohn's disease and ulcerative colitis), peptic stomach ulcers, candida albicans overgrowth, cancer, aphthous ulcers, varices (dilated submucosal veins in the stomach, which can be a life-threatening cause of bleeding), hernias, inefficient sphincters, diverticulosis, parasites, tropical diseases, side effects of medication, haemorrhoids, polyps, malabsorption, coeliac disease, pernicious anaemia, bacterial infections (including food poisoning), viral infections
THERAPEUTICS	Support elimination (kidneys, liver, lymph), work on nervous system (strengthening, relaxing), adrenal support, promoting gut flora
HERBAL ACTIONS CONSIDERED	Choleretic, cholagogue, bitter, hepatic, carminative, mucous membrane restorative, mucilaginous, nervine, relaxant, thymoleptic (mood lifting)
OTHER TOOLS	Stress management, exploring nutrition and trigger foods, exercises, massage, diet, counselling

* **Rosemary**, a mild bitter with warming circulatory actions, supports digestion after a heavy meal. Also a nervine stimulant, it may be indicated if there is lethargy linked with digestive insufficiency.
* **Dandelion** root is a gentle liver-supportive herb that is useful for digestive issues. It is particularly indicated where dips in blood sugar are being experienced.
* **Horseradish,** a powerful bitter, hot herb, helps to break down fats and supports movement of food through the digestion.
* Try Belly Blend Tea: chamomile, fennel, mint, meadowsweet and dandelion root.

NUTRITION
* Include bitter leaves, herbs and teas to stimulate digestion.
* Include fermented foods, e.g. sauerkraut, kimchi, kefir, yogurt, to encourage

prebiotics, probiotics and friendly gut flora.

* Eat prebiotics such as garlic, onions, chicory and Jerusalem artichokes.

LIFESTYLE

* Slow and mindful eating
* Thorough chewing
* Reduced intake of processed foods
* Meditation
* Regular exercise
* Keeping a food diary (if you suspect food intolerance).

TONGUE

In Traditional Chinese Medicine, tongue diagnosis is a tool used to assess various connections within the body, both to the meridians (energy lines) and the internal organs. The tongue can provide strong visual indicators of a person's overall harmony or disharmony. The tongue is also said to have a special relationship with the heart; it is an "offshoot" of the heart, or the "flower" of the heart, a beautiful analogy. Heart chi (or energy) is expressed through the tongue. It is said that if the heart is normal, then a person will be able to distinguish all five tastes. The tongue's colour, especially the very tip, gives an indication of the state of the heart chi.

A healthy tongue is pink, clean and covered in papillae, which contain taste buds. An inflamed, red, black or white tongue, or deep fissures (cracks), can be a sign that a person's health is compromised.

It is quite common to see tongues with a very thick white coating. This may indicate that there is an overgrowth of fungi, such as candida, or excess sugar in the diet. We have also seen green-coated tongues with heavy coffee and cigarette consumption. Aphthous ulcers, on the tongue or on the gums or lips, are a common sign of immune-system deficiency. If you'd like further information on this fascinating subject, there are many good books on both TCM and Ayurvedic tongue diagnosis.

Try making the dandelion root tincture on page 206. Take 23 drops of the tincture every morning and evening for one lunar cycle, watching your tongue every couple of days to note any changes that may occur. Perhaps try eliminating refined sugars or caffeine while you are doing this.

When examining your own tongue (in a mirror) or someone else's, ask:

* Does it have a coating (white, yellow, green, black)?
* Is it red, pale, pink?
* Is it serrated at the edges?
* Does it have a line down the middle?
* Are any areas particularly red?
* Are there any unusual dots, bumps or raised areas?
* Are there any ulcers, blisters?
* Is there anything else to note?

ROOT

Roots and rhizomes are lovers of dank, dark, moist soil, of the rich, fertile nourishment that brings with it promise of ancestral knowledge. Everything eventually returns to the soil and is absorbed into the energy of roots. The roots are the beginning of the vascular system – the pipeline that moves water and minerals from the soil up to the leaves and fruits. Roots generally make up around a quarter of the total dry weight of a plant. New moon energy draws everything down deeply into the darkness of the earth, so this is the perfect time for harvesting roots.

TYPES OF ROOT

A taproot is a main downward-growing, straight-to-tapering root with limited branching. The milky, slightly bitter, nutty-tasting white dandelion is a great example, burrowing down, strongly grounded.

A fibrous root is a profusely branched root that occupies a large volume of shallow soil around a plant's base usually formed by thin roots branching from the stem.

A rhizome is a thick horizontal underground stem, as found in mint, whose individual buds develop roots and shoots.

Storage or tuberous roots are enlarged roots that store a portion of the energy and nutrients gathered or produced by a plant.

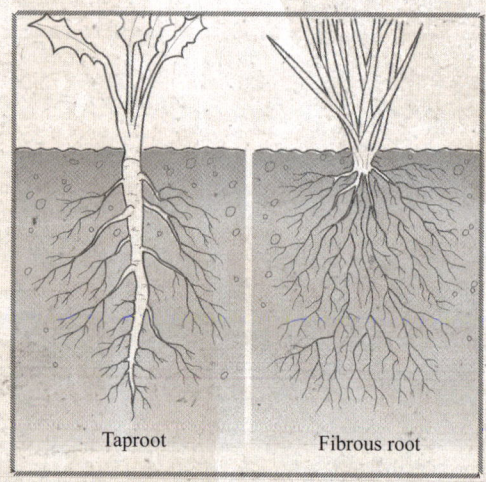

Taproot   Fibrous root

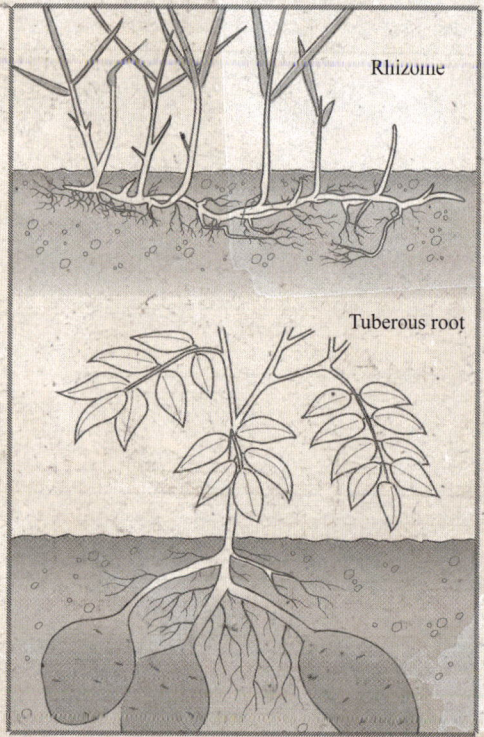

Rhizome

Tuberous root

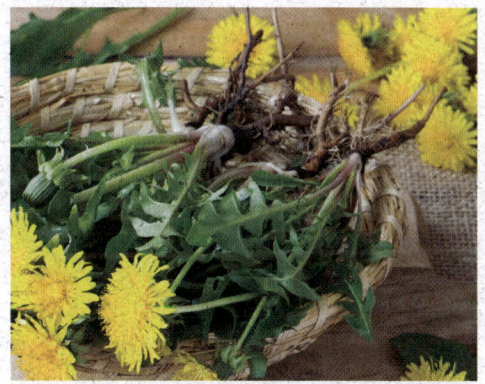

I AM ROOTZ

I am sweet nourishment,
Connected carrier
Full of grounded gifts of ancestry
Lover of the dark moon
Stabilizing
Supportive
Structure
Dig deep in the dark to discover
        secret labyrinths;
Hands dirty
Fingers sensing me pulsating in time
        with the rhythm of the earth

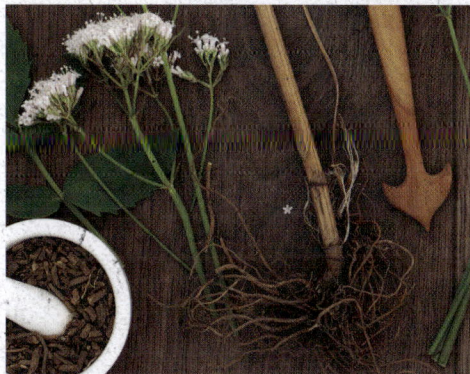

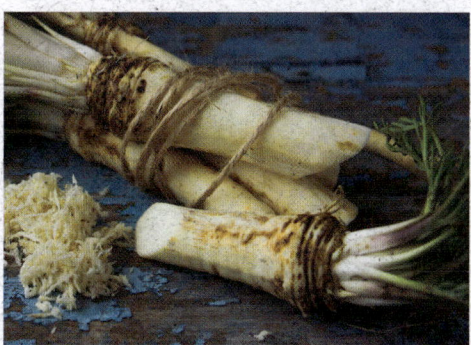

Root shapes of dandelion, valerian and horseradish

THE HERBS
THREE WINTER ROOTS: DANDELION, VALERIAN, HORSERADISH

DANDELION

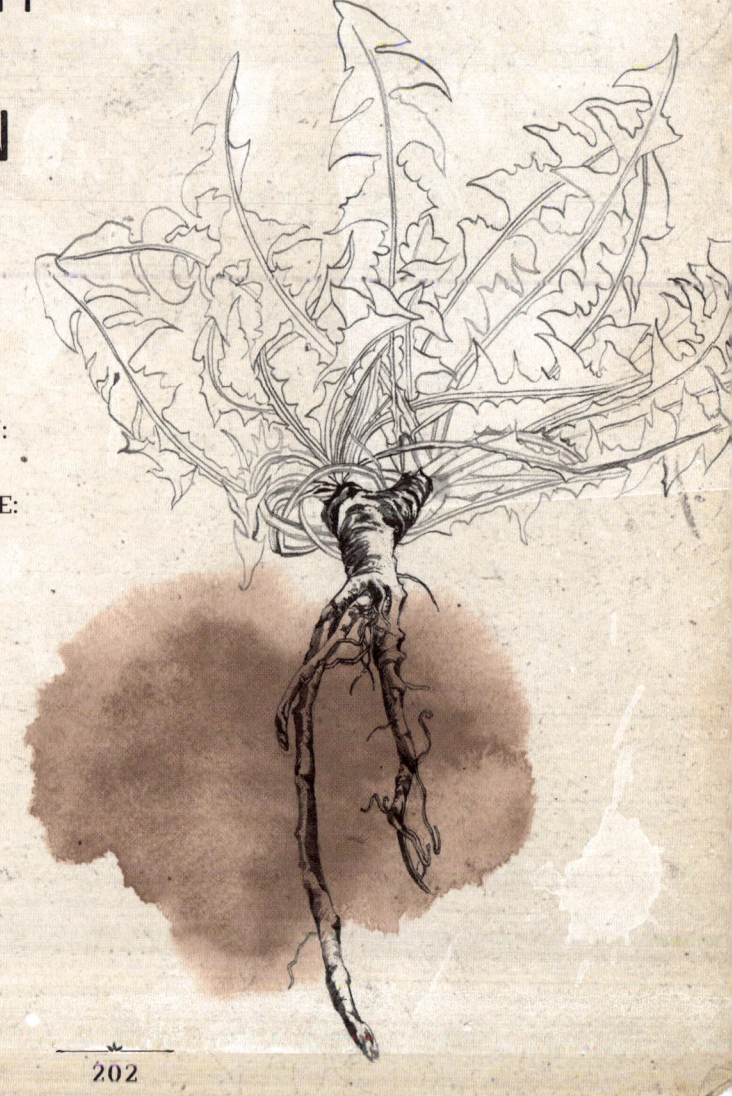

LATIN NAME:

Taraxacum officinale

FAMILY:

Asteraceae, Compositae,
Daisy family

ASTROLOGICAL SIGN:

Jupiter

SENSORY EXPERIENCE:

sweet, nutty, bitter,
milky, sticky sap

This globally growing herb travelled to the Americas from Europe in the early days of exploration. It loves gardens, waste grounds and cracks in the pavement or roadside. There is early reference to its medicinal use in the works of the Arabic physicians of the 10th and 11th centuries and in the early Welsh medical texts of the 13th century. The name dandelion has its roots in the French *dent-de-lion* (lion's tooth).

The root, while nutty in flavour, has a recognizable sweetness that indicates it is beneficial in regulating blood sugar levels. It is specific for post-prandial dips (feeling sleepy after a meal) or getting shaky when hungry (hypoglycaemia).

Dandelion root contains inulin, which is a polysaccharide (a long chain of sugars used as a food source for the plant). It is found in the milky sap that leaks from the base of the stem when broken. It is thought inulin is responsible for the blood sugar regulating actions of dandelion root. This implicates this plant in supporting a person with diabetes.

Dandelion is one of the most prolific plants, found on every continent. The taproot grows deep down into the earth, which is indicative that on an emotional level dandelion will help to get to the root of an issue. These roots contain bitter principles (namely, the bitter glycoside taraxacin), which stimulate and promote bile flow, and encourage the breakdown of fats in the body.

The detoxifying nature of the root helps to indicate the root cause of a "dis-ease".

In our experience dandelion root is balancing. It helps with a tendency to either hard or loose stools, and is indicated when there is a feeling of incomplete defecation. This is a gentle liver-supporting herb, so can be used if feeling weak or fragile. This staple of the medicine cupboard has stood the test of time, never going out of fashion as a valuable nourishing liver tonic. Considered as a weed by many, it aids in weeding out unwanted toxicity and emotions from the body.

Dandelion is a plant in perfect balance, each of the parts beautifully reflecting its elemental counterpart. It's a plant that wonderfully illustrates Sensory Herbalism's elemental view of plant medicine: the root is linked to the earth element; the leaf to water; the flower to fire; and the seed to air.

HOLISTIC VS. MECHANISTIC MEDICINE

Dandelion medicine helps us get to the root of any issue, as symbolized by the taproot, which buries deep down in the soil. Also, with its powerful digestive properties, it is a wonderful representation of holistic medicine. Digestion is a key component in so many ailments. Holistic treatment seeks always to treat the person and not the disease. Looking at the whole system, and supporting the individual, begins at the gastrointestinal tract.

DANDELION ROOT RITUAL FOR LAYING
TO REST A NEGATIVE HABIT

By grounding yourself and connecting to Mother Earth, you will have greater awareness and willpower. In this ritual, you make and bury a representation of yourself that holds a negative pattern or habit. As you bury it, you ask the earth to take your habit and lay it to rest. In return you make a promise to the earth to create a new habit, something nourishing.

On the new moon, locate and harvest a good number of dandelion roots. Wash the roots. Choose a root you feel drawn to, to represent yourself. Set this one aside and chop all the others up and lay them out on newspaper to dry. Consider what habits or patterns you have that are negative or no longer serve you well.

At full moon, start to carve your root into a representation of yourself. They are often very human-like with legs and arms. You may want to add facial features or symbols of you. Take your time over this; you have until next new moon to bury it.

Decide what aspects of yourself and your internal processes you'd like to be absorbed by the earth. What would you like to lay to rest? The earth can absorb anything you want to offer her.

At new moon, prepare a space where you'd like to bury your figure. What's growing there? Why have you chosen it? It is good to represent each of the elements in your ritual. A candle nearby could represent fire, with perhaps a shell for water, stones for earth and a feather for air. We like to burn mugwort to welcome in the element of spirit.

Once your candle or fire is lit, dig a small hole big enough to take your root character. Sing the Sensory Song (see page 82), then blow your old negative pattern/habit into the root.

Place your root into the hole and say the poem "I am Rootz" (see page 201) over it before asking for grounded connection, clarity and absorption of anything you've experienced and want to let go.

Simmer 1 teaspoon dried roots in 3 cups of water for ten minutes each morning, thanking the dandelion for its help in grounding you and helping to digest your thoughts. Drink this throughout the day.

The philosopher René Descartes (1596–1650) introduced the idea of a mechanistic reality to the medical establishment. This idea completely separates mind and body, suggesting that everything in life happens in a predictable and sequential way, like a mechanical clock. Modern medicine adopted Descartes's philosophy, as well as the ideas of Isaac Newton (1643–1727) about classical mechanics, and started to fit the human body into this mechanistic paradigm. If a part of the body became broken in some way, physicians were trained to fix it with medicines or surgery. This began to take the healing potential out of the person suffering and placed the responsibility in the hands of the physician – and marked the separation of mechanistic and holistic medicine. This idea has lived on ever since as the main medical model in the Western world.

In the meantime, traditional medicine philosophies have held on to the more creative outlook of holism. The word "health" is of Germanic origin from the word *hael*, which means whole or to be made whole. Taking a holistic viewpoint means incorporating the emotional, physical, spiritual and mental planes of an individual, while acknowledging the environment and wider community around them. Holism links all these elements and attempts to understand the root causes of illness by investigating them.

DANDELION ROOT COFFEE

If dandelions have done well in your garden, self-seeded and produced a bountiful crop of weeds, why not use the roots to make a delicious caffeine-free coffee? Wait until the plants are about 9–12 months old so that the roots are a good size. Dig, wash, cut, dry and then slowly roast in the oven until the pieces are a coffee colour. Grind when ready to use. A pinch of salt helps to heighten the flavour and the coffee may be drunk with milk and sweetened with honey. Older roots and a longer roasting time will create a more intense coffee flavour.

Dandelion reminds us of the importance of this approach, in which the focus needs to be on the imbalance that has created the issue rather than on relieving the symptoms. We do have the power to change and affect our health through the choices we make, the food we eat, and the way we care for ourselves and others. In holistic practice, we look beyond the individual to their environment, family, network and wider community.

DANDELION ROOT TINCTURE

This is a beautifully grounding and nourishing remedy. Try taking it for a couple of weeks with an affirmation of feeling nourished and grounded, and record your responses in a journal. Take a few drops three times a day, about ten minutes before food, to allow the bitter action to start to work.

1. On a new moon around the time of the winter equinox, create a clear intention for harvesting dandelion roots. For example: "I am harvesting the taproot of dandelion to keep me grounded and to aid with the digesting of information and nutrients."

Or: "I am exploring the root cause of my uncontrollable anger." Use something that resonates with you and your needs at this time. It can be simple and non-specific: "Supporting the health of myself and my family." However, expressing an intention is important; it focuses and potentiates the effects of your potion.

2. After digging out your dandelion roots, wash them and chop them as small as possible. As you do so, repeat your intention as a mantra in your mind. Say it out loud if you wish.

3. Fill a glass jar with the chopped roots and cover with good-quality vodka. Label with the date. You may also want to look up the sign of the zodiac through which the moon is moving at the time of harvesting and record that, as well as the place where you harvested the roots, and your intention.

4. Leave the jar out of direct light and heat. Agitate every few days, moving the jar about in a figure of eight while repeating your intention. Study the wonderful milky fluid that is in the jar, tasting and smelling it throughout the creation period.

5. After one lunar cycle, strain the roots from the liquid through a muslin or something else fine enough to remove all the dandelion root from the vodka.

6. Bottle and label the finished tincture. You can reuse the jar in which you produced it, but wash it out thoroughly so that none of the plant remains.

We witness how everything functions as a whole organism, and often as a microcosmic reflection of a bigger picture.

Dandelions rarely live in isolation. They choose to cluster in groups, surviving throughout the world and providing grounding, balancing medicine.

There have been recent trials into dandelion's promotion of apoptosis, the timely death of cells at the end of their life cycle, thus ensuring that healthy new cells can replace them. It is proposed that cancer cells can take hold when apoptosis fails to occur and the cells subsequently become old and change or lose their function. Research has started to see how dandelion root can promote apoptosis of cancerous cells.

In a study published in *Evidence-Based Complementary and Alternative Medicine*, a treatment of melanoma skin cancer made from a dandelion root was explored. Melanoma skin cancer, which has become one of the leading cancers, is oddly resistant to chemotherapy. Treatment, then, is limited to surgical excision of the primary tumour site followed sometimes by immunotherapy, radiotherapy and (the mostly ineffective) chemotherapy for metastasized melanomas. The dandelion root targets the mitochondria of the cancer cells, the site of cellular respiration, and generates reactive oxygen species, molecules which damage the cell, causing apoptosis. It clearly acts as a "natural

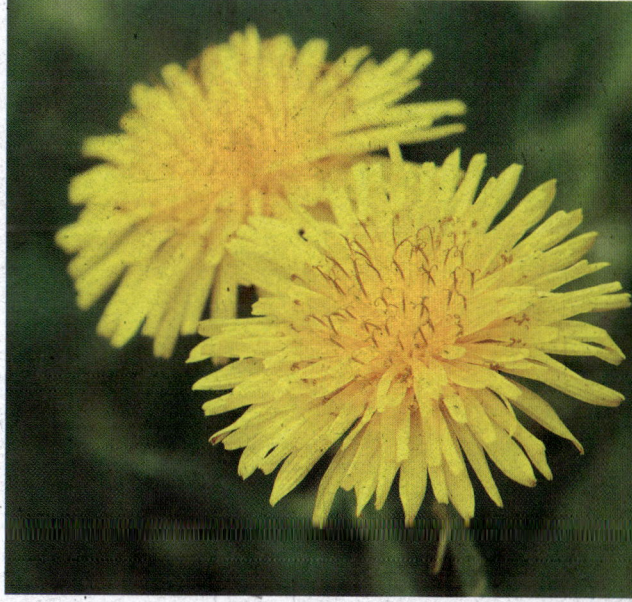

Linked to fire, dandelion flowers glow like the sun.

chemotherapeutic agent that may be extended to other chemo-resistant cancer lines", wrote the authors.

It seems, therefore, that the effects of dandelion are multi-faceted. This amazing herb helps regulate blood sugar levels, digestive secretion and enzyme production, normalizing the digestive function. It can cool an overheated system, supporting the emotional body with a grounding quality, and helps us explore the root causes of disease. And now it appears dandelion is also possibly a potent antitumour medicine.

PLANT CHARACTER: DANDELION

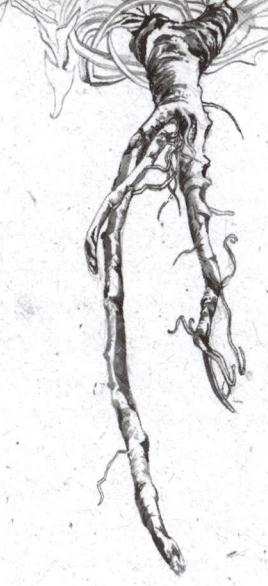

I AM DANDELION

From my low-down dirty roots
Cool, moisture-loving
To flights of fancy
Away with the breeze

The tips of my tappety taproots rarely
    see daylight
In their sweet, nutty nourishment
My bitter, milk-filled leaves
Serrated lion's teeth – water flowing
    freely
My bright sunlight blooms turning
    to time
Time that flows – freely

I grow everywhere
Globally
Detoxing the earth

Plant Character

Dandelion is our humble gardener, known as Doug. He is lion-hearted, salt of the earth, whistling to his plants as he breaks up the soil for the coming season. Folk are unsure how to take him – some love him and some hate him! He is quiet in his ways, getting on with any job at hand in a stolid, diligent way. Those who join him in the garden are given abundant baskets of sweet, medicinal, nourishing roots to take home.

You wouldn't think it to look at him, but he holds secrets to your past. He'll dredge up dirt without even knowing he's doing it, just a small passing comment or facial expression that'll remind you of something long forgotten. But after it is all revealed you'll feel clear, calm and settled with renewed energy to carry on.

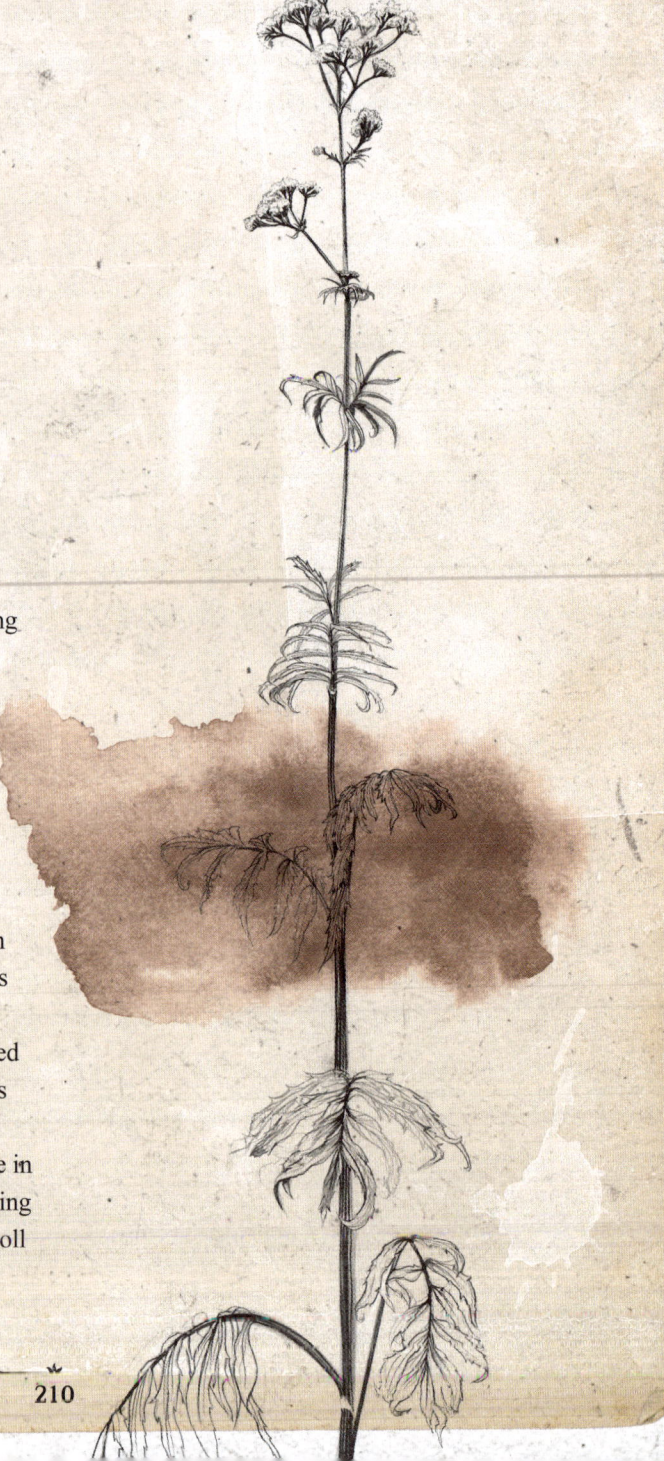

VALERIAN

LATIN NAME:
Valeriana officinalis
FAMILY:
Valerianaceae
ASTROLOGICAL SIGN:
Mercury
SENSORY EXPERIENCE:
Nutty, sweet, pungent, warming, numbing

The name "valerian" comes from the Latin *valere*, which means "to be in health". This Mercurial plant is found all over moist grasslands and spreads quickly if introduced to a garden. It is easily cultivated and loves nutrient-rich soil. We grew some in an old lorry tyre where it flourished, looking huge in comparison to its wild cousins. Neighbouring cats are the only problem, as they love to roll around in valerian, being driven wild by the heady scents. The roots have a pungent odour, reminiscent of cheesy feet, which many consider unpleasant. The odour is apparently attractive to rats; legend has it that the Pied Piper of Hamelin used valerian to lure the rats out of town.

The roots are ready to harvest after a few seasons; let the plant get established then divide the roots and keep some back to replant. The more the roots stink the better, for it is those volatile oils that hold most of the herb's relaxing qualities. We like to harvest the roots between September and November. You can smell their pungent soporific odour as soon as you start digging.

We use valerian for nervous conditions, particularly ones that involve high anxiety. It is very useful in any afflictions caused by physical or emotional tensions such as period pains, tension headaches, intestinal spasm, colic, flatulence, asthma, muscular spasms or where there is pain such as from toothache, broken bones, operations or heartache. As a Mercurial herb it is valuable in all nervous system complaints and as a root of the winter months it has great worth for the musculoskeletal system. Made into an oil, it is useful for sprains, muscular tension and spasmodic pains, but the smell can put some people off.

It is a central nervous system relaxant, while being uplifting for the spirits, but has very different effects on people. Some people can get hyper-stimulated as it kicks their body into compensating for its relaxing effects. A highly stimulated person who finds it hard to relax can overcompensate when given something to relax them, pushing them into worse anxiety. Valerian can help to improve concentration, reasoning abilities, energy levels and motor coordination, especially in hyper states where people have lost the ability to relax and sleep well.

ADHD (attention deficit hyperactivity disorder) is an example of a condition that overstimulates the system. ADHD and its core symptoms have been associated with abnormalities in the neural systems that govern release of neurotransmitters such as dopamine and noradrenaline. The conventional treatment is Ritalin, a stimulant rather than a relaxant.

In Europe, for around the past two decades, valerian has been studied as a treatment for learning disabilities and youth behaviour problems such as hyperactivity. In one study undertaken in Germany, valerian extract was administered to 120 children with an assortment of behavioural problems. The results were impressive. Three out of four children studied displayed an improvement after just three weeks of using the herb.

As with all herbs there will be differing effects on different people, depending on

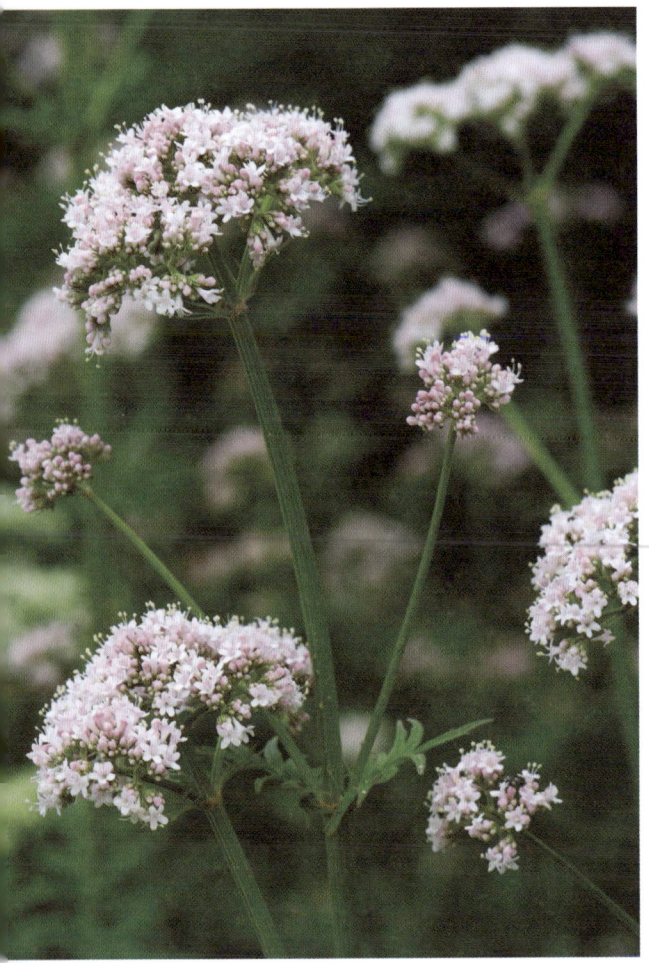

Valerian's delicate flowers give way to a mass of seeds proliferating the root medicine.

support of the system. We use it when digestive issues are linked with the nervous system, when anxieties are rife and when inhibitions need to be removed.

For a lot of people, small drop doses of valerian help to take away inhibitions that may be preventing them from experiencing life to the full. This is why we chose to use it in our Passion Potion, which emerged from giving small doses of valerian to many people in combination with daisy and chilli and watching how powerful the effects were. Research later confirmed the historical use of valerian as an aphrodisiac.

Daisy is a brilliant lymphatic and respiratory herb, which gives its natural gift of resilience to folk who use its wonderful medicine. We pick the daisy flower heads in early spring and make syrup to add to the other tinctures in Passion Potion.

Chilli plants create the hot and spicy element of Passion Potion. We harvest the chillies, chop them up, fill a jar with them and cover them with brandy to make a tincture, leaving it to infuse for one lunar cycle – powerful!

Valerian's stinky, cat-attracting roots are harvested on a dark autumnal moon, tinctured up and left to macerate for one lunar cycle.

Passion Potion makes people feel more sensual and sexier. A special blend of age-old aphrodisiacs put together in a new combination, it really ignites the passions.

the individual's terrain. In general, valerian is a herb that relaxes tension in the muscles, creating a gentleness to the structure and

The warmth of the chilli releases feel-good endorphins and heightens the senses. The valerian allows the blood vessels to relax so the chilli can reach every finger and toe, while daisy gently lifts the spirits and brings an element of joy and play to the experience of lovemaking. The drops can be taken every hour during a night of passion, or a smaller dose each day over a longer period of time to really get to grips with your intimate desires.

VALERIAN MILK SLEEP DECOCTION

Around the new or dark moon, uproot a well-established valerian plant. Wash the roots well, then chop them up finely and lay them out to dry in a warm place with plenty of ventilation for about seven days. Store in a jar away from direct sunlight. This recipe, using the dried root, is a wonderful calming sleep aid for children and adults alike. Drink a cup half an hour before bed; repeat dose if needed.

500ml (8 fl oz/generous 2 cups) almond/ rice milk / 2 very thin slices of ginger 1 cinnamon stick / 2 tsp finely chopped dried valerian root / honey, to taste

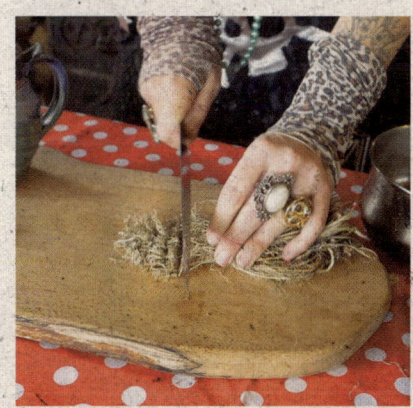

1, Place the almond/rice milk, ginger and cinnamon stick in a pan with a lid over a medium heat.
2. Bring to the boil and immediately turn the heat down and simmer for 10 minutes.
3. Add honey to taste.

PLANT CHARACTER: VALERIAN

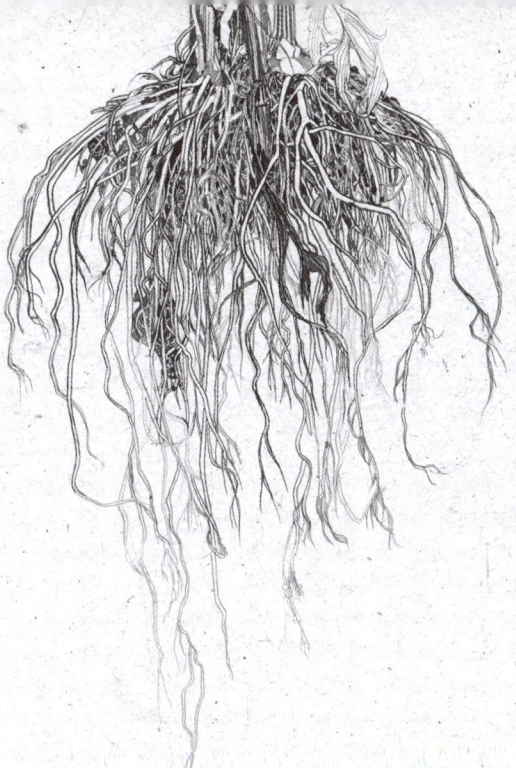

I AM VALERIAN

The stuff of dreams

Adored by feline goddess faces
Mercurial purrs
Which way to turn?
Watch and learn
Agitation?
Come to me
Swaddle in sedation

Musty, dark cupboard
Heady buzz
Retreat to my silent world
With not a care
Relax
Allow dilation
Blood vessels opening
Enhancing feeling
Releasing every inhibition

Passion through the slumber rising
Bone-white tangled, rooty locks
Spreading a vast network of sensual,
    radical romance
The evening dance
I am valerian

Plant Character

Grounded, pungent earthy
valerian will lull you to
sleep in her deep embrace.
She will relax your tensions
with experienced healing
hands, instantly warm on
your skin. With tales to tell
of journeys to far-off lands,
she compels you to sit and
listen, be mesmerized, be
in the moment. No cares
or worries here. Just pure
enjoyment. Release your
inhibitions as you drift.

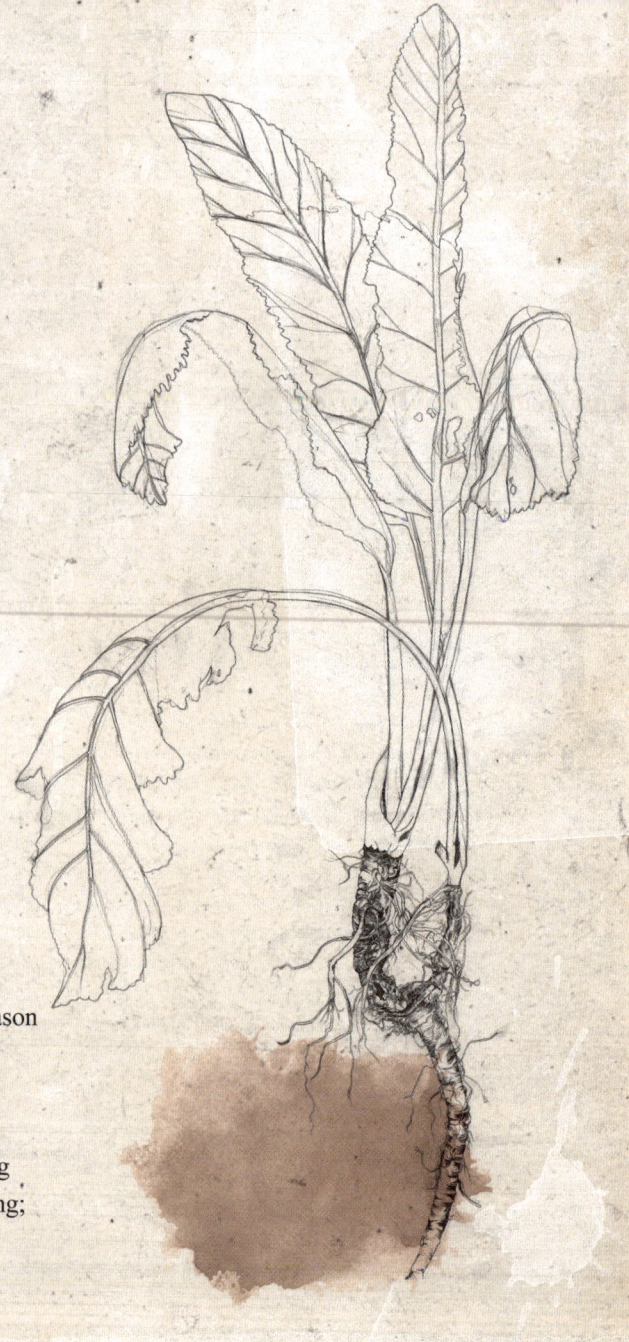

HORSERADISH

LATIN NAME:

Armoracea rusticana

FAMILY:

Cruciferae

ASTROLOGICAL SIGN:

Mars

SENSORY EXPERIENCE:

Hot, pungent, clearing, bitter

At the start of the winter months all things
warming and spicy are the order of the season
and horseradish is a great accompaniment
to the heavier foods usually eaten at this
time, facilitating the breakdown of fats in
the digestive system. We always keep a big
lump of horseradish back to use for cooking;
a small amount is tasty grated into stews
or sandwiches. The root needs to be kept

wrapped up so that the air doesn't get to it (this stops it from losing its spicy volatile oils and going bitter). Horseradish can be kept over the winter, stored in the fridge and used as a great spring-cleaning herb, fantastic for revitalizing the body after winter. It is a bitter digestive and circulatory stimulant and a powerful anti-inflammatory, a herb of Mars, with a heating nature.

Horseradish's heat is primarily created from the mustard oils in the root. When the cell walls become damaged through chopping, grating or chewing, an enzyme is activated and mustard oil is released, protecting the plant against animals that might eat it. The mustard oil released is so caustic to the eyes and mucous membranes of the nose that we always wear protective glasses or swimming goggles while processing a horseradish harvest!

When you chew a small amount, once the heat has subsided the taste is distinctly bitter. This promotes digestion by stimulating the liver and pancreas. By improving gastric secretions, the horseradish can give instant relief from indigestion and griping pains. Improving peristaltic action of the intestines also helps to relieve flatulence. Its gnarly, prolific roots are also used to ease the aches and pains of damp weather.

We harvest the roots of horseradish on a new moon, sometime between October and December. This herb loves to grow near watercourses and will usually be found in bulk. The large leaves are sometimes mistaken for dock, but tearing one a little to smell it will make identification easy as they also contain the volatile or essential oils. Horseradish can be invasive, so grow it in a large container in your garden.

Horseradish is super active and acts as an antibacterial, antibiotic, antiparasitic with its strong volatile oils. It is stimulating to the bowels, acting as a mild cathartic agent, creating movement with its fiery nature. Its aromatic bitters work as digestives, and it can stimulate many systems of the body. It helps treat water retention with its diuretic action, acting as a circulatory tonic and coronary vasodilator, and clearing the lungs with an expectorant action. It has been shown that the volatile oils – the mustard oils in particular – are excreted through the lungs and urinary systems (which is why we can smell it on our breath and in our urine), where it imparts antibacterial effects for both lung and urinary infections.

The Delphic oracle, the most important in Greek mythology, told Apollo that the radish was worth its weight in lead, the beet its weight in silver, and the horseradish its weight in gold.

Smelling the freshly cut root of the herb often produces tears due to the content of the caustic mustard oils. It becomes obvious how easily it clears the sinuses as breathing

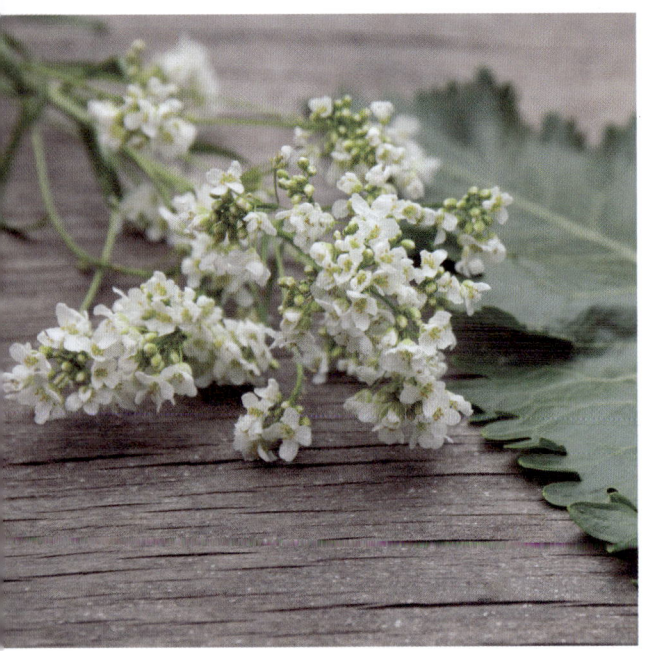

The term "cruciferous" describes the four-petalled cross-shaped flowers of this plant family.

channels become totally open and free. When used with other herbs, horseradish medicine rivals pharmaceutical antibiotics in treating many infections, such as bronchitis, cellulitis, influenza, impetigo, gastric infections, pneumonia, sinusitis, staphylococcal and streptococcal infections and UTIs.

THREADWORMS

Horseradish is a key ingredient in the glycerite we make to treat threadworms (see page 220). The threadworm, also known as pinworm, is one of the most common human intestinal parasites in Britain, resembling thin white threads that wriggle unpleasantly about in the stools of the infested host. Children are especially prone to this, with 39 percent in the UK said to have had a threadworm infestation. Soil and unwashed fruit and vegetables can harbour worm eggs.

As well as an itchy bottom, especially at night, symptoms of threadworms may include digestive disorders, bedwetting, mouth blisters, anaemia, grinding teeth, hyperactivity, insomnia, irritability and nervousness. Symptoms are often worse during new and full moons because the threadworms breed more at this time.

One time one of our daughters had caught worms that we just couldn't eradicate with our usual treatment which included a strong tea of chamomile and cinnamon; she was still displaying symptoms and the adults had also become re-infected. So we went to the doctor feeling defeated and were given mebendazole, the standard prescription for people aged over six months. All household members, including adults and those without symptoms, take a dose at the same time. This drug stops the worms' ability to utilize glucose, while also inhibiting their microtubular transport system. However, it has several possible side effects, including abdominal pain and diarrhoea, rash and even convulsions.

HORSERADISH OIL

Combine with other oils of your choice, such as a calming, soothing lavender-infused oil, to make an excellent rub for tired muscles.

1. Chop the horseradish up into pieces as small as possible soon after harvesting. If too dry, it is nearly impossible to chop.

2. Leave in a paper bag in the airing cupboard or other warm area for three to four days to get most of the moisture out.

If you put the root in the oil when it's still moist, the oil will go rancid.

3. When the horseradish root is dry, pack it into a sterilized jar and cover with oil. Almond oil is preferable, but any oil will do.

4. Open the lid every couple of days to release the sulphurous gases that form as the horseradish absorbs the oil.

5. After two weeks, strain the horseradish out of the oil through a muslin cloth.

In the event, mebendazole didn't work either, so finally we tried a horseradish glycerite, which we administered along with the other methods described on page 220. All of us were worm free within two weeks of this treatment.

PROTECTIVE POWER OF BRASSICAS

The Brassicaceae plant family includes cruciferous vegetables such as cabbage, broccoli, watercress and horseradish, amongst others. Medical studies have found that diets high in plants from this family are associated with a reduced risk of a variety of cancers.

For example, it's been found that the risk of suffering from colon cancer can be cut in half by eating more cabbage, horseradish and kale. It's also been shown that indoles, plant compounds present in cruciferous vegetables, can halt the growth of breast cancer cells. The Roswell Park Cancer Institute in New York found that just three servings a month of raw broccoli, cauliflower or cabbage reduced the risk of bladder cancer by 40 percent. The Netherlands Cohort Study on Diet and Cancer – a large-scale study with data collected from 100,000 people over six years – found that people who ate at least three servings of cruciferous vegetables per week lowered their

HORSERADISH GLYCERITE FOR THREADWORMS

This very effective treatment for threadworm uses glycerine to extract the constituents from the herbs. Glycerine is both a solvent and a preservative, which is good for preparing children's remedies because of its sweet taste and lack of alcohol. It's obtained by the hydrolysis of plants, usually coconut oil. You can buy organic glycerine online or in most chemists. Cloves are pain-relieving, antiparasitic, antifungal, antiviral and anti-inflammatory. They kill the eggs and stun the worms. Horseradish's bitter action increases stomach acidity and bile production. Caraway and fennel seeds both act as sedatives to the parasites, and garlic is an astonishingly effective remover of "nasties", helping to destroy many unwanted and harmful microorganisms. Making the preparation is a simple process, but it needs to be stored for three or four weeks before use.

1.5 litres (2½ pints) glycerine
100g (3½oz) cloves
100g (3½oz) dried horseradish roots
100g (3½oz) caraway seeds
100g (3½oz) fennel seeds
5 cloves garlic, chopped

1. Fill a glass jar with the glycerine, then add all the other ingredients.
2. Leave the glycerite mixture to brew in a darkened cupboard for one lunar cycle, then strain out all the herbs and spices.
3. Take a teaspoon of this mix at bedtime and first thing in the morning for two weeks, and again around the full and new moons for the following two months. Use drop doses for children.

To help pass out the threadworms, try eating porridge with desiccated coconut, as well as grated carrot and ground pumpkin seeds, which immobilize and expel intestinal worms and other parasites. Cucumber seeds are also anti-worm. And eat as much raw garlic as possible. If this is not palatable, infuse oil with crushed garlic for a day or two and then smother over the soles of the feet, cover with socks and leave overnight. The carrier oil prevents your bare skin from being burnt by the garlic. Make a fragrant essential oil mix from 3 drops each of lavender, lemon, peppermint, thyme and black pepper, added to 30ml (2 tbsp) of sweet almond oil. Rub on your abdomen before bed.

risk of developing colorectal cancers by a huge 49 percent. A study done in Singapore found that regular consumption of brassica vegetables lowered lung cancer risk in non-smokers by 30 percent, and in smokers by 69 percent! And in Seattle, researchers at the Fred Hutchinson Cancer Research Centre found that men eating three or more servings of brassica family vegetables per week lowered their risk of prostate cancer by 44 percent. Brassicas are true superfoods!

As a member of this family, horseradish can play an important part in preventative medicine. Like onions and garlic, the pungent, oil-rich root contains high amounts of sulphur, giving us a clue to its antimicrobial gifts. In tests it has been shown to be antibiotic and active against a variety of bacteria, invaluable given today's growing antibiotic resistance.

EU DIRECTIVE ON HERBAL MEDICINE

In 2004 an EU directive put strict guidelines on the type of herbs and the way that herbs can be sold over the counter to the public, discounting most of a modern *Materia medica* (list of medicinal herbs) and causing confusion by classifying many herbs as foodstuffs. Horseradish, for example, is one of our oldest and best-loved condiments yet is still a valuable medicinal herb. There are many problems associated with this

legislation. Because it is now forbidden to market herbs classified as foodstuffs on the basis of their healing properties, unless under expensive licensing, the public is in danger of becoming less well informed about these plants' important medicinal benefits.

The one main benefit to the EU herbal medicine directive is that it is bringing herbal medicine back into the home. People are having to learn about the growing and harvesting of their own herbs to obtain the remedies they need. This can be very empowering. Herbal medicine is a grass roots art form that should be accessible to all those who have a desire to learn. There will always be a need for more in-depth expertise for deep-rooted or acute health issues. However, huge pressure could be taken off public health services if people became more confident and adept at treating simple health complaints, nourishing themselves with food and herbal medicine and recognizing that not every health problem needs to be referred to a doctor.

We can creatively move forward in response to this legislation by ensuring that we have the knowledge we need to keep ourselves and our communities safe and healthy and to help our children grow up with herbalism in their lives.

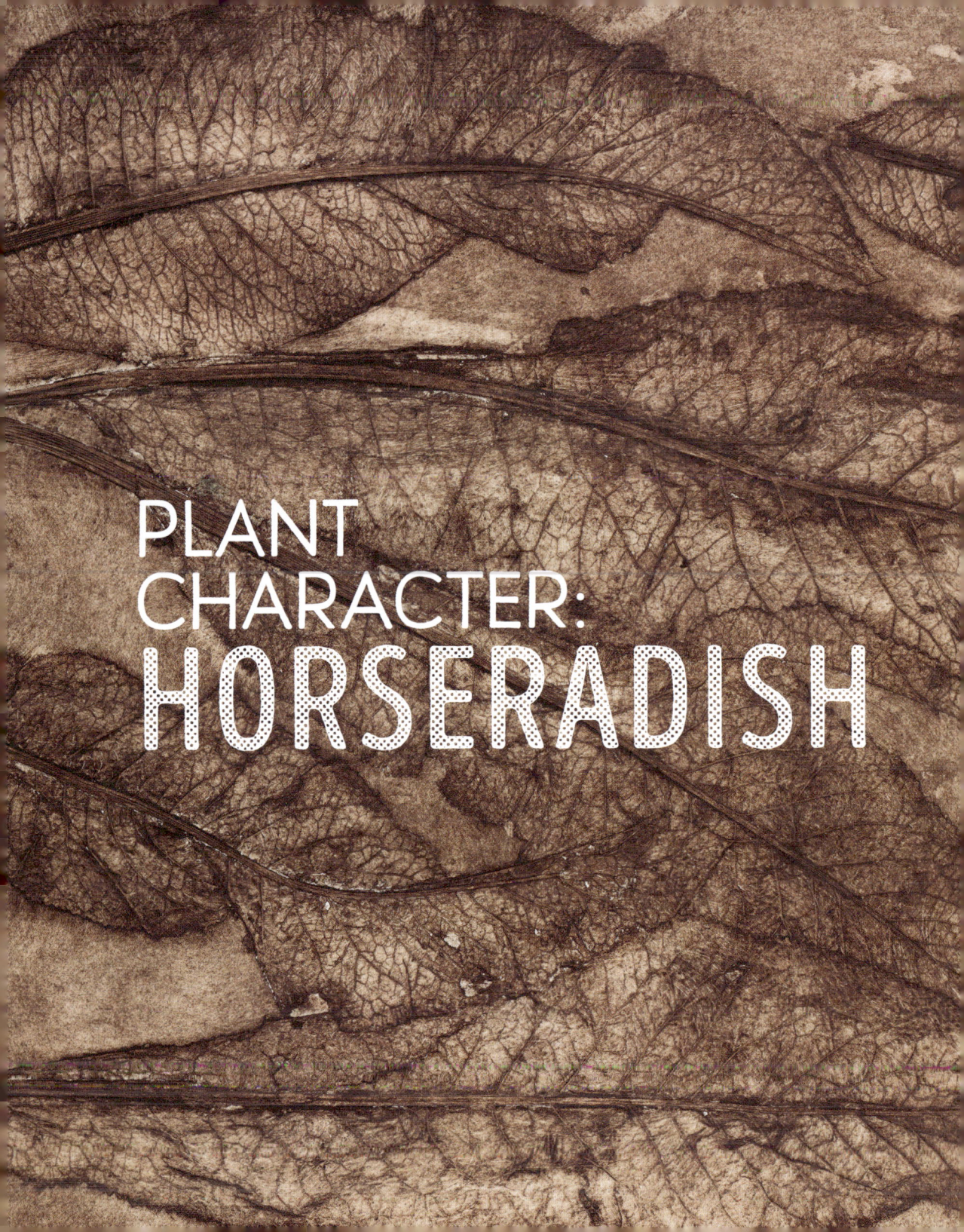

PLANT CHARACTER:
HORSERADISH

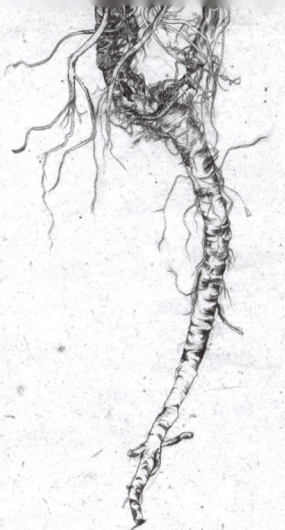

I AM HORSERADISH

Plugged into the earth
I will be your spark
Blazing
Clearing
Heroic medicine

Care to dine from my condiment pot?
Transform your ills
With my sharp tongue

Waves of heat radiating
As we dance
You will never be the same again
Twisting, turning, discoing through
    digestion

From my burning oils
Rivers of unemotional tears will
    stream
Never quenching the fire
Of the warrior horseradish

Plant Character

Hector Horseradish is super
strong, a real workhorse.
Often carrying a heavy
load, never tiring, as big as
a house. His deep, resonant
voice, always uttering
wisecracks, and his edgy
laugh can make people
feel very uncomfortable
if they aren't used to lewd
humour. His pungent scent
has people reaching to cover
their noses, and often they
sneeze at the first whiff of
his strong aroma.

NUTRITION AND RITUAL WITH ROOTS

ROASTED PARSNIP AND BURDOCK ROOT IN APPLE-SOY GLAZE

This recipe, to serve four people, is a delicious and easy way of bringing root vegetables into your everyday diet.

200ml (7 fl oz/scant 1 cup) unsweetened apple juice / 3 tbsp soy sauce / juice of 1 lemon / 4 tbsp honey / 1kg (2lb 4oz) burdock root, scrubbed, peeled and sliced into 5mm (¼in) rounds / 1kg (2lb 4oz) parsnips, scrubbed, peeled and sliced into 5mm (¼in) rounds / 1–2 tbsp olive oil 50g (1¾ oz/generous ½ cup) flaked (slivered) almonds, lightly toasted salt and pepper

1. Preheat oven to 220°C/425°F/Gas Mark 7. To make the glaze, heat the apple juice, soy sauce, lemon juice and honey in a saucepan over a medium heat, stirring slowly. When the mixture begins to bubble, reduce the heat to medium-low and cook until it has thickened and reduced. Remove from the heat and allow to cool slightly. 2. For the roasted roots, toss the burdock root and parsnip rounds in olive oil until coated. Spread in a single layer over two lipped baking sheets and roast for 30–35 minutes, turning it at the halfway point, until tender and lightly browned.

3. Place the roasted roots in a large bowl and toss with the apple-soy glaze until evenly coated. Season with salt and pepper. Serve immediately, topped with some lightly toasted sliced almonds.

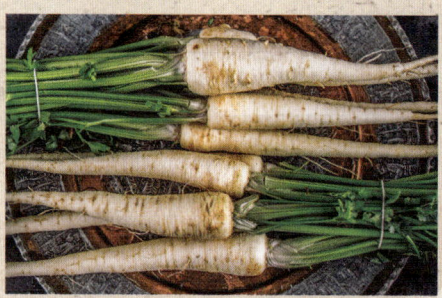

The colder and darker winter months invite us to enjoy the warmth and nourishment of the root vegetables, which lend themselves so well to soups and stews. By connecting with winter's rituals and roots, we enhance our lives with introspection and contemplation. Harvesting winter's roots connects us with this energy of slowing down, patience and self-reflection. The roots featured here offer us a variety of qualities – dandelion with its earthy, solid energy, warming valerian with calming air energy and horseradish with its hot, fiery, circulatory nature.

With the support of the digestive dandelion root tincture (see page 206), you can create healthy boundaries that will help with practical ventures. Using valerian milk (see page 213) will support your nerves as it gently lulls you into a relaxed state, creating a sense of stillness that is so important at this time of year. Horseradish oil (see page 219) offers rewarding warmth and movement where frozen physical or emotional issues are leading to stagnation.

Make the time to reflect, create the space to be still and cultivate an attitude of acceptance and surrender. Use these dormant months to connect with the deep energies of the earth and to reflect on the function of the digestive and musculoskeletal systems.

As nature slows, the trees lose their leaves and the light departs, we can focus on letting go of anything that no longer serves us. The table below highlights some of the rituals we practise during winter to tap into this energy. Consider: what patterns of behaviour do you dislike and wish to let go of? What makes you feel angry and frustrated?

Winter Rituals

MARKERS	Winter solstice, root, bulb
NATURE REFLECTIONS	Death period, stillness, introspection, darkness, grey, black, white
FOCUS	Planning and surrender
MOON ASPECT	Dark
RITES	Releasing into the earth any anger and asking to transmute it into creativity. Burying stones with a mantra of trust in nature. Honouring the ancestors.

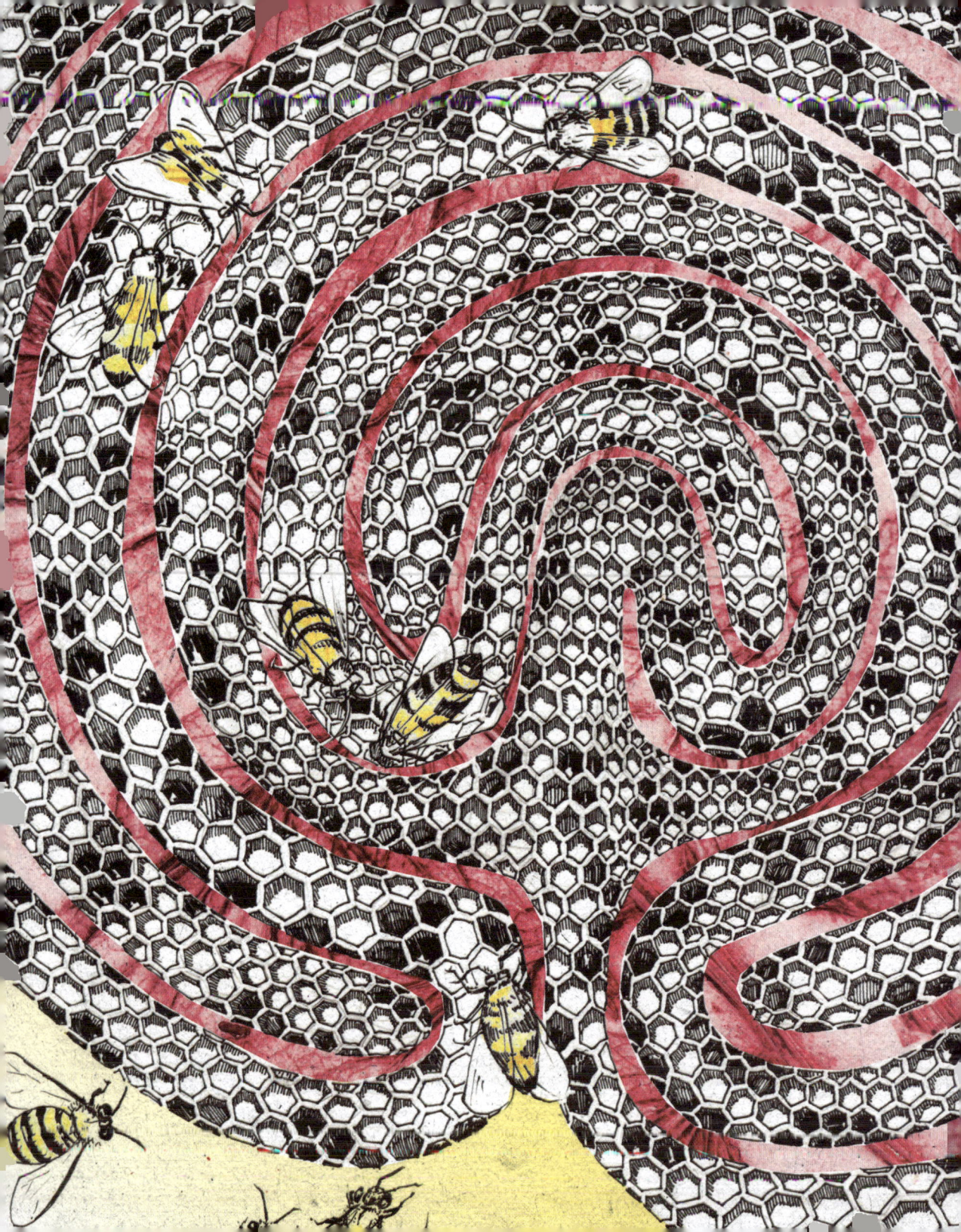

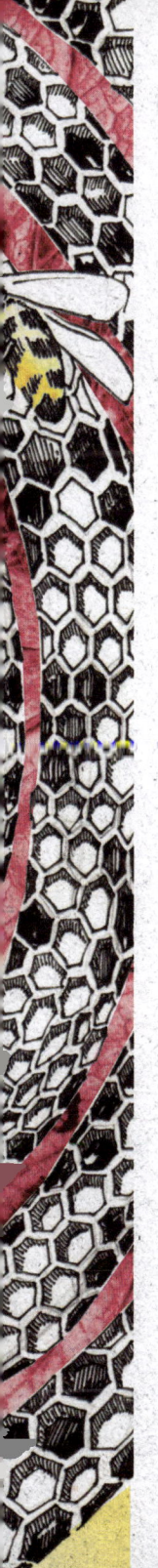

13 MOONS SPIRIT WHOLE PLANT

OPENING OUR HEARTS TO SPIRIT, TO GUIDE OUR FEET THROUGH THE DANCE

The element of spirit, found throughout the plant world, has the potential to initiate profound personal discoveries. Spirit permeates all parts of a plant and cannot be confined to one season. It is part of the changing of the seasons and is affected by the fluctuations of the lunar cycle. Sensory Herbalism therefore associates spirit with the entire plant in all its parts and across the 13 lunar cycles of the year. Connecting with spirit brings up-lift, meaning and support in day-to-day life.

13 MOONS / SPIRIT

The moon waxes and wanes approximately 13 times in a year, exerting strong influence in every season. The energy is palpably different as she moves through her cycle. Insomnia and lucid dreams are more common at full and new moons. More babies are born on the night of a full moon and psychiatric institutions are renowned for being more "lively" when the moon is at her brightest. The moon directly affects the plants and the movement of water within them. The tides become higher and lower with the full and new moons. Spirit is ever present.

Sensory Herbalism takes note of the lunar cycles in all aspects of working with plants, from the germination of seeds to the final harvest. Respect for the power of the moon permeates herbal culture: planting, growing, harvesting, creating and taking medicines. The moon is extremely influential in the design of our rituals. Lunar cycles exert a strong influence over the magnetic energies of attraction and illumination, and honouring the moon is part of our spiritual practice.

The day becomes the night and once more the day, the moon waxes and wanes in our skies; the light lengthens and darkens and we watch the changing seasons as we transit through them year after year. The only constant is change and the opportunity to celebrate that change is ever present when harnessing the power of the moon. Many magic treasures can be found in each season to bring into the home to create an altar: lush leaves to make a mandala or a Green Man (a symbol of seasonal renewal), vases of colourful flowers, special stones, shells or seed pods. Slowing the pace down and observing nature is healing. Collecting from the outside world and creating an altar in your home is a marvellous way to welcome each season and bid farewell to the last.

As the element of spirit permeates each season, connecting with nature through rituals that reflect the cycles of the turning year brings us closer to nature and ourselves. The element of spirit informs the design of the herbal rituals we use throughout the year. Spirit helps us to find the resources deep within ourselves and to unearth personal healing tools in the pursuit of balance, health and happiness. You will find the rituals summarized in the table opposite at the end of each seasonal chapter.

SPIRIT

An understanding, or a definition, of spirit comes with subjective experience. It can be an emotional response to the environment, a feeling of awe or wonderment or something

A Year of Sensory Herbal Rituals

MARKER POINT	REFLECTIONS FROM NATURE	FOCUS	ASPECT OF THE MOON	RITE
Spring equinox, bud, shoot	Growth and new life, greens	Leaving the dark behind, welcoming new light and ideas, clearing out the old	Waxing	Using running water to cleanse and wash away old habits to leave room for positive growth. Planting a particular seed with an intention of growth for a new project.
Summer solstice, blossom	Full energy and attraction, pollination, light, bright yellows, oranges, reds	Celebration and passion	Full	Burning negative habits in the flames of the fire. Celebration and gratitude for all the gifts of nature. Attraction spells. Dancing/ movement to create rising energy.
Autumn equinox, seed, fruit	Harvest time as nature begins to die down, fruits are ripe. Planning ahead ensures stores for the winter months. Perfect balance. Muted reds, browns, yellows.	Inspirations, preparations and organization for the dark months (making chutneys, dried fruits, etc.)	Waning	Seed saving. Preparing dried fruits, jams or syrups with intentions of protection over the dark months. Celebration of abundance. Spells of preparation and planning.
Winter solstice, root, bulb	Death period, stillness, introspection, darkness, grey, black, white	Planning and surrender	Dark	Releasing into the earth any anger and asking to transmute it into creativity. Burying stones with a mantra of trust in nature. Honouring the ancestors.

that affects how we feel inside without really knowing why. Think about the deeper meaning of expressions such as "my spirits are low" or "they're a spirited one".

Spirit is the subtle energies of the universe, palpable but not necessarily explicable. It is the magic of cell fusion when sperm meets egg. It drives the stem cell phenomenon or meristematic cells in plants, where cells "know" what needs to be created – an ear or toe, a root or leaf. Spirit is the blueprint of life.

It is the interaction between people, the shared breath of millennia, the constant cycle of air breathed in and out by people and plants – the same air that was breathed by the dinosaurs. The electromagnetic energy is measurable, radiating out, beating rhythmically from the human heart. This electromagnetic frequency is also emitted from plants, sometimes known as the aura. Spirit is the power of nature and the driving force of belief, activism and hope. It can power us to fight injustice.

Sensory Herbalism is a dedicated spiritual practice and brings the element of spirit into all areas of the work with herbs. It uses various rituals and tools to improve wellbeing and to support the health of the planet. Spirit is inextricably linked to the creativity needed in a challenging world, to drive social change, especially where personal and social healthcare is concerned.

Spirit comes in many forms and can be nurtured, encouraged and celebrated throughout our lives. Gathering together as communities to connect and honour the spirits of the plants can bring great inspiration and strengthen bonds, whether through growing a medicine garden or celebrating the apple harvest. Spirit offers opportunities for creativity – pure magic.

SPIRIT OF STORYTELLING

The creation of folklore needs to be revived as a carrier for important knowledge. In Sensory Herbalism we create personal contemporary tales that promote health and herbal education. Humans absorb and learn in a visceral way through stories.

A storyteller is so much more than simply a teller of tales. Storytellers are educators and healers and help us to understand the world around us, both real and imagined. Creating stories and folklore about the herbs is fundamental to Sensory Herbal practice. It weaves new threads into plant stories and carries their spirit on to the next generation.

SPIRIT EXPRESSED ENERGETICALLY

On each step of the journey through our lives we have an opportunity to take stock of all the tools available to us to support us in spiritual growth. We can do this by focusing and directing our energy, "counting our blessings" and fostering a sense of wonder at the gifts we have around us. When spirit is expressed energetically in a person they will have a deep sense of peace and calm, a gift of putting others at ease, and they are often naturally gifted at giving to, and uplifting, others. Some people are born with this inner state but others choose to practise or study to achieve it. Meditation, yoga, t'ai chi, gardening, singing, dancing, drumming, walking and being in nature, are all routes to spiritual enhancement.

Connecting with nature, with others and with our own subtle energies are all energetic expressions of spirit. Excess and lack cannot be so clearly defined in this context, as spirit is such a personal and ethereal experience. Someone may appear manic or spaced out or disconnected and low. They may need more community, more time with their hands in the soil, more connection to story and magic.

Spirit is about a sense of balance and holism. Even if one element dominates, the power of spirit can be adopted to ensure that this is expressed in balance and celebrated.

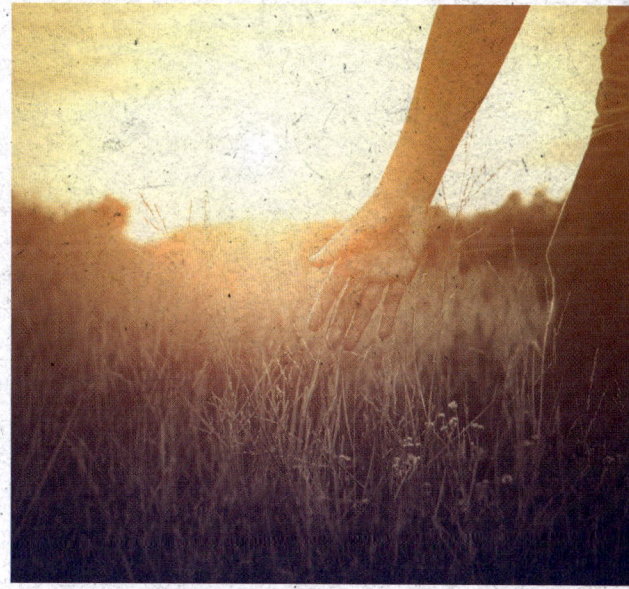

Spirit asks us to focus on the wonder of being alive.

SPIRIT EXPRESSED IN THE PHYSICAL

Spirit is connected to the wonders of the male and female reproductive systems. This does not mean just the act of creating new life, but also the potential power that can be harnessed when the womb and the prostate are cared for throughout life. The prostate is thought to be a centre of intuition and power, and shares the same brain relay system as the womb, at the brainstem level. The womb has been seen as an organ of perception, somewhere from which we can intuitively sense.

At the pivotal moment of conception, a great deal is determined about the future life of each human being, the merging of DNA. Although we know much about the process of fertilization, the miracle of new life still has an ethereal, magical nature. For this reason Sensory Herbalism associates the womb and ovaries, and the testes and prostate with the element of spirit.

FEMALE REPRODUCTIVE SYSTEM

WOMB

Many wisdom traditions have tales of how spirit comes into a growing foetus, referred to as "the quickening". This is also the term used for a mother's first sensation of the baby's movement in her womb. In Greece in the time of Aristotle, it was thought that this happened differently for males and females, with a boy ensouled at day 40 and a girl at day 90. Muslim scholars teach that the soul enters the foetus at 120 days. The yogic guru and scholar Paramhansa Yogananda said that the uniting of sperm and ovum begins the creation of the medulla oblongata, the seat of the ego. He states that a flash of light occurs in the astral world when the moment of conception occurs. There are also beliefs that a soul can already be waiting for the moment of conception, choosing to enter the world through particular parents, at particular times.

The womb holds the amazing potential for bearing the creation of life. Then, once the fertile years of a woman decline, her womb becomes a void, filled with the echoes of a pulsing, cyclical life. A void with the power to amplify perception and support social evolution through creative insight. The womb (like mugwort, featured here) is aligned with the moon energies: reflective, obscuring and illuminating, darkness and light in the space of a cycle. Acceptance and surrender to the ending of each cycle with a bleed, and then rebirth as the womb lining flourishes again, are innate within women, their fertility playing this cycle out regularly for 25–45 years. Don Juan is said to have called the womb "the perceiving box". He wrote about the uterus and ovaries as being tools of perception and even suggested that they can become the epicentre of evolution!

FEMALE REPRODUCTIVE SYSTEM

Fallopian tube

Uterus (womb)

Ovary

Cervical canal

Endometrium

Vagina

OVARIES

The ovaries contain all the eggs that will be released through the monthly cycle during a woman's life. Ovaries develop the eggs in utero. This means that half of the DNA that made us was carried in the womb of our grandmothers as our mothers developed. We are directly connected to and affected by our female ancestry through the food they ate while pregnant and the experiences and emotions they had and this determined much about the eggs which then become the chance of new life.

Every month of the fertile years (in a regular cycle without hormonal intervention), an egg is released, often accompanied by a sense of possibility and a surge of energy.

COMMON SYMPTOMS OF FEMALE REPRODUCTIVE IMBALANCE

These include: pre-menstrual tension (PMT), period pains, menstrual irregularities (such as scant periods, spotting and sustained heavy periods).

SUPPORTING THE FEMALE REPRODUCTIVE SYSTEM

HERBS

* **Yarrow** aids blood flow to the pelvic area, promoting and supporting healing and the natural functions of the female reproductive organs. This herb has a strong affinity with psychic protection, as indicated by its powerful essential oils, protecting the plant from disease. Menstrual issues can relate to feelings of safety around sexual encounters and/or a disconnection to the womb due to past trauma or negative associations. Yarrow supports healing on many levels of menstrual and reproductive health, but is not recommended in pregnancy.
* **Rosehips** have a gentle nervine quality, which encourages nurture and relaxation. Ruled by Venus, rose embraces the power embodied in the feminine and in free sexual expression.
* **Rosemary** is a stimulant with a powerful nervous system action, enlivening the spirit. It also acts as a hepatic on the liver, which is key in processing sex hormones such as oestrogen (present in any gender) and testosterone (present in any gender). If the liver is compromised in any way, the build-up of hormones can have a profound effect on the body (think of the spots of puberty and pre-menstruation). Rosemary invigorates the spirit and supports the excretion of hormones.
* **Mugwort** is a nervine relaxant and womb herb extraordinaire. It initiates a waking-dream state, connecting us to our innate wisdom and intuition so we can tap into the medicine we really need. Relaxing the muscles of the womb (not recommended in pregnancy), this herb tones and supports the whole pelvic region.

Conditions of the Female Reproductive System with Treatment Strategies for the Practising Herbalist

CAUSES	Exogenous hormones such as the contraceptive pill, hormone-replacement therapy (HRT), and corticosteroids, diet, stress, maternal line issues – mother-child relationship or ancestral
CONDITIONS	Endometriosis, infertility, fibroids, menstrual irregularities, mittelschmerz (one-sided pain on ovulation), period pains, premenstrual tension (PMT), cancer
THERAPEUTICS	While treating any womb imbalances it is important to explore creativity, how they feel emotionally and what they believe the root causes of the "dis-ease" are. Promote blood flow to the womb, in order to encourage movement in the area and help to eliminate waste. Symptomatically, herbs to relieve pain (anodyne) and cramping (antispasmodics) are useful.
HERBAL ACTIONS CONSIDERED	Lymphatics, womb tonics, circulatory agents, detoxifiers, nervine tonics/relaxants, antispasmodics
OTHER TOOLS	Meditation and breathing, exercise, connection to nature and time spent outside, massage including womb or sacral massage, diet, counselling and ritual around relationships with mother/grandmother, women's groups

NUTRITION
* Increase intake of omega oils: flax, pumpkin and sunflower seeds.
* Eat lots of leafy greens for iron and general high mineral content.
* A diet low in refined sugars helps to decrease inflammation.

LIFESTYLE
* Womb/pelvic massage to encourage circulation to the area
* Gentle exercise (take extra care with heavy lifting or overexertion around menstruation when ligaments are more relaxed).

MALE REPRODUCTIVE SYSTEM

PROSTATE AND TESTES

The prostate is primarily responsible for the release of seminal fluid into the semen for ejaculation. It has been referred to as the seat of a man's power and indeed seems to be particularly vulnerable to disease when a fast-paced, excessive work life has been the norm. Alakananda Devi writes that the prostate reflects the physical, emotional and spiritual relationship an individual has with their reproductive capacity. Disease in the prostate can reflect the overall relationship with the entire body. A diet high in rich foods, alcohol and cigarettes has been shown to lead to prostate complications in later life. These factors could be said to represent a lack of awareness around self-care.

The testes produce the sperm that contains half of the DNA that merges with the female egg to initiate new life. When the sperm and seminal fluid of the prostate merge, they produce a substance that in Chinese medicine is said to be high in *jing*, a finite form of energy with which we are born.

Sperm is produced daily but takes weeks to mature and is reabsorbed if not utilized. The testes have long been a symbol of male power and potency. Phrases like "grow some balls" and "he's got serious balls" exemplify what the testes culturally represent.

Tantra focuses more on the idea that male potency and power is preserved if there is less ejaculation, controlling the release of his essence or *jing*.

COMMON SYMPTOMS OF MALE REPRODUCTIVE SYSTEM IMBALANCE

These include: problems with sexual function, difficulty with ejaculation or small volumes of fluid ejaculated, reduced sexual desire, difficulty maintaining an erection

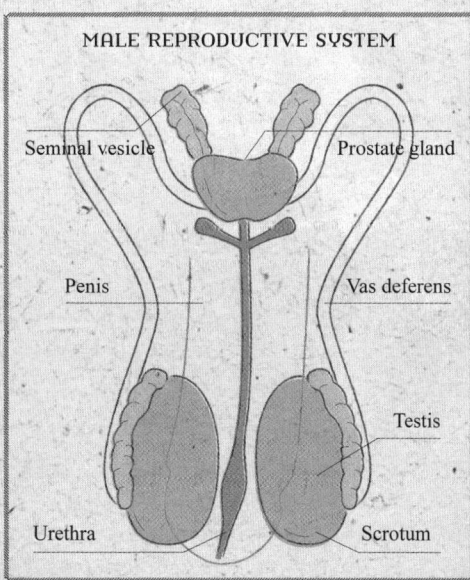

MALE REPRODUCTIVE SYSTEM

Seminal vesicle

Prostate gland

Penis

Vas deferens

Testis

Urethra

Scrotum

(erectile dysfunction), pain, swelling or a lump in the testicle area, abnormal breast growth, decreased facial or body hair, having a lower than normal sperm count, difficulty with urination (can be from occlusion of urethra from benign prostate enlargement)

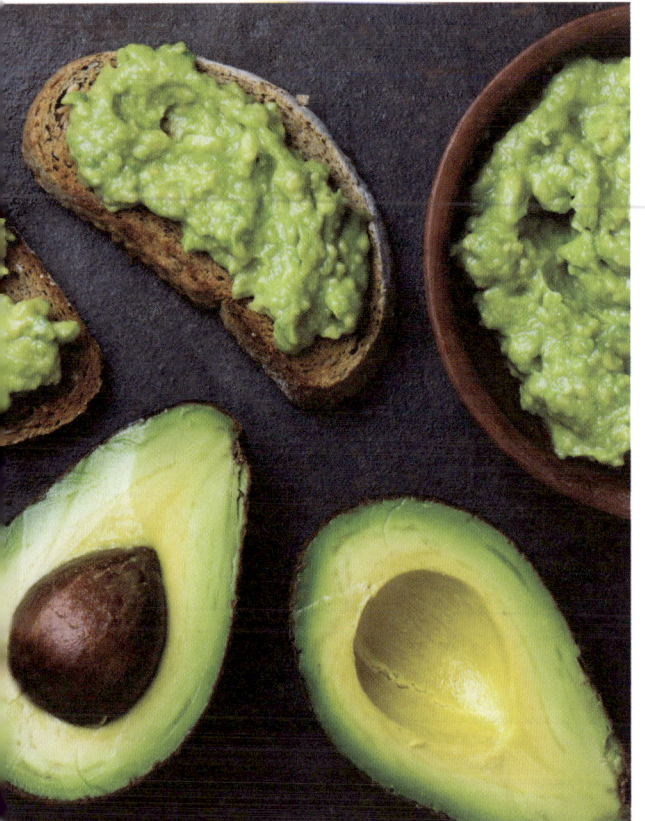

Avocados, rich in beta-sitosterol, support the prostate.

SUPPORTING THE MALE REPRODUCTIVE SYSTEM

HERBS

* **Yarrow** is a circulatory herb, especially useful for circulation to the pelvic region, encouraging blood flow as well as increasing the removal of unnecessary hormones from the area.
* **Nettle root** has been shown to be particularly effective in supporting the urinary issues involved in the case of an enlarged prostate. It's anti-inflammatory, diuretic and radiates out encouraging emotional connection and softening. It is also tonifying for the whole area.
* **Cleavers** is a lymphatic, supporting the system when dealing with infection, inflammation and detoxification.
* **Valerian** is a nervine relaxant and very useful if there are any anxiety-related issues connected to sexual health and reproduction.

NUTRITION

* Tomatoes contain lycopene, a phytonutrient that has been shown to be beneficial for prostate health.
* There are studies showing that zinc is very important for the health of male hormones, therefore increasing the intake of zinc-rich sunflower seeds in the diet can be beneficial.

Conditions of the Male Reproductive System and Treatment Strategies for the Practising Herbalist

CAUSES	Exogenous hormones (such as corticosteroids), diet, stress, self-esteem
CONDITIONS	Loss of libido, benign prostate hypertrophy, cancer (e.g. prostate, testicular), chromosomal or hormonal abnormality, gynecomastia (abnormal breast growth), low sperm count
THERAPEUTICS	Consider liver clearance of endogenous hormones, overall toxicity of the system, diet, alcohol etc., as well as nervous system involvement, stress, self-care and self-esteem
HERBAL ACTIONS CONSIDERED	Lymphatics, circulatory agents, detoxifiers, nervine tonics/relaxants, antispasmodics, anti inflammatories, hepatics
OTHER TOOLS	Meditation and breathing, exercise, connection to nature and time spent outside, massage including self-perineal massage, diet, counselling, men's groups

* Avocados are rich in beta-sitosterol, a plant sterol thought to reduce symptoms associated with benign prostate hypertrophy (BPH).
* Increase omega oils: chia, flax, pumpkin and sunflower seeds.
* Eat lots of leafy greens for iron and general high mineral content.
* Cut out caffeine.
* A diet low in refined sugars helps to decrease inflammation.

LIFESTYLE
* Pelvic massage to encourage circulation to the area
* Exercise
* Counselling or emotional support

WHOLE PLANT

Spirit governs the entire plant, permeating the roots, leaves, flowers and seeds. It is the life force that ignites the cycles of death and rebirth. The element of spirit offers excitement and challenges when working with the plants. Each plant can bring deep insights and guidance, eureka moments and sometimes a sense of acceptance, of being at peace in the world. Each has the ability to open particular states of being that can lead to synchronicity; signposts pop up as you follow your heart and trust your intuition. Some plants shout louder than others, but all have the potential to connect you more deeply with yourself and the nature that surrounds you.

Many of the plants have a strong ability to alter perception and deepen connection to spirit. Some of the stronger mind-altering herbal medicines have been demonized over centuries, thus access to information and research is limited. Despite these plants offering great gifts and connection, they are often surrounded by fear and stigma.

We have used mugwort to enhance our spiritual medicine practices through its gentle perception-altering effects. Plants that alter perceptions create curiosity. Some, such as mugwort and datura, have an energy that can lead to us questioning society, the status quo and the world around us. They also hold the

possibility for greater self-awareness when approached with respect and knowledge. The plants of spirit represent the right to stand up for our beliefs and to resist injustice, helping to achieve what our heart feels is true and just.

Datura is a powerful antispasmodic, used for asthma in Western Herbal Medicine. But governments have instilled fear about this plant and even encouraged its destruction. For this reason, it can symbolize the struggles of herbal medicine as a whole. Herbalism has been embraced, viewed with suspicion, embraced again and then fallen out of fashion.

The third of our spirit plants is a herb vital to allopathic medicine, supplying morphine for pain relief in hospitals worldwide, but it is also at the heart of much armed conflict. Poppy has inspired much of our own political cause through being such an impactful and powerful prescription medication and a street drug that has taken over many a creative soul over the years. It is a plant that enhances any garden, with its intricate heads that become full of delicious seeds as they dry out. These can be collected to use in cooking.

We would like to invite you to get to know these three wonderful, powerful plants more intimately, through understanding their history, by growing them and by recognizing their power and beauty.

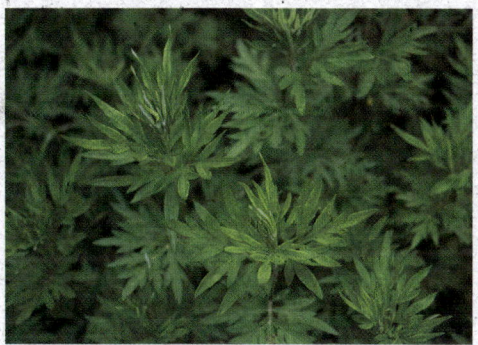

I AM SPIRIT

Catch sight at the change of light
Playful wisdom, deep insight
Boundless freedom
Free flow
Where the only constant is change

Wondrous new journeys
Ages old
The wisdom of generations holds
Movement through familiar lessons
Playfulness in death
Birthing freedom through discipline
Seek inside to discover the divine

Blowing on the winds
Deep down in the soil
Flowing with the currents
Burning in flames
Pulsing through your veins
I am spirit

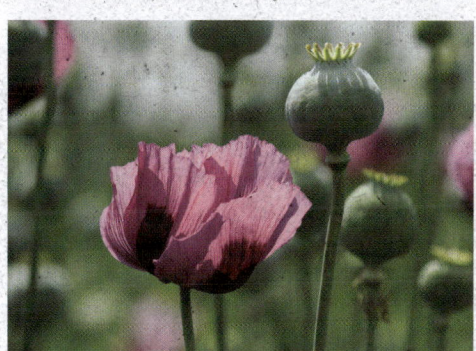

Plants of the 13 moons: mugwort, datura and poppy

THE HERBS
THREE MYSTICAL PLANTS: MUGWORT, DATURA, POPPY

MUGWORT

LATIN NAME:

Artemisia vulgaris

FAMILY:

Asteraceae

ASTROLOGICAL SIGN:

Moon or Venus

SENSORY EXPERIENCE:

Aromatic, astringent, dreamy, sage-like

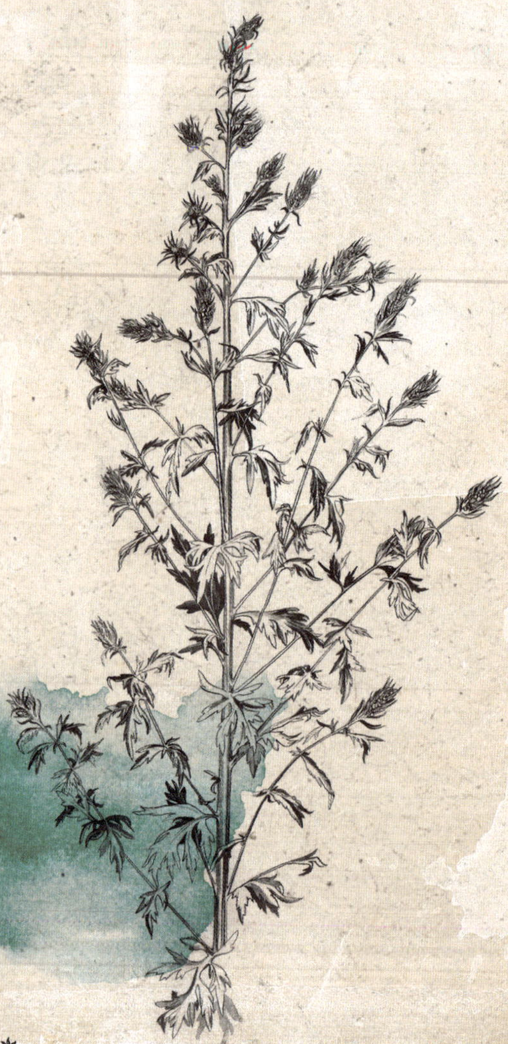

Mugwort, also called Una ("one"), is cited as the oldest of all plants in the *Lacnunga*. This 10th-century Anglo-Saxon manuscript, its name meaning "remedies", is a collection of texts about plants that includes the Nine Herbs Charm, in which mugwort is praised as a powerful treatment for poison and infection.

Mugwort holds the secrets and mysteries of the ancestors in her incarnation. In myth and story, she is the huntress, poised with bow and arrow, the protectress of the young; she is holder of creation with the gifts she brings to birthing mothers. Mugwort is named *Artemisia vulgaris* after Artemis the moon goddess, twin sister of Apollo; she holds the cycles and duality of the moon's magnetism, the full bright light and pitch darkness are all contained within her. This duality of the light and dark is both the mystery and the clarity, all aspects of the feminine dancing in time with the moon's rhythms, clearing and opening channels to our dreams, connecting right and left hemispheres, rebalancing our pineal and pituitary gland activity.

Growing up to 1.8m (6ft), mugwort is often found in dense bunches, with strong stems in hues of purple and red that can grow fat and hollow. The small, bobbly, pale-green and silvery flowers bloom in late summer, and are pungent in their flavour, with a heady aromatic scent. The deep-green leaf tops and silvery undersides indicate this herb's association with the moon, and the flowers reflect moonlight, a wayside guide to travellers at night. The Romans brought mugwort from Europe to the British Isles and famously filled their shoes with the herb to support aching feet.

Mugwort tastes slightly bitter but not as intensely as wormwood and southernwood. It is more ethereal, with gentle sweetness and mild astringency.

Connecting with mugwort encourages a liminal state in which the boundaries of the self start to dissolve and a sense of connectedness to the realm of dreams becomes palpable, encouraging intuitive insights. In these states, past, present and future weave together. Mugwort has influence over the pineal gland, located near the centre of the brain and shaped like a pine cone. It releases the hormone melatonin at night. This is thought to trigger the experience of dreaming. The pineal gland is said to be the "seat of the soul". Carl Jung believed that our soul is revealed to us as we dream.

We use mugwort in guided exploration to enhance and aid dream work. Dreaming, when we lose consciousness and dive into the deep waters of sleep, is one of our most mysterious and intriguing states. Dreams provide insights into our aspirations, hopes and fears. They reveal unconscious processes, unlock intuition and offer an opportunity for the dreamer to recognize the mind's own power to heal itself. In ancient Greece, patients went on pilgrimage to visit healing dream temples, and Hippocrates is said to have received his medical training in one such temple: the Asclepeion on Kos.

Mugwort can be drunk or burned to help enter into a dream state and harness the power of dreaming. It can also be used before harvesting a herb, so that you might more easily connect with it on a vibrational level. It promotes a waking-dream state and conscious attention to what our subconscious is trying to tell us. It also encourages the processing of emotions that come forth. The lady Artemisia has the power to work her magic in our dreams, sending us both coded and clear insights to grasp as we wake from slumber.

We like to invoke Artemis to open our harvesting rituals. We burn or smoke a little mugwort to initiate a connection with nature. We also leave offerings of a pinch of its greenery to the plant spirits after picking other herbs for our medicine making. This is a custom that many earth-loving peoples have used around the world with gateway plants such as mugwort or tobacco.

Before the beer purity law passed in the duchy of Munich in 1497 (adopted across Bavaria in 1516), mugwort was one of the chief brewing herbs used to make ale. This may be where the name mugwort arose – a mug of wort. The 1497 law restricted the use of mind-altering substances such as mugwort and henbane in beer, stating that only water,

barley and hops were to be used. This law can therefore be seen as the very first drug law passed – the beginning of the "war on drugs".

BIRTHING

Giving birth is a deeply primal and natural event, but over the centuries many women and their newborns have died in childbirth. One of the gifts of modern medicine is that today there are far fewer childbirth-related deaths in the West. However, because of increased medical intervention, as well as deskilling within midwifery for cases such as supporting natural breech birth and delivering twins, we also see greater numbers of unnecessarily medicalized births. In response to this, the number of home births in the UK has been rising, with funded and dedicated home-birth teams around the country.

Mugwort is a wonderful birthing herb that supports uterine contractions, aids with pain relief and helps connect us with the strength of Artemis. We have both had the pleasure of giving birth at home with the use of herbs and the loving support of each other; we have even caught each other's babies. We know first-hand how hot mugwort tea drunk in labour is a powerful supportive force, aiding contractions and providing vital energetic bolstering at this time when access is needed to your deepest spiritual reserves. We used mugwort as part of a syrup and tincture blend, but it can also be drunk as a tea during birth.

CLEANSING SMOKE

People the world over use plants to generate smoke to produce beneficial effects, such as driving off insects or preventing the airborne transfer of disease. Smoke is deeply symbolic. It ascends to the heavens, as if bringing prayers and intentions up to the gods. The smoke generated by plants has a rich history of use as part of spiritual practice.

There are many words for the practice of using smoke to clear a space. Difference censers or incense burners for the use of herbs and resins have been used throughout time worldwide from ancient Egyptian to the Aztecs. There is "smudging" used by tribes of native America, the practice of "saining" in Scotland.

We have re-adopted the word "reeking", an Anglo Saxon term for creating smoke. We make reeking rods form local herbs, mainly mugwort. Reeking, sometimes called sacred smoking, is a powerful spiritual cleansing technique that calls upon the spirits of sacred plants to clear, clarify, purify and restore balance. It initiates an opening to subtle spiritual energies. The practice allows you to wash away all the emotional and spiritual negativity that gathers in your body and your space, a bit like taking a spiritual shower! The effects of using smoke are instantly noticeable, banishing stress and providing energy and peace. The air often twinkles with vibrancy after a good smoke cleanse.

MAKING A REEKING ROD

There is nothing more powerful than using sacred tools you've made yourself and reeking rods are no exception. You can put all your energy and thought into the herbs during the harvesting, the tying of the twine around them, the drying and then finally the burning. These herb bundles are great for gifts, or to use with clients if you are a practitioner.

While you are harvesting and making the reeking rods remember to use the intentions of uplifting, purification and protection.

We use mugwort as our base herb as it is abundant and enables the smudge stick to burn without going out. Find a good patch with lots to give and watch out for the perfect time to harvest, just as the plant has flowered and, ideally, when the moon is full, as mugwort is so connected to the moon. We had been keeping an eye on a huge patch of mugwort up a pedestrian country lane, waiting for the right time for the plant and the moon. We finally harvested on a beautiful sunny day when the flowers were silvery and fluffy. The next day, the farmer came and mowed down the whole wayside. Close call – but the moon was looking out for us.

Depending on the plant size, we usually harvest from about halfway down the stem, above where it looks like it could divide off and keep growing if the weather is right. You

The Smoking Herb

Native to South America, the tobacco plant is in the Solanaceae family with the potato, the chilli pepper and datura. As early as 5000 BC, native South Americans began using tobacco in religious and medicinal practices, to dress wounds, and as a painkiller. The use of tobacco spread north, and in 1492 Christopher Columbus was offered dried tobacco leaves as a gift. Not long after, the plant was being grown all over Europe. Up until then, however, the smoking herb in England had been mugwort (also known as "the traveller's smoke" or "the sailor's smoke"), which was not physically addictive.

Tobacco, on the other hand, is highly addictive, because it contains the alkaloid nicotine. We now are all aware of the negative health implications of cigarettes. Mugwort is still available in plentiful supply on waste grounds, a free source of smoking herb for those who may want to break the habit of addiction to nicotine.

need pieces at least 30–40cm (12–15in) long to make nice fat reeking rods.

To choose the herbs to go with mugwort, we usually head to the garden for yarrow or rosemary. Aromatic herbs tend to burn well and provide the most cleansing and protective actions. These herbs are high in essential oils, which are the plant's defence system. The oils burn well and produce lovely aromas.

Lay a bunch of your herbs out in front of you, including a bigger proportion of mugwort. The thickness of the smudge stick is up to you, and the weird and wonderful shape of the finished product often reflects the character of the person who made it! Ideally the bunch should fit snugly between your thumb and first finger joined tip to tip to make a round.

Match up the stems approximately (you can trim them afterwards) and then, holding the base of the bunch in one hand, slightly twist the bunch with the other hand, bending it over so that the end comes back down to where your first hand is.

Now place some cord (green garden twine or coloured embroidery threads) around the end of the bunch and wrap it aound a couple of times before starting to work up toward the top end. Be careful to include all the ends of the herbs as you go. It needs to be bound tightly as the herbs will shrink as they dry, but there should also be enough air in the bunch to allow the herbs to dry properly.

MUGWORT RITUAL: REEKING CLEANSE

To reek or cleanse your house with smoke, first clean, tidy and have a good clear out. Put some music on, light a candle in each room and ask for support from your spirits. Light your reeking rod by pushing back some of the thread and holding a flame to the end. When it starts to take, gently blow on the herbs until embers form and the stick smokes. Start in the north top corner of the house and work through each room, moving through each nook and cranny north, east, south and west. As you go, say an intention such as, "clear the old vibes and make space for new energies." Pay special attention to the doors, saying, "Let all who enter do so with peace in their hearts and exit filled with love."

To energetically cleanse a person, start at the feet and gently blow on the reeking rod or waft it with a big feather. Then work up and around the body, saying a suitable intention as you go. Pay special attention to the womb or pelvic area, the heart, the third eye and the crown. Finish here.

Work up and then down again, criss-crossing the thread so that the herb bundle does not separate as the thread starts to burn. Do a few tight rounds at the bottom before knotting the loose ends of thread secure. Place an intention on each knot as you tie it.

Hang your reeking rod in a warm place to dry (next to a wood burner or in an airing cupboard are ideal). Feel it from time to time to check if it has dried. The length of time that it needs to dry will vary depending on how thick your bunch is, how tightly you've tied it and where you hang it. The quicker the drying the better, as the herbs can become mouldy in the middle where they are most dense.

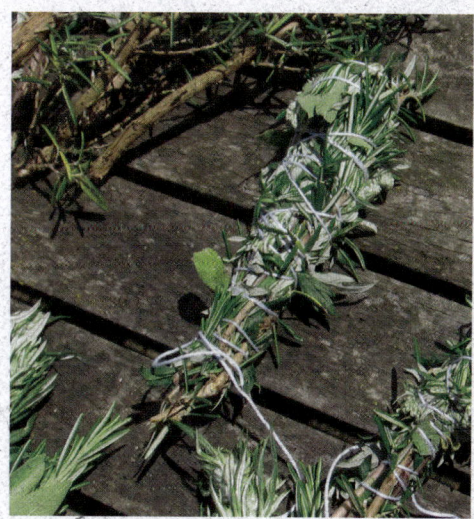

Bundles of fresh mugwort; hang these up to dry.

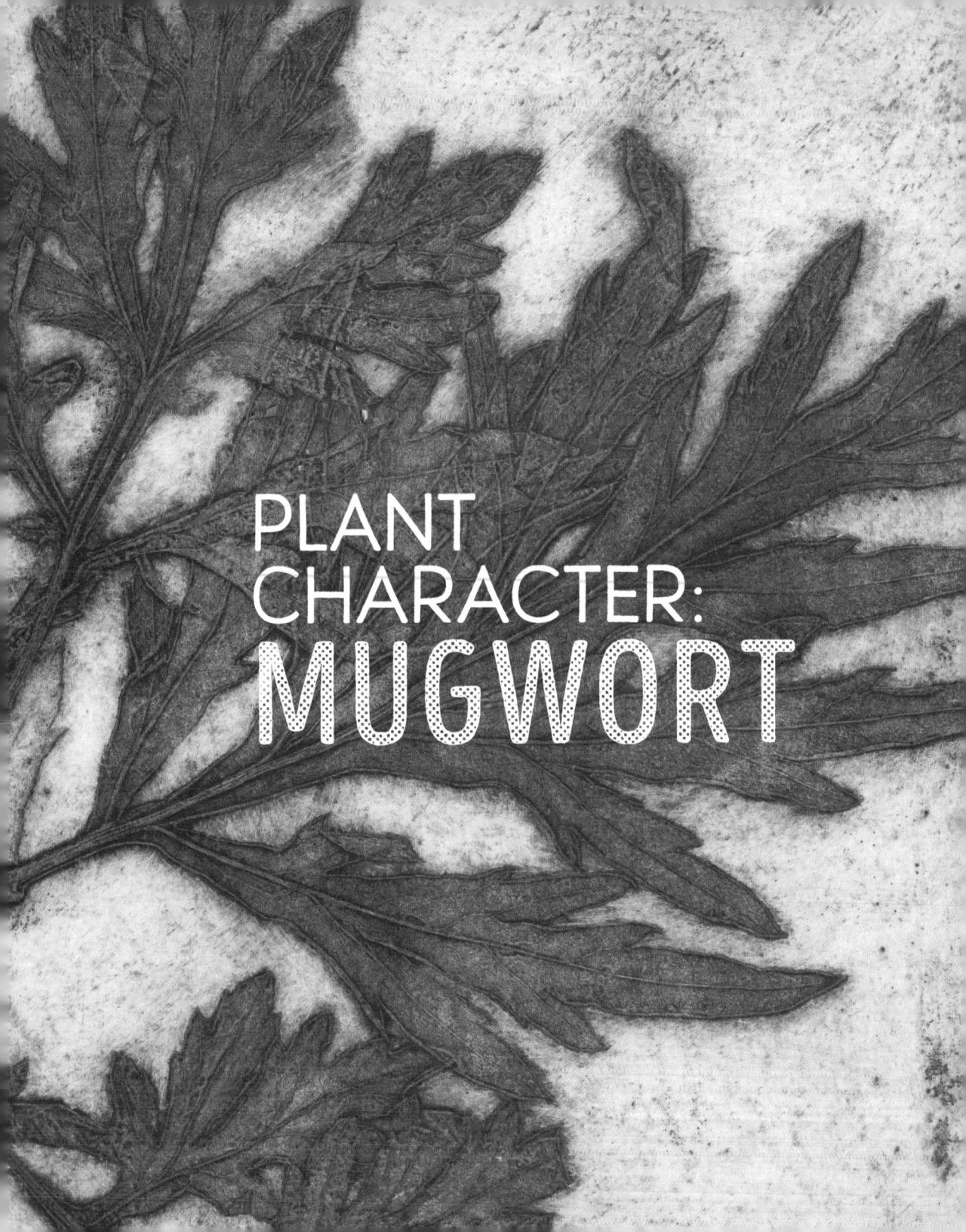

PLANT
CHARACTER:
MUGWORT

I AM ARTEMISIA VULGARIS

Travelling in silver lights
The halo of the moon at night
Clear insight
Supporter of weary feet
In the lucid realm we meet
Oldest of all
Huntress of your wildest dreams
Oily aromatic balance
Lining the way
From darkness to day
Cleanser of spaces, many faces
Fierce protectress of all that births
Filigree greens
Stuffed in gypsy pipes
Smoking vapours
Accessing heights
Pleasure pineal gateway crossing
Libation brewing
Eros wooing
Paradoxical dichotomy
Psychic synchronicity

I am mugwort

Plant Character

Artemis is goddess of the
hunt, of small children and
of the creatures of the forest.
She is a moon goddess
living in the silver light
of dusk, she speaks to our
dreams filling our minds
with belief in ourselves.
Gifting us with powers
of psychic abilities to see
clearly into our futures
and read our pasts, she wafts
a deep-scented aroma in
her wake.

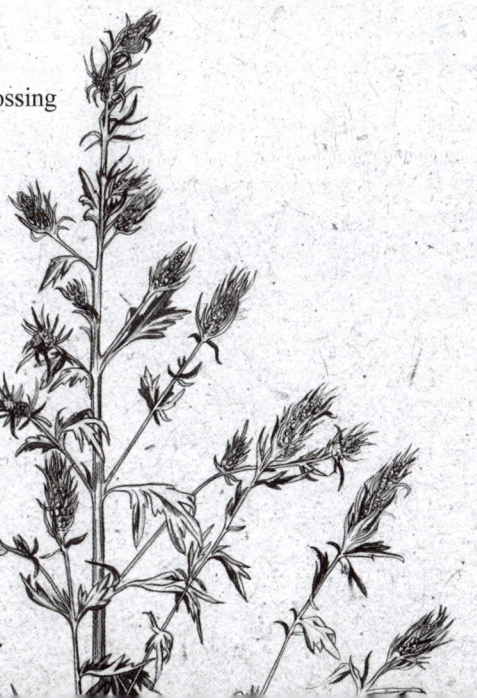

DATURA

LATIN NAME:
Datura stramonium
FAMILY:
Solanaceae
PLANET:
Saturn
SENSORY EXPERIENCE:
Complex, bitter, pungent, sweet,
fetid smell

Part of the Solanaceae or nightshade family, datura, also known as angel's trumpet, thornapple and moonflower, has sticky stems, deep-green leaves, elegant trumpet flowers and spiky seed pods. It flowers at night, a luminous trumpet that appears like the full moon when looked at directly. It beckons the moths with its moon-like appearance and sweet, sweet smell to pollinate its trumpets.

Some of the plants of the Solanaceae family, such as datura, are referred to as the witching herbs. They have powerful connotations and symbolize, among other things, personal responsibility, freedom and feminine wisdom. These herbs are often misunderstood. Fear of the unknown is strong in societies that focus on measurable and predictable outcomes, and we are not encouraged to accept the invisible world. But with lack of research, we are in danger of losing important knowledge from the past.

This favourite plant of ours is found growing on wasteground and where the soil has been turned up, in building sites, at the edges of fields and in any garden. There are 13 main species of datura throughout the world, as well as sub-species. *Datura stramomium* (an annual that grows in northern climates) and *Datura inoxia* (a perennial that grows in warmer climates) are the species that we have mainly worked with for medicine, but we have grown many species along with the closely related brugmansia or "tree daturas" of South America, whose huge trumpet flowers hang down instead of pointing skyward.

After flowering, *Datura stramonium* gives up its seed and then begins to brown to a beautiful dried skeletal form, the seed pods hanging on the ends of the branches. *Datura inoxia*, on the other hand, goes on to flower each year and cannot survive the chilly winters of the northern countries without being brought indoors.

Medicinally, herbalists use datura for the lungs, specifically as a bronchodilator. By opening tight or restricted lungs, it helps us to breathe more deeply, take in oxygen and fill ourselves up with life.

Unfortunately, many a trippy explorer of the 1970s dabbled in datura without knowledge of the correct dosage and found themselves psycho-emotionally burned, often returning with tales of madness and lost days. The stories travelled throughout the alternative scene and spread fear among those experimenting with psychotropic plants. A residue of fear still surrounds the beautiful moonflower, associated as it is with death and madness. Datura does not come without risks, but heroic doses are not the order with this beautiful and mysterious plant, which demands careful consideration and respect

Datura has a shadowed history, a tale that needs to be told. It has long been associated with werewolves, as many "psychenauts" (we prefer psyche to psycho) have found out in their journeys to other realms. Feelings of morphing into a wolf, of growing hairier and of hands turning into paws are common when under the influence of datura, especially when it is imbibed during the luminous full moon. Interestingly, when used as a mind-altering agent, datura often produces similar experiences in different people. This phenomenon has been documented since the mid-1500s when Andrés Laguna, who served

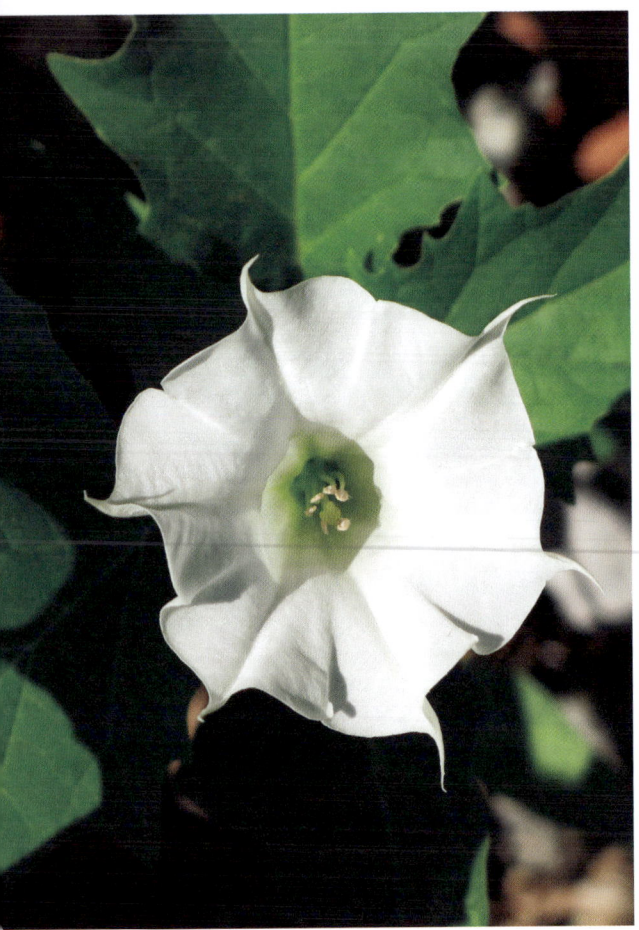

The lovely trumpet-like flower of datura

were having came from the plants and not from direct communion with the devil. He showed that even the wife of the executioner had similar experiences to those who were deemed witches. His work was swiftly shut down under pain of death.

A POWERFUL HERB

Datura acts, in part, on the cholinergic pathways of the nervous system. The nerve cells of this pathway respond to the neurotransmitter acetylcholine (ACh), which has been associated with several cognitive functions, including memory, selective attention and emotional processing. ACh is therefore associated with consciousness. There is an aspect of the cholinergic pathway that connects the cortex (to do with conscious awareness and making sense of the world around you, as learned in this lifetime) to the deeper regions of the brain. When we interfere with this pathway, as with datura intoxication, we can access more ancient, primal and animalistic aspects of the brain. We can, in effect, reveal our ancient selves.

In heart tissue, ACh acts in an inhibitory way, reducing the heart rate. In skeletal muscles, however, it is excitatory and has a function that aids the movement of muscle and the mobilization of joints.

Datura acts as an anticholinergic. It can, therefore, induce extreme torpor, paralysis and even coma with stronger doses.

as a physician to the Spanish king, started to look more deeply into the effects of the plants that were being discussed during the witch trials. A scholar of medicine, Laguna set about trying to prove that the visions people

Anticholinergics, such as the tropane alkaloids, are present in variable amounts in the classic witches' flying herbs: datura, belladonna, henbane and mandrake.

Atropine, one of the tropane alkaloids found in relatively large amounts in datura, sits on the receptors in the cholinergic system, which means that heart rate increases and muscle activity decreases, and as a result, a still, trancelike state known as torpor, characterized by sluggishness, is induced.

Atropine is found in much higher amounts in belladonna (atropa), which is used to dilate the pupils before eye operations

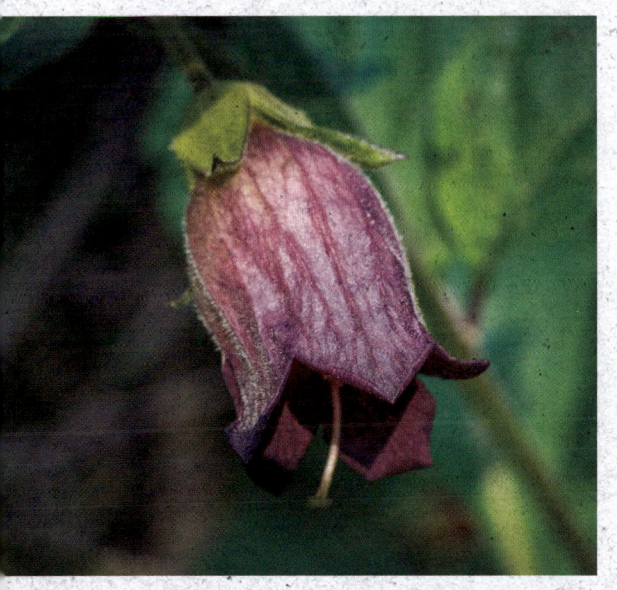

Belladonna, another of the fabled witching herbs

and as an anaesthetic. Overuse of the tropane alkaloids results in anticholinergic syndrome, with symptoms including thirst, the sensation of extreme heat and delirium. In Chinese medicine, this is seen as an indicator of yang separating from yin and a precursor to death.

In the case of an excess dose of Datura you will see the symptoms described above, usually starting with an unquenchable thirst. The pupils also become dilated. In some large doses, the muscular effect means the body will be very still but the heart will be racing. There is a very descriptive ditty describing the symptoms of this syndrome:

Blind as a bat,
Mad as a hatter,
Red as a beet,
Hot as Hades,
Dry as a bone,
The bowel and bladder lose their tone,
And the heart runs alone.

If experienced in minute doses, however, this beautiful medicine can bring deep insights and wonderful experiences. Even just growing the herb is often enough for it to enter our dreams and take hold of us in a truly magical way.

We always teach that these herbs must be explored in very small doses. It really doesn't take much to connect with and experience the spirit of a plant, especially one so powerful.

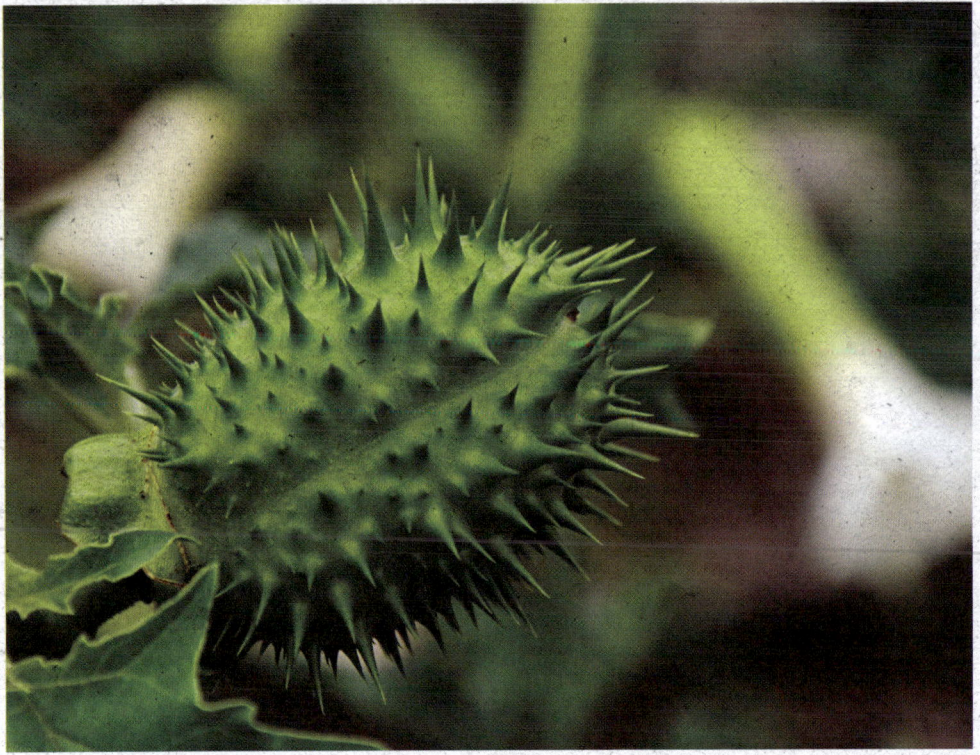

The name "thornapple" derives from datura's spiky seed head.

Datura has had a long history of persecution due to its powerful nature and is currently classed as a Schedule 20 herb, which puts it on a practitioner-only register. The effects of this plant can be extremely harmful when taken without consideration but we feel that restricting access to knowledge about its safety, preparations and uses makes it potentially more harmful, and removes the opportunity for deepening our understanding of how this amazing medicine can be used for spiritual awakening, transformation and health.

As clinical herbalists, we have used minute doses of datura for anxiety, with brilliant results. Datura has also shown useful effects for the treatment of tremors of Parkinson's Disease.

PERCEPTIONS OF ALTERED STATES

Datura can induce hallucinations. The word "hallucination" is defined in the *Oxford English Dictionary* as "an experience involving the apparent perception of something not present". The origins of the word are from the Latin *aluncinari*, to wander in mind – which is a lot less negative than the usual connotations of hallucinating.

Altered states of consciousness and indeed so-called hallucinations can, in other cultures and certain situations, be perceived as messages for healing from our own subconscious or influences outside our own experience. However, in a culture that views altered states, and more specifically hallucinations, as a "mental health issue", it can be isolating trying make sense of these experiences. We need to seek ways of creating safe spaces to connect with other realities and encouraging cultural acceptance of differing viewpoints about these topics.

Attitudes to psycho-emotional health are culturally led. Where you live in the world determines how you are perceived and subsequently treated, especially in cases of anxiety, depression, schizophrenia or degenerative brain conditions. The mental state induced in people seeking spirituality or just a connective high when out with some friends would be considered as signs of madness in the orthodox medical model. Hallucinations are deliberately sought out or induced in some cultures that have maintained some of their ancient traditions. A hallucinatory state is seen as an opportunity to commune with the spirit world and accessing it is perceived as a skill.

By contrast, in the West, it is perceived as a danger. People are effectively banned from accessing altered states of consciousness. This is not only detrimental to the health of the individual, but to society as a whole, lessening our ecological resilience and our ability find novel solutions to the big problems of the era.

In the West, people are often negatively labelled if they access altered states. The ensuing isolation and paranoia can lead to panic attacks, phobias and other negative states, which effectively act as methods of social control. Internalizing stigma creates not only a diminished sense of self, but also a diminished sense of what it means to be fully human and co-creative in this wonderful world and larger ecosystem.

It is our belief that lunar flower essence of datura (see page 130 for how to make lunar flower essence) can be safely used to make connection to the spirit world or altered states more accessible. We do this to live more fully within the ecosystem; it is a part of our manifesto for planetary wellness.

PLANT
CHARACTER:
DATURA

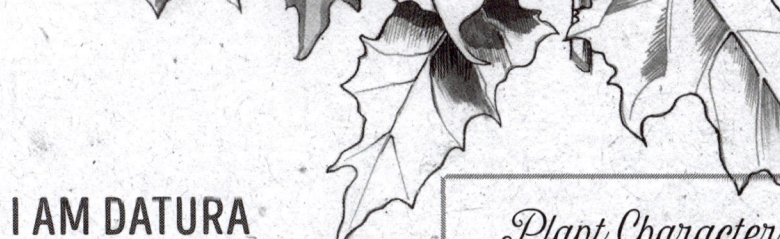

I AM DATURA

I am datura

Dilating with hip hop stripes of white
Trumpeting light
Sexual being
Attracting the night
Thorny geometric alchemy
Protecting the black seed
The future potential
Down the tunnel
Reptilian brain revealing
Self-to-self
I am the mistress of the thin spaces
Deep dark places
Syncope races
Surface calm and dreamy sleep
Still body
Chaotic soul
Schismed in entirety
Dose balancing act
Tippety tip tap
My heart beats fast
Tachycardiac
My lips
Through full moon trumpets blast
Hypnotic scents

Plant Character

A temptress with snow-white skin and jet-black hair, Datura lives at the edges of a shady world that she beckons you to enter. In the dark she blossoms into a moon maiden bursting with light, alluring the creatures of the night. A sexy storyteller trickster, full of soporific horror and delightful forgetfulness, she invites you to explore your dark inner world and reveals ancient secrets. At full moon she transforms into a wolf, scouting the night for love.

Attracting night creatures to my zombie twisted paradise
Alien desire
Creator of fright
Mistress of the night

I am datura

POPPY

LATIN NAME:
Papaver
FAMILY:
Papaveraceae
PLANET:
Saturn
SENSORY EXPERIENCE:
Cooling, cold, bitter, sweet

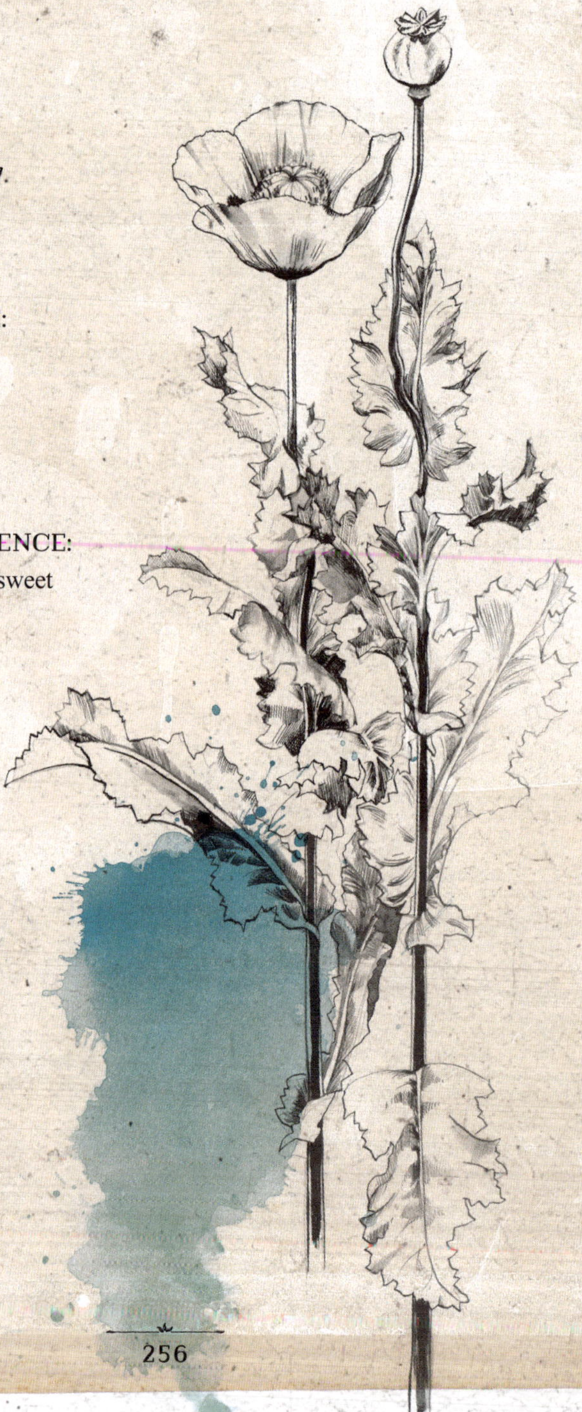

We have chosen to feature poppy in this chapter because of this plant's incredible analgesic qualities, alleviating pain while creating a deep sense of peace. It is the opium-rich sleep inducer, with great power over us humans.

Poppy alters perceptions, having the power to alleviate pain and enhance pleasure. But this enhancement of pleasure and absence of pain is compelling and delicious. Poppy, when abused, casts a spell over humanity, and is associated with both addiction and war.

The dried seed heads, which make excellent shakers, contain prolific potential for life. The seeds can lie dormant for decades, perhaps as long as a century, denoting the longevity and tenacity of poppy's life force. This explains why poppies are one of the first plants to appear on battlegrounds, where the soil becomes disturbed and dormant seeds have a chance to grow. Consequently, field poppy has become associated with the remembrance of those killed in battle; this connection also represents the dark history of this plant. All the poppy species contain opiates in some degree, but the highest concentration is found in the namesake of the drug opium, the opium poppy.

As poppy is such an amazing analgesic medicine, it has been utilized in countless medical remedies over the years. It was a key component of the famed "soporific sponge",
which was used extensively during the medieval period as an anaesthetic whilst surgical procedures were undergone. First written about by Nicholas of Salerno in the 12th century, a sea sponge would be soaked in the plant juices of poppy, henbane, mandrake and other soporific narcotics and then dried and stored until needed. When it was used, the sponge was dampened and placed over the patient's nose and mouth, which resulted in the inhalation of the herbal narcotic fumes. It is said that the fumes induced a sleep lasting up to five days so that the body had the opportunity to recover from the trauma of surgery as well as rendering the patient insensible during the procedure.

Poppy is also a key ingredient in laudanum, a very famous and widely used medicine up until the 20th century. The height of laudanum's consumption was in the Victorian period, when many writers seem to have been under its intoxicating spell. But it is a much older remedy, the name laudanum (from the Latin *laudare*, meaning "to praise") having been coined by the 16th-century Swiss-German physician Paracelsus. The most important ingredients for his laudanum recipe were poppy, henbane root, coriander seeds and cloves.

In the 1800s laudanum became a medical standard. It was cheaper than alcohol and widely available – you could buy it on any high street, in pubs, grocers, sweet shops, barber shops, tobacconists and, of course, pharmacies. It was prescribed almost as a panacea, for everything from relaxing a fraught baby to treating depression, women's "troubles", persistent cough, rheumatism, diarrhoea and anything painful!

By 1868 laudanum was known to be an addictive narcotic with many people suffering when their supply ran out. The first restriction of its use came about in this year. From then on, it could only be sold by registered chemists in England and, because of its dangers, had to be labelled as a poison.

OPIUM

The opium poppy is so called because opium is extracted from the seed heads. Opiates are analgesic, or painkilling, compounds found naturally in the highest quantities in the opium poppy, *Papaver somniferum*. Psychoactive compounds found in the opium plant include morphine and codeine, which are widely used in allopathic medicine across the globe today. The poppy has given humanity many medicines and has largely driven the modern fixation with "feeling no pain". However, the poppy also highlights human greed. This greed has generated and sustained terrible levels of addiction across populations, resulting in wars. The search for non-addictive painkillers has led to the creation of one of the most addictive, destructive drugs: heroin (diamorphine).

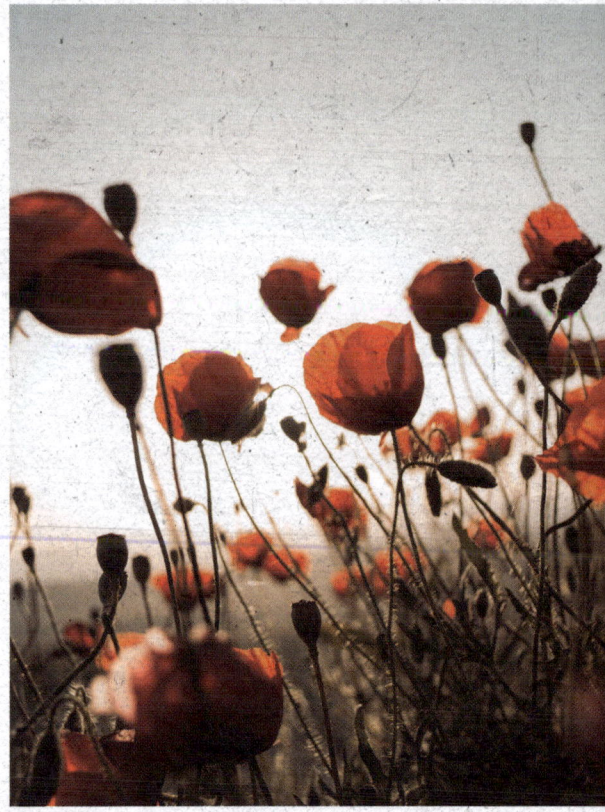

Field poppies remind us of the war dead and the poppy's long link to armed conflict.

Opium is concentrated from the sticky, dark latex of the opium poppy. The traditional method of obtaining the latex is to score the immature seed pods, releasing the latex. The sticky, yellowish residue is scraped off and collected the next day. The word "meconium", which today is used to describe a baby's first, sticky, dark-green/black poo after birth, is derived from the Greek word for "opium-like". The word was historically used for preparations made from other parts of the opium poppy, and from other species of poppies, in which the latex would be boiled down until it became a tarry, black paste, looking just like opium.

Every single important medical text from the ancient world documents the use of opium. Grown for food, anaesthesia and ritual purposes since at least the Neolithic period, the human experience of pain, surgery and addiction has evolved with the opium poppy.

Chinese history is in part the history of this plant. Medicinal use of opium was commonplace since the 700s and evidence of recreational use dates from the 1500s. In 1729 the Chinese emperor banned smoking opium and opium dens. At the time, the British were cultivating their own addiction to Chinese tea (*Camellia sinensis*). The Chinese would only trade tea for silver bullion and were uninterested in the British modern "tat" that had been sent for the interest of the Emperor. The British East India Tea Company saw an opportunity to trade opium from India in exchange for the prized tea. They participated in this illegal trade despite the Emperor's decree, creating widespread opium addiction in the country that guaranteed repeat sales. In the 19th century, there were two Opium Wars over this trade. The first resulted in the transfer of Hong Kong to the British Empire after 1842 and the trading port was subsequently used as a centre for the sale of more opium. While only 69 British soldiers died during these wars, over 20,000 Chinese lost their lives.

There has been much speculation over the role of the opium poppy in the recent war in Afghanistan, and in Taliban rule there. Access to morphine was at an all-time low before the 2001 US and UK invasion of Afghanistan. A new wave of heroin (made from morphine) reached the streets shortly after the invasion, medical stocks of morphine were also replenished and it was reported at the time that troops were protecting the opium fields in the mountains. Governments denied having any control of how much heroin was brought to the West, but there was an increase around this time in deaths on the streets from heroin overdose.

With the rampant growth that capitalism and globalization has fostered, we now seem to be stuck in a "more more more" culture of limitless greed, expansion and consumerism, on a dark path of decline, climate change and societal suicide. Where does this addiction to greed come from? We are taught to consume from a very young age, influenced by advertising and marketing that prey psychologically on our insecurities. Scratching the surface of these insecurities often reveals our deepest fears and traumas.

Addiction has a root in personal feelings of lack and inadequacy. We are currently seeing this play out in the "death economy" of modern Western society – in our addiction to consumption and hoarding wealth that is destroying the very ecosystem we rely on for life.

GREATER CELANDINE

The Papaveraceae plant family is a large one with over 800 different species, of which quite a few are utilized in herbal medicine. One very useful and commonly found plant from the poppy family is the greater celandine (*Chelidonium majus*). This friendly

POPPY SEED CAKE

Poppy's tiny, medicine-packed seeds, which offer contrast, flavour and a crunchy texture, are the star of this cake recipe. We use this cake in a special celebration to remember the dead; poppy is associated with end-of-life medicine and an ability to lie dormant in the earth, and so represents the turning cycle of life and death. We bake this cake and sit around a table with a candle lit for each family member or friend we wish to remember. We say their name, talk about them and eat some delicious cake in their memory.

55g (2oz) butter / 100ml (3½fl oz/scant ½ cup) maple or date syrup / 2 eggs
300g (10½oz/3¼ cups) ricotta cheese / 1 tsp vanilla extract juice of 2 lemons zest of 1 lemon / 210g (7½oz/generous 1½ cups) almond flour
2 tbsp poppy seeds / 2 tsp baking powder

1. Preheat oven to 180°C/350°F/Gas Mark 4. Grease a 20cm (8 inch) round cake pan or use baking parchment. In a blender or food processor, mix the butter, syrup, eggs, ricotta cheese, vanilla, lemon juice and lemon zest until smooth.

2. Fold in the almond flour, poppy seeds and baking powder until evenly incorporated.

3. Transfer to the cake pan and smooth out the top. Bake for 40 minutes, or until the top browns nicely. Cool before slicing.

looking perennial plant, which can grow to about 80cm (2½ feet) high, is often found in gardens and parks. It has bright yellow flowers in the spring and summer months, and bushy foliage.

Greater celandine contains an alkaloid called chelidonine, which is very similar to the papaverine found in its cousin, the opium poppy (*Papaver somniferum*). Chelidonine is an antispasmodic with mild tranquillizing properties. Because of this the herb makes a wonderful remedy as a tea for irritable bowels, gallbladder spasms and bronchitis.

When the stems are broken, an intensely coloured orange/yellow sap bleeds out, which makes an excellent remedy for getting rid of warts or verrucas. Simply go to the plant once or twice a day and apply this sticky, colourful sap onto the wart, continuing for 2–3 weeks.

The sap is corrosive so it dissolves the wart, and, because of this, caution should be taken when working with this plant. Don gloves when harvesting and be careful not to get the sap anywhere else on your skin. The warts go black before dropping off.

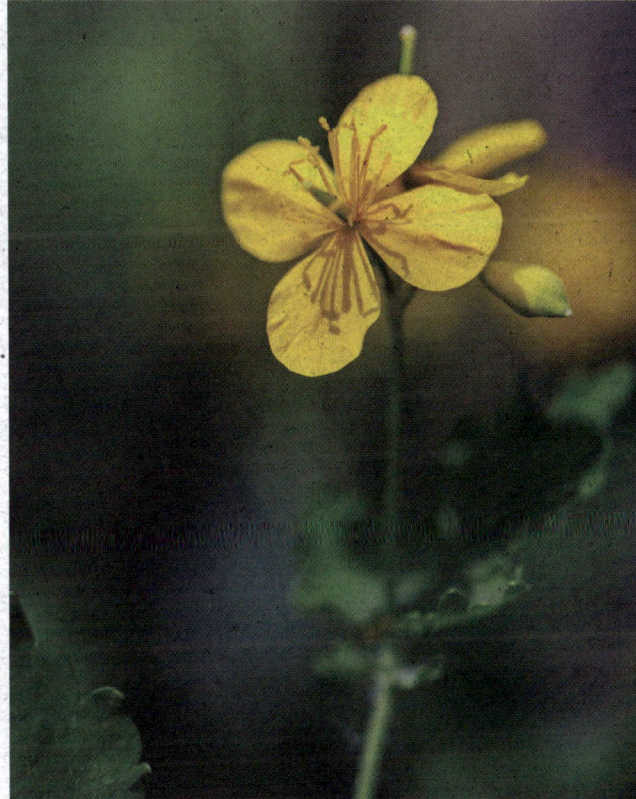

Greater celandine can be used to remove warts and as a remedy for irritable bowels and bronchitis.

CALIFORNIAN POPPY

Eschscholzia californica, with its bright orange flowers, is an incredibly visually uplifting and useful plant that grows prolifically and is often found in gardens and public parks. It is a good treatment for nervous anxiety in children, symptoms such as bed wetting, night terrors, nail biting and insomnia can be gently soothed with a tea of this plant. Drink sips of tea made from a heaped teaspoon of the dried herb per cup and leave brew for 5–10 mins. This heartening beauty of a plant is also super helpful as a toothache reliever.

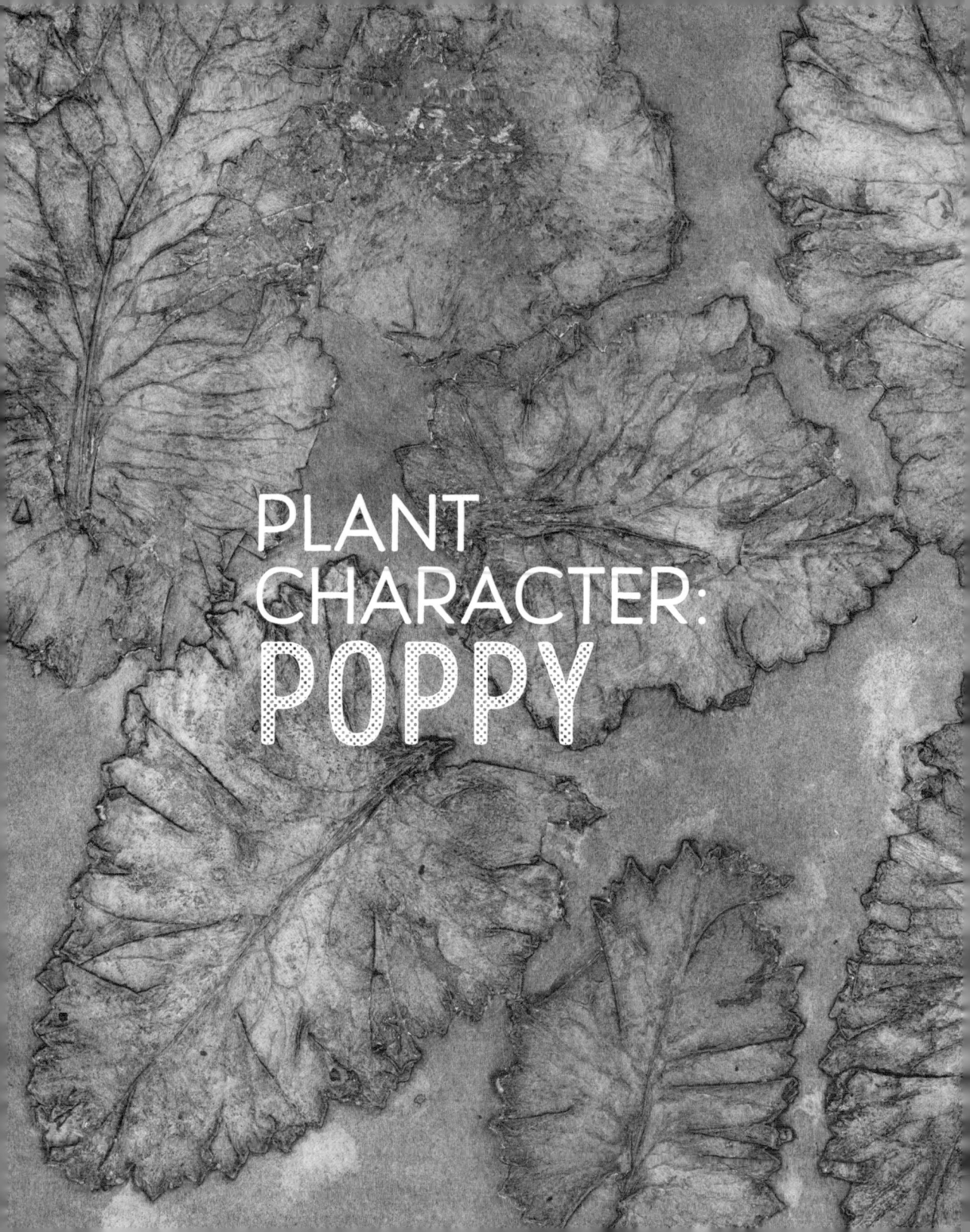

PLANT CHARACTER: POPPY

I AM POPPY

Pale enchantress
Blowsy paper thin
Attracting you to my resinous calming
    pain relief, saviour of fear
God of slumber holding hypnotic
    states of bliss.
While wars rage over my bounty
White bitter tears I cry for lives spent
Mountain cultivation protected by
    soldiers
Each of my trillion seeds in rattle
    headed percussion
Capable of sleeping one hundred years
Remembrance of those armed men
Glorified as winter death returns

I am poppy

Plant Character

Madame Poppy is as old as
time, her papery, delicate
skin looks translucent and
you can visibly see her blue
veins just underneath

She never wears perfume
but always smells of
baked goods as her oven is
always fired, full of seed
filled treats. When you
are in her presence there
is a wonderful calm and a
stillness that she emanates,
this relaxation permeates all
who spend time with her and
she is an incredible healer
of pain. Queues of folk often
line up to receive treatment
from her healing hands.

Madame Poppy is a singer
she is famed for her gentle
sleep-inducing lullabies and
often sings the multitude of
her children, grandchildren
and great-grandchildren
to slumber.

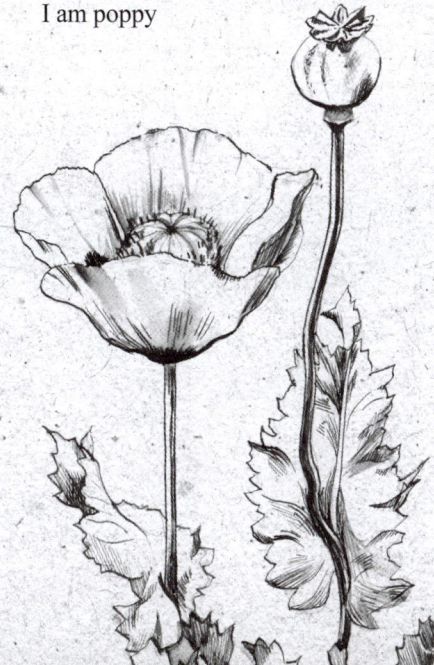

THE SPIRIT OF NUTRITION

The foods of spirit are any that are grown, harvested or prepared with LOVE. One very special recipe that embodies the element of spirit is the friendship cake. The spirit of love, kindness, abundance and community travels with this sweet treat through groups of people passing on a sense of connection. The yeasty dough just keeps proliferating, so sharing it out makes complete sense. And you have cake to share too, once it's ready!

FRIENDSHIP CAKE

250g (9oz/1¼ cups) brown sugar / 6 tbsp warm water / 2 tbsp active dry yeast
600ml (20 fl oz/2½ cups) milk / 500g (1lh 2oz/3¾ cups) plain flour

1. Sprinkle 1 tbsp of the sugar and the yeast over the warm water.

2. Leave in a warm place for 10 minutes.

3. Mix the milk, remaining sugar, flour and the yeast mixture in a large bowl.

4. Cover loosely, leave in a warm place for 24 hours. Follow these instructions, and give them to friends and families along with the starter dough:

Day 1: Congratulations, you have a friend. Pour her into a bowl to continue to grow.

Day 2: Stir 3 times with a wooden spoon.

Day 3: Stir, talk to her, say an affirmation of supportive community so your circles grow with the dough.

Day 4: Feed her 300ml (10 fl oz/1¼ cups) milk, 200g (7oz/1 cup) brown sugar and 250g (8oz/1¾ cups) sifted self-raising flour.

Days 5–8: Each day, stir well, repeating your affirmation.

Day 9: Feed as for Day 4. Then split into five portions and give four away.

Day 10: Time to make your cake with the starter dough. Add 150g (5½ oz/1 cup) self-raising flour, 3 beaten eggs, 150g (5½ oz/¾ cup) brown sugar, 2 tbsp cinnamon powder, 100g (3½oz) chopped nuts or dried fruit, 2 finely chopped apples, 100ml (3½fl oz/scant ½ cup) of sunflower oil. Cook in a lined 18cm (7in) cake pan for about an hour at 180°C/350°F/Gas Mark 4. Once cooled, personalize with toppings of your choice.

WHERE TO NOW?

Our aim in this book is to make information and knowledge accessible so you can reach informed decisions about your healthcare. Having read it, you should know a little more about yourself, your health and the plants that grow around you. We also hope that you feel inspired to connect with others to pass on things you've experienced and learned.

The next step is to look again at the Sensory Herbalism tools and techniques of plant connection. Then, turn to the season you're in, and start using the book as a manual for working with herbs. Take the time to go outside and meet your local plants. See if you can focus on the three featured in the current season and really get to know them individually. Look at the exercises and rituals and start to work with the elements as they dance through the year.

* Be super observant when walking around your area; carry a plant ID book in your pocket or basket and get to know your local medicinal herbs.
* Make a list of 10 herbs within walking distance of your home.
* Start collecting and saving seeds, planting and germinating some plants for your garden or windowsill.
* Connect with local growing projects; check out if you have a community garden project near your home and go meet some fellow earth lovers.
* And most importantly start sharing and showing people the herbs that you are learning about; it is important to proliferate the knowledge that you are acquiring.

Imagination and creativity permeate all our work. Through the stories of the plants, characterization, drawing, making remedies and discovering new recipes, we can reignite our ancestral knowledge of plant medicine.

By using our senses, we can re-engage with earth magic and become emissaries between the human and plant worlds.

We are living in interesting times. Many people have completely forgotten what was common knowledge during the lives of their own grandparents. We have become increasingly dependent on chemical medicine and more and more people are spending less and less time outside. Technology has burst through into all our lives and we are still learning to manage what all these screens have to offer and at what cost. And yet we are increasingly aware that it is vital to revive the old knowledge before it is forgotten. Herbal medicine will play a major part in the survival of the human species, it always has! And you can play your part in this revival.

REFERENCES AND FURTHER READING

Adams, Patch with Mylander, Maureen. *Gesundheit! Healing Arts Press*, Vermont, 1998.

de Bairacli Levy, Juliette. *Common Herbs for Natural Health*. Ash Tree Publishing: New York, 1997.

Batmanghelidj, F. *The Body's Many Cries for Water: You're Not Sick; You're Thirsty*. Global Health Solutions: Virginia, 2007.

Brooke, Elisabeth. *A Woman's Book of Herbs*. Aeon Books: New York, 2018.

Culpeper, Nicholas, *Culpeper's Complete Herbal*. Various editions.

Devi, Alakananda. *Prostate Cancer*. Available at: docplayer.net/20847773-Prostate-cancer-by-alakananda-devi-m-b-s-lond.html

Hedley, Chrisopher and Shaw, Non. *Herbal Remedies*. Parragon Book Service: Bath, 1996.

Hoffman, David. *The New Holistic Herbal*. Element: London, 1994

Kindred, Glennie, author of 11 books on Earth wisdom, native plants and Earth cycles, including *Earth Wisdom*. Hay House: London, 2011

Maciocia, Giovanni. *The Foundations of Chinese Medicine*. Elsevier Churchill Livingstone: London, 2005.

Mcintyre, Anne. *Flower Power: Flower Remedies for Healing Body and Soul Through Herbalism, Homeopathy, Aromatherapy, and Flower Essences*. Henry Holt and Company, 1996.

Mills, Simon. *The Essential Guide to Herbal Medicine*. Arkana: London, 1993.

Newson, RB, Shaheen, SO, Chinn S, Burney, PG (2000) "Paracetamol sales and atopic disease in children and adults: an ecological analysis", *European Respiratory Journal* 16: 817–823.

Pert, Candice. *Molecules of Emotion: Why You Feel the Way You Feel*. Pocket Books: London, 1999.

Soni, P, Siddiqui, A A, Dwivedi, J, and Soni, V (2012) "Pharmacological properties of *Datura stramonium* L. as a potential medicinal tree: An overview", *Asian Pacific Journal of Tropical Biomedicine*, 2(12), 1002–1008. www.doi.org/10.1016/S2221-1691(13)60014-3

Trompetter I, Krick B, Weiss G (2013) "Herbal triplet in treatment of nervous agitation in children", *Wien Med Wochenschr*. Feb;163(3-4):52-7. Available at: www.doi.org/10.1007/s10354-012-0165-1

Warner, Felicity. *A Safe Journey Home: A Simple Guide to Achieving a Peaceful Death*. Hay House: London, 2011.

Warner, Felicity. *The Soul Midwives' Handbook: The Holistic And Spiritual Care Of The Dying*. Hay House: London, 2013.

Worth, Jennifer. *In the Midst of Life*. W&N: London, 2012.

RESOURCES

Sensory Herbalism Apprenticeship For many years, we have shared our passion for plants through our Sensory Herbalism trainings. The seasonal study takes the participants on a journey into their own health and wellbeing, explains how to apply their skills to others and how to create beautiful, handcrafted potions and lotions. It is through our wonderful apprentices that we continue to learn and be challenged. A strong, inclusive community of grounded, open-hearted individuals, with a common goal to protect the Earth and heal each other with herbs, has developed.

Sensory Solutions Community Interest Company (CIC) was born in 2004, underpinned with a political ethos, in response to the trend in herbal medicine to use plants from across the globe. It was set up as a herbal, health and arts education company, focused on native or naturalized plants. There is emphasis on optimizing community health and on teaching the art of herbalism, seed saving and medicine growing. We work to encourage the collection, saving and also cultivation of local seeds, for food and for medicine. Plants have developed for thousands of years to be able to cope with the specific environment local to them. In saving seeds we are tapping into an ancient practice and protecting local diversity. For more information, see: www.seedsistas.co.uk

For more information on herbalism, see:

Heartwood *heartwood-uk.net/home/team*

Herbalists without Borders *herbalists without borders.weebly.com*

For more information on psychedelic medicine, see:

Breaking Conventions *www.breakingconvention.co.uk*

INDEX

A

acetylcholine 155, 250
Achilles 17, 141
Achillea millefolium (see yarrow)
Ache-Ease Balm 135
acids 53
aconite 29
adaptogens 156–157
addiction 32
additives 142
adrenal glands (adrenals) 28, 93, 156
adrenaline 156
affirmations 66–68
air (element) 152–153
Alchemilla vulgaris (see lady's mantle)
alcohol 191
aldosterone 156
alkaloids 54
allopathic medicine 10, 18–19, 70–71, 203–205
altar, making an 228
altered states 253
Armoracia rusticana (see horseradish)

amylase 196
androgens 156
animism 15
anticholinergic syndrome 250–251
anxiety 32, 33, 155, 173, 211, 252
apoptosis 152, 207
Aquarius 24, 29, 42
Aries 24, 28, 42
arbutin 135
aromatic oils 53, 54
Artemis 16, 27, 241
Artemisia (genus) 16–17
Artemisia vulgaris (see mugwort)
artemisinin 16
arthritis 32
aspirin 16, 19
assimilation 79
asthma 142, 211
astrology 10, 24–29, 73
Astronomica (epic poem) 24
atropine 250
attention deficit hyperactivity disorder

(ADHD) 211
aucubin 52, 99
aura 144, 230
autonomic nervous system 154, 159, 161
autumn 152, 162, 184–185, 229
avocados 236, 237
Ayurveda 10, 15, 36–37
azulene 140
arrow capes 365, 387–8
arrows 228, 298–9, 316–17, 345
arson 40–1, 102n
artificial hills 39
artisans 21–2
arts 27
  see also martial arts
ashigaru formation 304–5
ashiuchi trays 264, 266
auspicious achievements 321–2
auspicious direction 248, 258–9
auspicious times 249
aversions 58–9
awasu term 232

B

Bach, Dr Edward 12, 68
Baïracli Levy, Juliette de 112
Batmanghelidj, Dr Fereydoon 89
bearberry 135
beer 242
bees 135
belladonna 29, 251
Bellis perennis see daisy
Belly Blend Tea 198
Beltain 34

beta-carotene 193
beta-sitosterol 237
bites, insect 99, 101
bitters, herbal 53, 196–197
bladder 95
blackberry 28
blood 125
body brushing 91, 193
bones *see* musculoskeletal system
borage 69

brain 154
brassica vegetables 219–221
bread, rye soughdough recipe 148
breastfeeding 174
breathing 159, 161
bruises 129, 192
Buhner, Stephen Harrod 68
burdock 28
burns 105

C

caffeine 95, 111, 158
  see also coffee, alternatives to
calcium phosphate 190
calendula 90, 192
California poppy 261
Calluna vulgaris see heather
Calpol® 141–143
cancer 24, 27, 207, 219–221
Candida albicans 36, 195
Candlemas *see* Imbolc
Capricorn 24, 29, 42
caraway 220
carbohydrate 53
cardiovascular system 44, 79, 83, 122–125, 141
cat power 213

catecholamines 156
celandine, greater 260–261
celery 192
cellulose 55
Centuary 28
chakras 30–33
characters, creating plant 61–62, 65
chelidonine 261
chi 36, 93, 153
chickweed 27
childbirth 242
children, treating 71, 261
chilli 212
Chinese medicine 10, 15, 37–38, 92–93, 251
chlorophyll 96, 125

cholesterol 156
circulation; poor 32; as a therapeutic idea 79
Clear Vision Drops 135
cleavers 26, 27, 45, 53, 89, 90, 94, 96, 104–109, 236
clothing, plants as 14
cloves 220
clumsy 33
co-dependency 32
coffee, alternatives to 105, 111, 189, 205
colds 83, 180
colic 174, 211
colitis 32
collagen 190
colours 30–33, 126

INDEX OF RECIPE TITLES

AUTHOR ACKNOWLEDGEMENTS

We wish to thank our super-supportive families and friends for their incredible encouragement and help with the creation of this book. So thank you to our parents, partners and children for understanding the passion that drives us in this work. Huge love to Meg and Rachael for your unwavering belief and support. Thank you to our proofreaders Hannah, Jane, Liz and Katie for your amazing input, dedication and diligence. Thank you to our herbal-content readers, Marcos and Jules, and to Caroline for the five element theory advice. Thank you to the wonderful Brigitta of Nux Photography and for the Seed SistA portraits and leaf images. Thank you to all our apprentices. Thank you Dieter, for providing the bread recipe. Thank you to Martyn and John Howard Print Studios for your support with the artwork. And above all, thank you to the plants that guide us in this wonderful exciting life.

PHOTOGRAPHIC CREDITS

Front cover (leaves) Brigitta Scholz Mastroianni/Nux Photography; Inside cover Brigitta Scholz Mastroianni/Nux Photography; 6–7 MVP/Unsplash; 11 Brigitta Scholz Mastroianni, Nux Photography; 12 Diana Baliuk/Shutterstock; 15 waldenstroem/Shutterstock; 17 Zhen Hu/Unsplash; 22–3 Annie Spratt/Unsplash; 25 Alamy/Zodiac Man; 35 Scharfsinn/Shutterstock; 41 David Dibert/Unsplash; 44 Bystrov/Shutterstock; 46–7 Dylan Nolte; 52 Manfred Ruckszio/Shutterstock; 57 Popova Valeriya/Shutterstock; 62 janaph/Shutterstock; 64 Sarah Biesinger/Shutterstock; 69 (top) Madeleine Steinbach/Shutterstock, (middle) Michael Gromov/Shutterstock, (bottom) sergios/Shutterstock; 70 Elena Veselova/Shutterstock; 74 Chamille White/Shutterstock; 77 Chamille White/Shutterstock; 80–81 Jeremy Thomas/Unsplash; 85 Foxxy63/Shutterstock; 97 (top) milart/Shutterstock, (middle) Belle Benfield & The Seed Sistas, (bottom) tomertu/Shutterstock; 101 (left) Belle Benfield & The Seed Sistas, (right) Belle Benfield & The Seed Sistas; 106 Lapis2380/Shutterstock; 113 Nataliia K/Shutterstock; 116 Belle Benfield & The Seed Sistas; 121 Vadymn Lebedych/Unsplash; 124 Nick Fewings/Unsplash; 127 (top) Kurlin Cafe/Shutterstock, (middle) lek2481/Shutterstock, (bottom) Mark Herreid/Shutterstock; 130 Belle Benfield & The Seed Sistas; 131 mizy/Shutterstock; 137 bernashafo/Shutterstock; 143 LFRabanedo/Shutterstock; 145 petratrollgrafik/Shutterstock; 153 Saad Chaudhry/Unsplash; 163 Elena Schweitzer/Shutterstock; 165 (top) Tim Shapcott/Unsplash, (middle) Igor Pushkarev/Shutterstock, (bottom) Will Metts/Shutterstock; 169 Marina Khrapova/Unsplash; 174 Belle Benfield & The Seed Sistas; 175 Belle Benfield & The Seed Sistas; 180 Belle Benfield & The Seed Sistas; 181 zetat/Shutterstock; 195 Morinka/Shutterstock; 197 Kuttelvaserova Stuchelova/Shutterstock; 201 (top) Madeleine Steinbach/Shutterstock, (middle) Marilyn Barbone/Shutterstock, (bottom) Sokor Space/Shutterstock; 207 Nedim Bairamovic/Shutterstock; 212 Andris Tkacenko/Shutterstock; 213 Drew Star Crow; 218 Oxik/Shutterstock; 224 Marian Weyo/Shutterstock; 231 TAVEESUK/Shutterstock; 236 Larisa Blinova/Shutterstock; 239 (top) Simona Pavan/Shutterstock, (middle) LFRabanedo/Shutterstock, (bottom) Sonja C/Shutterstock; 245 Belle Benfield & The Seed Sistas; 250 Belle Benfield & The Seed Sistas; 251 footageclips/Shutterstock; 252 ZayakSK/Shutterstock; 258 Milos Tonchevski/Unsplash; 261 Sergey Chayko/Shutterstock